Hearing Research and Theory

VOLUME 2

Contributors to This Volume

HEWITT D. CRANE
ELLEN M. DANAHER
ROGER HAMERNIK
DON HENDERSON
JOHN H. MILLS
J. M. PICKETT
SALLY G. REVOILE
RICHARD SALVI
BERTRAM SCHARF
RICHARD A. SCHMIEDT
J. C. WEBSTER

Hearing Research and Theory

VOLUME 2

Edited by

JERRY V. TOBIAS

Auditory Department
Naval Submarine Medical Research Laboratory
Groton, Connecticut

EARL D. SCHUBERT

Hearing and Speech Center
Stanford University Medical Center
Stanford, California

1983

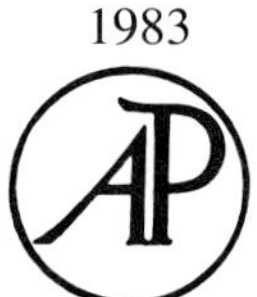

ACADEMIC PRESS

A Subsidiary of Harcourt Brace Jovanovich, Publishers

New York   London
Paris   San Diego   San Francisco   São Paulo   Sydney   Tokyo   Toronto

ACADEMIC PRESS, INC.
111 Fifth Avenue, New York, New York 10003

United Kingdom Edition published by
ACADEMIC PRESS, INC. (LONDON) LTD.
24/28 Oval Road, London NW1 7DX

ISSN 0730-1480

ISBN 0-12-312102-7

PRINTED IN THE UNITED STATES OF AMERICA

83 84 85 86   9 8 7 6 5 4 3 2 1

Contents

Loudness Adaptation

Bertram Scharf

Speech-Cue Measures of Impaired Hearing

J. M. Pickett, Sally G. Revoile, and Ellen M. Danaher

Applied Research on Competing Messages

J. C. Webster

IHC–TM Connect–Disconnect and Mechanical Interaction among IHCs, OHCs and TM

Hewitt D. Crane

Physiological Bases of Sensorineural Hearing Loss

Richard Salvi, Don Henderson, and Roger Hamernik

Frequency Selectivity: Physiological and Psychophysical Tuning Curves and Suppression

John H. Mills and Richard A. Schmiedt

List of Contributors

Numbers in parentheses indicate the pages on which the authors' contributions begin.

Hewitt D. Crane (125), Sensory Sciences Research Center, SRI International, Menlo Park, California 94025

Ellen M. Danaher (57), Sensory Communication Research Laboratory, Gallaudet College, Washington, D.C. 20002

Roger Hamernik (173), Callier Center for Communication Disorders, University of Texas at Dallas, Dallas, Texas 75235

Don Henderson (173), Callier Center for Communication Disorders, University of Texas at Dallas, Dallas, Texas 75235

John H. Mills (233), Department of Otolaryngology, Medical University of South Carolina, Charleston, South Carolina 29425

J. M. Pickett (57), Sensory Communication Research Laboratory, Gallaudet College, Washington, D.C. 20002

Sally G. Revoile (57), Sensory Communication Research Laboratory, Gallaudet College, Washington, D.C. 20002

Richard Salvi (173), Callier Center for Communication Disorders, University of Texas at Dallas, Dallas, Texas 75235

Bertram Scharf (1), Auditory Perception Laboratory, Northeastern University, Boston, Massachusetts, 02115, and Laboratoire de Mécanique et d'Acoustique, CNRS, 13277 Marseille, France

Richard A. Schmiedt (233), Department of Otolaryngology, Medical University of South Carolina, Charleston, South Carolina 29425

J. C. Webster (93), Communications Research Department, National Technical Institute for the Deaf, Rochester Institute of Technology, and National Academy of Sciences, Academies of Science, Institute of Psychology, Moscow, USSR and Prague, CSSR

Preface

In this second volume of *Hearing Research and Theory* we again present short monographs on problems in auditory science. The underlying objective is to provide a forum in which authors can combine broadly based reports of their research with enlightened speculation. To that end, we have offered each contributor space enough to pull together a mass of research on a single topic and to comment on it, to interpret it, and to guide the reader through its intricacies.

In the first article, Scharf analyzes the responses of listeners to low-level signals that decrease in perceptual strength as a function of exposure time, and considers the mechanisms that could account for the auditory system's adaptive behavior.

Pickett *et al.* consider the question of speech perception by the hearing-impaired listener unfamiliar with high-fidelity reproductions of sound, who might, accordingly, perform badly when tested with high-fidelity signals. These authors look into the acoustic structure of speech to find useful factors for the treatment of hearing-impaired people.

Webster examines a major problem in selective attention—the analysis and interpretation of simultaneously presented speech signals. Among other things, he reports some novel work with multilingual subjects who respond to messages presented in two languages at a time. His results improve our grasp of the underlying cognitive process.

Crane develops a theoretical framework that can account for the functions of a number of confusing structural and physiological aspects of the mammalian auditory system. He speculates on the effects of mechanical and neural connections of the hair cells and offers explanations of why efferent stimulation does not affect some kinds of neural firing and of how the cochlear structure permits sound perception throughout a broad dynamic range despite the atomic dimensions of basilar-membrane activity.

Based on their studies on sensorineural hearing loss, Salvi *et al.* provide a clear exposition of the relations between sensory-cell damage and hearing-sensitivity changes. They deal with such problems as threshold and pitch shift, recruitment and tinnitus, and summation and inhibition. The scope of their coverage makes the work valuable to laboratory researcher and clinician alike.

The volume concludes with a comprehensive paper on frequency selectivity by Mills and Schmiedt, who consider and test potential answers to such puzzles as why, despite apparent similarities in their auditory apparatuses, people vary tremendously in frequency-discrimination ability; and why, although the low and the high sides of a tuning curve consist of different processes, it is no longer obvious that the low side does anything at all. Mills and Schmiedt consider such issues, test potential answers to them, and point us toward the next steps that need to be taken.

Acknowledgments

When one puts together any stack of paper that is to be bound between hard covers, one is encouraged to write a sentence or a paragraph acknowledging the contributions of the handful of people without whom the work could not have been accomplished so swiftly or so thoroughly or so painlessly or so well. In the volumes in this series, most of the gratitude belongs to a small group of people who fit in a category that seldom gets mentioned in the same breath with ''we appreciate'' and ''we are grateful'': they are the authors of the monographs that constitute these hardbound stacks of paper. We have been and continue to be fortunate in being offered manuscripts of what we believe to be high quality and potential importance. Our thanks belong to our contributors. We appreciate them. We are grateful.

Contents of Volume 1

Loudness Adaptation

Bertram Scharf

Auditory Perception Laboratory
Northeastern University
Boston, Massachusetts
and
Laboratoire de Mécanique et d'Acoustique, CNRS
Marseille, France

I. DEFINITION OF LOUDNESS ADAPTATION

Loudness adaptation is used in this article to mean a decrease in the loudness of a steady sound over time. This definition is analogous to that used by phys-

HEARING RESEARCH AND THEORY, VOLUME 2

iologists to denote the decrease in the response of a single neural unit to a steady stimulus or, more generally according to Young and Sachs (1973, p. 1535), the "decrease in response magnitude" to a "constant stimulus level." When the response magnitude in question is loudness, the subjective itensity of a sound, its measurement must ultimately depend upon subjective judgments of one kind or another (Scharf, 1978). To demonstrate loudness adaptation, recourse is necessary to subjective judgments or at least to measurements closely correlated with such judgments. Accordingly, this article deals primarily with experiments in which listeners judged the loudness of a continuous sound as a function of time. Changes in threshold after a sound stops are considered only in connection with preceding loudness changes that may have occurred while the sound was still on. Generally, such poststimulus measurements tell us about residual masking and fatigue effects but reveal little about adaptation—which we treat as an ongoing process. In this vein, loudness adaptation has been called perstimulatory fatigue, the fatigue that accompanies stimulation, but fatigue is a word better reserved to designate a diminution of sensitivity. The term fatigue has the added disadvantage of implying the basis for any measured decline in loudness.

Ward (1973) in his review of adaptation and fatigue used the term *tone decay* to refer to the disappearance of a tone after a short period of stimulation. Since the loudness of the tone must decrease as an initially audible tone descends to threshold, tone decay entails loudness adaptation. However, in studies of tone decay, little or no attention has been paid to the change in loudness (either to the rate or amount of loudness change). Most attention has been paid to the exposure duration required to reach threshold and the amount of threshold increase. Tone-decay tests have become a standard clinical procedure, used especially when an acoustic neuroma is suspected (Carhart, 1957; Parker *et al.*, 1968).

II. DOES LOUDNESS ADAPT?

In most sensory modalities, a sensation is stronger at the beginning of steady stimulation than at the end; sensation magnitude declines over time.[1] Brightness, odor intensity, taste, and felt vibratory strength on the skin all become weaker while stimulation continues unchanged (see Marks, 1974, for a review). Loudness resembles pain in that it decreases as a function of time only under special

---

[1]Durations are assumed always to be longer than the duration over which temporal integration occurs. For brightness and loudness, sensation magnitude increases with duration up to several hundred milliseconds. Sensory adaptation, as distinct from physiological adaptation, is measurable only after at least several seconds of stimulation.

stimulus conditions as described below. For the most part loudness adaptation cannot be demonstrated. Nevertheless the psychoacoustical literature is full of studies, especially since the influential paper by Hood (1950), that have reported as much as a 50-phon decline in loudness level over a 2- or 3-min listening period. A 50-phon decline means the loudness at the end of 2 or 3 min was approximately one-thirtieth its value at the beginning.

Almost all of these studies used an interaural matching procedure to measure adaptation. A sound was presented steadily to one ear, and occasionally or intermittently to the other ear. The subject's task was generally to match the loudness in the unadapted ear to that in the adapted, that is, steadily stimulated, ear. After a few minutes the listener would set the intermittent sound to a much lower level to match the steady sound in loudness. In sharp contrast, most procedures that avoid interaural interaction reveal little change in loudness, except at low sensation levels. Thus the change in loudness found by interaural matching procedures seems to depend upon an interaction between the intermittent sound in one ear and the steady sound in the other ear. Since this interaction increases with stimulus duration, an appropriate term for the observed concomitant decrease in loudness over time may be *induced loudness adaptation*. So far such induced adaptation has been clearly demonstrated only by interaural matching procedures. Consequently, many authors have not considered it true adaptation. Bocca and Pestalozza (1959) were among the first to emphasize and provide evidence for the possible role of interaural interaction in this type of loudness change. Elliott and Fraser (1970) also pointed out the possible confusion of localization cues with loudness changes in simultaneous interaural matching. Ward (1973) goes further to imply that interaural procedures demonstrates some kind of time-bound change in the auditory percept owing to interaural interaction but not a decrease in loudness. Another possibility, supported by recent, preliminary evidence, is that it is the periodical, intermittent nature of the contralateral stimulus that induces loudness adaptation, and that, in fact, an intermittent sound induces some adaptation even when presented to the same ear as the steady sound. Interaural interaction enhances the adaptation but it may not be a necessary condition for induced adaptation. Since the data based on interaural matching have often been cited as evidence for simple loudness adaptation, simple in that it depends only upon time, a full survey of this paradigm is included in this article.

From the survey of experiments both on simple adaptation and on induced adaptation, we shall see that simple adaptation is found only for soft sounds whereas induced adaptation is found for strong sounds as well. The survey covers experiments in the literature and a series of unpublished experiments from the Auditory Perception Laboratory at Northeastern University.

III. PREVIOUS RESEARCH

A. Measurements without Recourse to Interaural Loudness Matches

Interaural loudness matches have often led us astray, seeming to demonstrate loudness adaptation where there was none, or at least not simple monaural adaptation. Hence, we first review those experiments that were based on other procedures: on absolute judgments of loudness (as in magnitude estimation), on cross-modality matching of loudness to vibration magnitude and duration, on tracking in which the observer is given control of the intensity of a steady sound which he is to keep at constant loudness, on absolute threshold measured as a function of duration (tone decay), and on two other possible monaural paradigms.

1. Absolute Judgments

When a person listens to a moderate-level, continuous tone for a few minutes, he notices little if any change in its loudness, hardly any decline. (Unless, perhaps, attention is diverted from the sound so that the person stops listening, but upon focusing once again on the sound, he hears it as loud as ever.) Some investigators who have claimed that loudness adapts dramatically over a short period, as measured by the simultaneous loudness matches described below, have suggested that a listener does not report a loudness decrease when simply listening because he cannot remember the loudness of a sound from one minute to the next. Except for one report by Lawrence *et al.* in 1949, I could find no experimental data based upon such a straightforward judgment. Lawrence *et al.* were primarily interested in measuring a listener's ability to detect a gradual change in the intensity of a continuous sound. They increased, decreased, or left unchanged the level of a 1000-Hz tone over a 30-sec listening period. At the end of the 30 sec, the observer's task was to say whether the sound "had increased or decreased in loudness." Nine observers with little training said 82% of the time that the loudness of an unchanging tone had decreased when it was 15 dB above threshold; they said 66% of the time that loudness had increased when the tone was 70 dB above threshold. The observers judged the loudness of a 15-dB tone as unchanged (i.e., half the judgments were that the sound had increased in loudness and half that it had decreased) when the tone actually increased at a rate of nearly 3 dB/min. At 70 dB SL, the tone had to be decreased at the rate of 0.5 dB/min for the loudness to be judged as constant. One interpretation of these results is that the loudness of a soft tone decreases over time but that of a tone at a moderate level may increase slightly. No one else appears to have published data based upon such a direct question.

In my laboratory, we have also asked for direct loudness assessments, but the observer's task is somewhat more complex (Fishken *et al.*, 1977; Scharf and Horton, 1978). Observers assign numbers to represent the loudness of a continuous tone at specified times during a 2- or 3-min presentation. This method of *successive magnitude estimation* is described in detail in Section IV. Like Lawrence *et al.* we find a decrease in the loudness of a 1000-Hz tone at low sensation levels and none at higher levels. Indeed, our method reveals no loudness adaptation at any frequency above about 30 dB SL.

2. Cross-Modality Matching

In two studies, observers adjusted the intensity of a nonauditory stimulus at specified time intervals in order to make it equal in subjective magnitude to the loudness of a continuous sound.[2] Gummlich (1971) had 30 observers press a button the length of time necessary for the perceived duration of the button press to match the loudness of a one-third-octave band of noise. Judgments were made every 5 min for 60 min. Results suggested a large increase in loudness over the first minute, as compared to a 2-sec noise, followed by the equivalent of a 12-dB drop during the next 55 min. The initial increase in loudness, equivalent to 20 dB, which is not found in loudness matching (nor in absolute judgments), is puzzling. Since even after 60 min the continuous noise was judged louder than a brief, 2-sec noise of the same level, Gummlich did not demonstrate loudness adaptation.

In the other cross-modality experiment, Gruber and Braune (1974) had 12 observers match the magnitude of a vibratory stimulus on the forearm to the loudness of a 75-dB narrow-band noise centered on 1000 Hz. Matches were made at regular intervals over a 31-min listening period. Figure 1 shows that the vibration amplitude was the same—within 1 dB—at the end as at the beginning of 31 min, indicating no loudness adaptation.

3. Tracking

In the tracking procedure, the observer is given control of the intensity of a continuous sound and told to keep its loudness constant. Harris and Pikler (1960) were apparently the first ones to use the method, not to study adaptation but to study the stability of loudness judgments. They gradually increased or decreased the intensity of the tone while the observer tried to keep loudness constant by compensatory tracking. The observers maintained nearly constant intensity for a 1000-Hz tone at 40 phons for up to 1 min. Had loudness been decreasing owing to adaptation, observers would have been expected to err by overcompensating

---

[2]Cross-modality matching has also been used to measure olfactory adaptation (Ekman *et al.*, 1967) and vibrotactile adaptation (Berglund and Berglund, 1970).

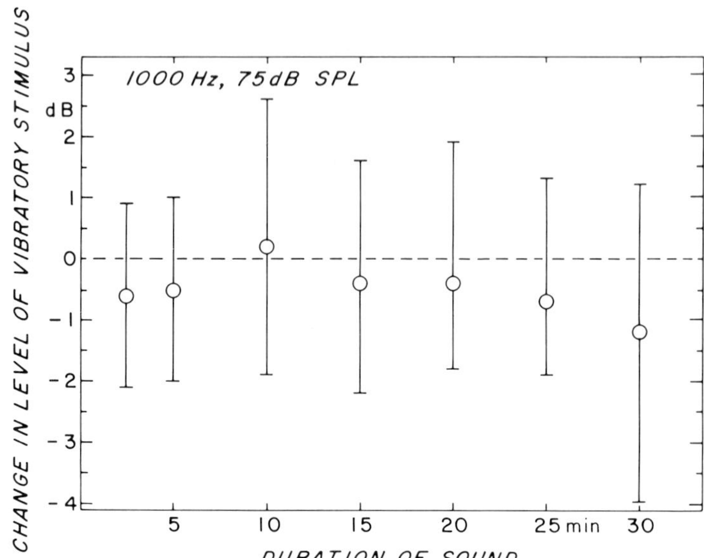

Figure 1   Change in level of a vibrating stimulus to the forearm needed to keep its perceived intensity equal to the loudness of a 75-dB narrow-band noise centered on 1000 Hz. plotted as a function of the duration of the noise. (Circles are averages for 12 observers.) (Adapted from Gruber and Braune, 1974.)

for a tone physically decreasing in intensity and undercompensating for a tone physically increasing.

A tone of continuously changing intensity may provide a poor test of adaptation. In subsequent studies by Mirabella *et al.* (1967) and Wiley (1972), observers increased and decreased the intensity of a tone, which otherwise remained physically constant, in order to keep loudness constant. This tracking procedure revealed little or no adaptation. The 72 observers of Mirabella *et al.* showed from 2 to 5 dB of adaptation for a 3500-Hz tone over a 10-min period at 70 dB SPL and reverse adaptation (increased loudness) at 90 dB. Results were similar for a 1000-Hz tone and for wide-band noise. Wiley (1972) measured no adaptation whatsoever between 10 and 60 dB SL at either 500 or 4000 Hz, over a much shorter, 30-sec period. Melnick (1967) used a similar tracking procedure except that every 30 sec, he interrupted the continuous tone to present a 5-sec, 1000-Hz reference tone at 60 dB SPL. Over a 4-min period, five observers kept the continuous 1000-Hz tone nearly constant at about 62 dB SPL as they tracked its loudness.

The tracking procedures alone may not yield entirely convincing outcomes because even small changes in stimulus intensity could conceivably disrupt adaptation. As soon as the observer increases intensity to compensate for a possible loudness decline, he may reduce or terminate the adaptation underway.

4. Tone Decay or Threshold Increase over Time

In 1882 Rayleigh noted that a steady high-frequency sound of "moderate intensity," which was probably close to threshold, disappeared within 3 to 4 sec. Interest in this phenomenon was stimulated much later when it was found that persons with a retrocochlear lesion such as an acoustic neuroma often show extreme tone decay (e.g., Carhart, 1957; Sorenson, 1960), although not all authors agree as to its diagnostic specificity (Palva *et al.*, 1967). The usual procedure is to set a steady tone just above the observer's threshold and have him signal when he no longer hears it, upon which the experimenter raises its level 5 dB; the observer again waits for the tone to disappear. The level of the tone must be increased as much as 60 dB over 1 min in order for some listeners with acoustic neuroma to continue to hear it. The level must be increased between 10 and 25 dB in order for normally hearing persons to continue to hear it (e.g., Hempstock *et al.*, 1964; Snyder, 1973; Sorenson, 1962; Stephens and Hinchcliffe, 1968). For the listener to signal that a steady tone at "threshold" is no longer audible, he must first hear something and that something must have some loudness. Thus the tone-decay test may be considered a measure of loudness adaptation in the vicinity of threshold. It suggests a great deal of adaptation near threshold where the steepening of the loudness function means that a 10-dB change in intensity corresponds to as much as a tenfold change in loudness (Scharf, 1978).

5. Other Procedures

Monaural measures of loudness adaptation yield evidence for significant amounts of adaptation only at low levels of stimulation. Exceptions are some papers by Weiler and colleagues (e.g., Davis and Weiler, 1976; Feaster and Weiler, 1975; Weiler and Gross, 1976) that report large amounts of adaptation at various levels and frequencies. Feaster and Weiler used a simultaneous monaural loudness balance. Their observers matched a 10,000-Hz comparison tone in loudness to a 500-, 1000-, or 2000-Hz test tone at 50 dB SPL before and after a 7-min exposure to the lower-frequency tone alone. Both tones were presented to the same ear; the 10,000-Hz comparison tone was presented intermittently (every 2.5 sec for 1.25 sec) during the postadaptation period while the test tone remained on continuously. To equal the loudness of the 500-Hz tone, the comparison tone was set 9 dB lower, on the average, in the postadaptation period than in the preadaptation period. Differences were smaller for the two other test frequencies. It is important to note that in the preadaptation matching both the test and comparison (10,000-Hz) tones were intermittent whereas in the postadaptation matching only the comparison tone was intermittent.

Weiler and Gross (1976) used a similar monaural matching paradigm. Again the comparison tone was at 10,000 Hz. The test or adapting tone was 500 Hz at 60 dB SPL. Prior to a 7-min presentation of the 500-Hz tone, the comparison and test tones—presented simultaneously every 25 sec for 10 sec—were matched in loudness. After the 7-min adaptation period, the 500-Hz tone remained on continuously while the 10,000-Hz tone was reintroduced, intermittently. The comparison tone was set 22 dB lower in the postadaptation period than in the preadaptation period. Differences in the intermittency, test-tone level, and subjects could account for the much larger drop in loudness reported by Weiler and Gross than by Feaster and Weiler. These results suggest that an intermittent or pulsed sound may reduce the loudness of a simultaneous, steady sound in the *same* ear.

In still another attempt to measure adaptation monaurally, Davis and Weiler (1976) reported that auditory reaction times were longer after a 7-min exposure to a pure tone than before. Reaction times were based on responses to a brief tone burst superposed on a prolonged 500-Hz "adapting" tone. Although the measured increase in reaction time, which is closely correlated with loudness (Chocholle, 1946), could reflect a decrease in the loudness of the prolonged tone, it could as plausibly reflect any one of a number of other mechanisms (such as a dulling of reflexes after 7 min of just listening to a pure tone).

In summary, measurements of adaptation made without recourse to interaural loudness matches lead to the following conclusion. The loudness of a steady sound presented alone does not decrease over time—there is no loudness adaptation—except near threshold.

B. Measurements of Adaptation Based on Interaural Loudness Matches

Loudness is most often measured by matching one sound to another, standard or *comparison* sound. Accordingly, experimenters have attempted to measure loudness adaptation by matching the loudness of a brief comparison sound in one ear—the unadapted ear—to that of the adapting or test sound in the other ear—the adapted ear; the match is made before and after continuous exposure to the adapting sound. Adaptation was thought to be demonstrated when the level of the comparison sound was set lower after exposure than before.

The postexposure match is made by presenting the comparison sound either after the test sound has been turned off or while it is still on. Figure 2 presents examples of the time course of delayed dichotic matching and two types of simultaneous matching. In Fig. 2A, the comparison is presented only once, just after termination of the adapting sound; in B, the comparison is presented also only once, but just *before* termination of the adapting sound; in C, the comparison is presented repeatedly throughout the adaptation period. In methods such as adjustment and tracking, the observer sets the comparison sound's level so that

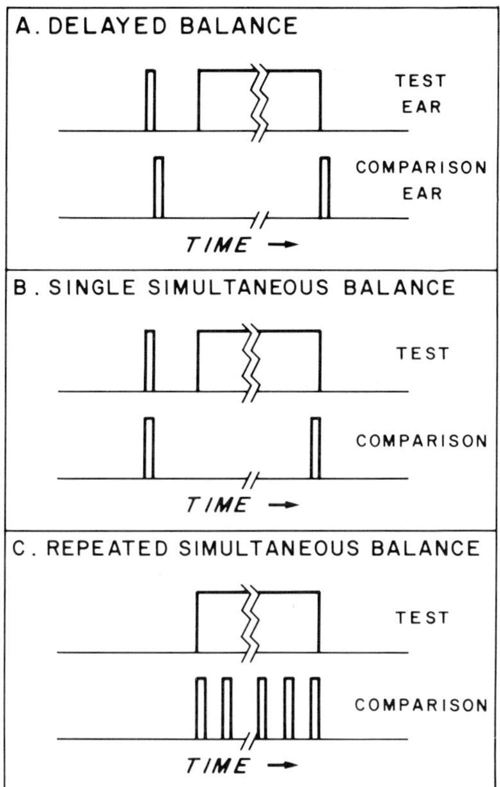

Figure 2 Schematic representations of three different procedures for measuring loudness adaptation by means of a dichotic loudness balance.

the comparison is as loud as the test sound in the adapting ear. In methods such as constant stimuli and limits, the observer judges the loudness of the comparison, whose level is set by the experimenter, relative to that of the test sound.

Until the late 1960s most measures of loudness adaptation were made with one form or another of simultaneous dichotic loudness matching. The results revealed large amounts of loudness adaptation, quite contrary to the monaural data cited above. It turns out, however, that the supposedly neutral comparison sound, brought in merely as a yardstick, often has a marked effect on the loudness of the test sound, a depressing effect that increases over time. Thus the simultaneous measures tell us about induced loudness adaptation, the adaptation that takes place in the presence of an intermittent or occasional comparison sound in the contralateral ear. (It seems that an intermittent sound in the ipsilateral ear—in the same ear as the steady sound—may also induce loudness adaptation.)

Two sections follow. The first reviews those experiments that have used a delayed dichotic balance and can tell us about simple adaptation. The second section reviews those experiments that have used a simultaneous balance and that tell us about induced adaptation.

1. Delayed Dichotic Loudness Balances

Reports from four different laboratories show that there is little or no adaptation of loudness when measured by matching the loudness of a brief sound in one ear to a long-duration sound in the other ear, provided that the match is made after termination of the long-duration sound as per Fig. 1A (Fraser *et al.*, 1970; Harbert *et al.*, 1968; Margolis and Wiley, 1976; Petty *et al.*, 1970; Stokinger and Studebaker, 1968; Stokinger *et al.*, 1972a). These six reports covered a frequency range from 500 to 4000 Hz, levels from 30 to 100 dB SPL, and test durations up to 7 min. Between 4 and 19 observers served in each study for a total of 52 observers. Generally, listeners judged the comparison and test sounds to be equally loud when equally intense, whether the test (adapting) tone had been on for a few seconds or for many minutes. Matches were made by various psychophysical methods, including constant stimuli (Margolis and Wiley, 1976; Stokinger *et al.*, 1972b), limits (Stokinger and Studebaker, 1968), tracking (Fraser *et al.*, 1970), and an adaptive up–down procedure (Petty *et al.*, 1970).

These papers were not the first to report the results of delayed dichotic loudness balances. Using approximately the same paradigm, Békésy (1929) had measured an average of 20 dB of adaptation for 10 observers, Wood (1930) approximately 12 dB for four observers, and Egan and Thwing (1955) 9 dB for one observer. Exposure intervals were of the order of 2 min. The discrepancy between the earlier and the more recent studies probably arises from subtle differences in procedure, which cannot be pinpointed from the sparse information provided in the earlier reports.

Except for a few early reports, the contemporary literature is consistent in showing, by delayed dichotic loudness balances, an absence of loudness adaptation. This conclusion agrees with that drawn from the monaural studies.

2. Simultaneous Dichotic Loudness Balances

Although data based on monaural procedures and *delayed* dichotic loudness balances show that loudness does not adapt except near threshold, many data based on *simultaneous* dichotic loudness balances show that the loudness of a steady sound does decrease. In simultaneous balances, the comparison sound is presented to the ear contralateral to that receiving the steady sound while the steady sound is still on; the comparison sound is presented either once as in Fig. 2B or repeatedly as in Fig. 2C. Many investigators (e.g., Egan, 1955; Hood, 1950; Palva and Kärjä, 1969) have interpreted the loudness decline measured under this paradigm as evidence for simple loudness adaptation. We now know that such an interpretation is wrong. The loudness decline is not the direct result of prolonged stimulation but is the result of interaural interaction with the simultaneously presented "comparison" sound. Support for this interpretation comes from a variety of experimental data, all of which show that eliminating interaural interaction eliminates the loudness decline and reducing the interaction reduces the decline. We have already seen how interaction can be eliminated and loudness adaptation avoided by monaural procedures or by delayed loudness balances. Reduced interaural interaction is achieved by manipulating the "comparison" signal. Several of these stimulus manipulations are considered.

Repetition. Presenting the comparison sound to the contralateral ear just *before* terminating the adapting sound—as in Fig. 1B—reduces the loudness of the adapting sound, but only a little (Fraser *et al.*, 1970; Petty *et al.*, 1970; Stokinger and Studebaker, 1968; Stokinger *et al.*, 1972a). The amount of loudness reduction is independent of how long the adapting sound had been on. However, if the comparison sound is repeatedly presented to the other ear, as in Fig. 1C, then loudness decreases more and the decrease becomes larger as the duration of the adapting sound lengthens (Egan, 1955; Harbert *et al.*, 1966; Hood, 1950, Kärjä, 1968, Palva and Kärjä, 1969, Petty *et al.*, 1970).

Data from Petty *et al.* (1970) and from Kärjä (1968) illustrate how the loudness decline depends on the experimental paradigm and stimulus parameters. Both experiments used a Békésy tracking procedure to achieve loudness balances between 1000-Hz test (adapting) and comparison tones, with the test tone set to 60 dB SL. The observer's task was to match the loudness at the two ears by varying the level of the comparison tone. To do this, he used a switch to increase the level of the comparison when it seemed softer than the test tone and to decrease the level when it seemed louder. The level was recorded continuously on the Békésy audiometer, and the midpoint of the excursions was taken as the equated level.

Figure 3 presents the means for 6 observers from Petty *et al.* and for 32 observers from Kärjä. The sensation level of the comparison tone at which it was judged equal in loudness to the test tone is plotted as a function of the duration of the test tone. A delayed 1-sec comparison tone (circles) was set only 2 dB lower than the continuous test tone, and this difference remained the same whether the test tone had been on less than 2 sec or more than 420 sec. A comparison tone (squares) presented 1 sec before termination of the test tone was set 6 to 10 dB lower, but the difference did not increase with test-tone duration. A comparison tone repeated every 60 sec for 15 sec (unfilled triangles)—while the test tone was on—was set lower and lower as the duration of the test tone increased, until at 420 sec, it was set 19 dB lower. Repeated every 400 msec for 200 msec (filled triangles), the comparison level was set nearly 23 dB lower than the test tone at the end of 180 sec.

The measured adaptation is ascribed to interaction between the steady tone and

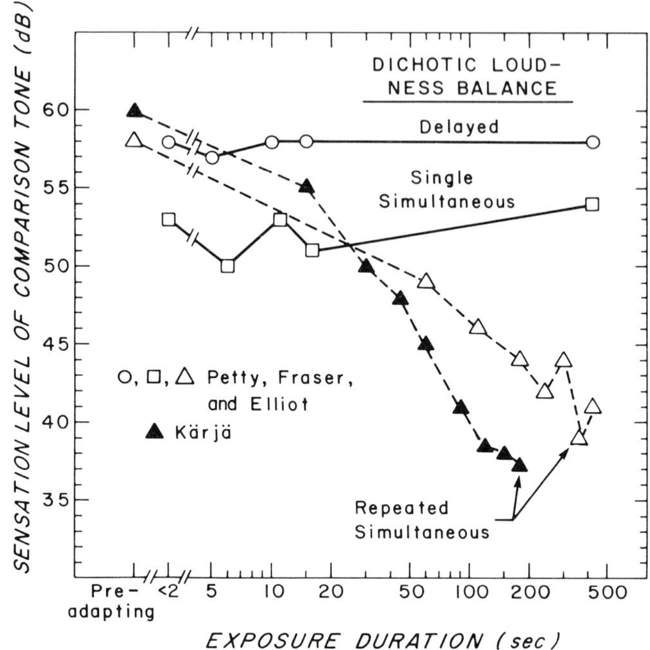

Figure 3   Sensation level at which a 1000-Hz intermittent comparison tone was judged as loud as a steady 60-dB 1000-Hz tone in the contralateral ear, plotted as a function of the exposure duration to the steady ear. [Data are for the three types of dichotic balance illustrated in Fig. 2 and are based upon reports by Petty *et al.* (1970) and Kärjä (1968).]

the comparison tone and is not assumed to demonstrate a decline in loudness that would have taken place simply as a function of time without the intervention of the contralateral comparison sound. We can be sure of this analysis for two reasons: (1) if interaction is eliminated, as in the monaural studies cited above, or if it is reduced by making the frequency of a comparison tone which is presented only once different from the test frequency (Fraser *et al.*, 1970; Morgan and Dirks, 1973; Bray *et al.*, 1973), then adaptation disappears; (2) if interaction is increased by lengthening the duration of the simultaneous comparison sound (Small and Minifie, 1961; Stokinger *et al.*, 1972a) or by presenting it intermittently throughout the period of the adapting sound (Hood, 1950; Kärjä, 1968; Palva and Kärjä, 1969; Petty *et al.*, 1970), or by both, i.e., by lengthening the on-time of an intermittent sound (Ahaus *et al.*, 1975), adaptation may reach levels as high as 30 or 40 dB. It would appear that the best way to study induced loudness adaptation is to present an intermittent sound to one ear and a steady sound to the adapting ear. Using a 200-msec tone burst that came on every 400 msec, Kärjä (1968) measured an average of 30 dB adaptation at the end of 3 min for frequencies of 2000 Hz and higher at 60 dB SL. Kärjä used a tracking procedure; his observers varied the level of the intermittent tone by means of a Békésy audiometer throughout the 3-min listening period. The decline in loudness level was generally exponential (decibels vs time) with the function approaching asymptote at 3 min. A remarkable feature of these data is that the listener reduced the level of the intermittent tone until it was some 30 dB less intense than the steady tone, yet the intermittent tone continued to cause the loudness of the steady tone to decrease. Since the effect required time to reach its full value, it may be considered a form of adaptation. However, it cannot be considered an example simply of lateralization. In normal lateralization, a tone 30 dB higher in one ear than in the other would totally suppress the apparent locus of the weaker tone, so that the listener would hear only the more intense tone to its side. The introduction of intermittency in one ear and continuity in the other wholly disrupts the normal lateralization which would be toward the more intensely stimulated ear. In general, time overides intensity in interaural effects. Further consideration is given below to Kärjä's data together with new data from my own laboratory.

The potency of the intermittent tone is also shown in its ability to overcome a frequency difference between it and the steady tone. (As noted above, introducing a frequency difference eliminates adaptation when the comparison tone is presented only once just before termination of the steady tone.) Egan (1955) obtained a loudness reduction equivalent to 23 dB when observers matched a 1000-Hz tone presented for 30 sec every 60 sec to one ear against a steady 800-Hz tone in the other ear. Thwing (1955) measured less adaptation with a comparable frequency difference, but his intermittent tone came on for only 15 sec every 120 sec, and he changed the frequency in the test ear to the same as that in the comparison ear during the 15-sec match. He thereby measured the spread of the effect across frequency, revealing patterns not unlike masking patterns but more symmetrical.

In an earlier, extensive series of experiments de Maré (1939) obtained sizable amounts of loudness decrease by presenting a 400-msec comparison tone every 3.5 sec to one ear and a nearly steady tone to the adapting ear, nearly steady because he turned it off during the 400 msec that the comparison tone was on. Moreover, he changed the frequency of the steady tone for the 400-msec interval just preceding presentation of the comparison tone. Despite these manipulations, loudness declined. Experiments by Sergeant and Harris (1963) show that even with an intermittent tone to one ear that repeats itself continually during a 5-min interval, adaptation takes place when a similarly intermittent tone is presented to the other ear for 10 sec every 30 sec. It is not clear whether their five observers judged primarily sound locus or loudness since the two experienced observers adjusted the interrupted tone to center the auditory image whereas the three inexperienced observers reported that they were matching loudness between the ears.

From all these measurements based on interaural loudness comparisons, we can conclude that loudness adaptation occurs when a steady tone (or continuous intermittent tone) is accompanied by an intermittent tone. Adaptation does not occur otherwise (except at low levels). Despite the many experiments on induced adaptation, our understanding of the phenomenon is poor partly because the intermittent signal, which induces the adaptation, was always varied in level. Unpublished experiments are reported below that kept the intermittent signal constant. Before turning to those experiments and to other experiments on simple adaptation, we review those measurements of adaptation based upon judgments of the locus of a binaural sound inside the head. Such lateralization experiments are germane to the often posited relation of induced loudness adaptation to lateralization and localization.

C. Measurements of Adaptation Based on Lateralization Judgments

Two equally intense sounds of similar spectra presented simultaneously to the two ears are heard as a single sound at or near the middle of the head. This percept corresponds to localizing a sound source directly in front (or back) from which direction the inputs to the two ears are identical. Since identical sounds presented separately to each ear produce about the same loudness, it would seem to follow that equally loud simultaneous sounds are always localized in the median plane, usually in the middle of the head in earphone listening or to the front in sound-field listening. Hence, if one ear is exposed to a steady sound whose loudness decreases over time owing to loudness adaptation, the introduction of an equally intense sound to the unadapted ear should result in lateralization toward that ear where loudness would be greater instead of to the median plane (i.e., the middle of the head). A quantitative measure of the amount of adaptation is obtained by adjusting the level of the comparison sound in the unadapted ear until the observer reports median-plane localization. The difference in levels between the ears has been taken as a measure of the degree of loudness adaptation.

Logical as it seems, this approach has been discredited as a measure of *loudness* adaptation, for two reasons. First, median-plane localization does not require equal loudness at the two ears. Second, even if it could be shown that loudness equality is required for median-plane localization, it does not necessarily follow that prolonged stimulation results in loudness adaptation; prolonged exposure could just as well fatigue or result in adaptation of a pure lateralization mechanism. Let us examine the empirical bases for these two objections and then discuss a possible basis for adaptation of the lateralization mechanism.

1. The Role of Loudness in Lateralization

For a sound to be centered must the inputs at the two ears be equally intense or must they be equally loud? Some of the ways to disassociate loudness and intensity include introducing a masking noise to one ear, shortening the duration in one ear well below 100 msec, introducing large frequency differences between the two ears, fatiguing one ear with an intense sound, and using observers with unilateral of unequal binaural impairments. Each approach has the disadvantage of leaving uncertain whether the manipulation has altered the lateralization mechanism so as to render meaningless loudness effects. More of a problem is that only lateralization under masking and by the hearing impaired seem to have been studied. (Urbantschitsch did report in 1881 that after exposure to a monaural fatiguing tone, a binaural tone is heard toward the nonfatigued side, but no comparison was made between loudness decrease and lateralization changes.)

Raab and Osman (1962) reported that in order to center the sound image observers set a brief tone burst in one ear, presented against a partially masking white noise, to somewhere between the same intensity and the same loudness as in the control, unmasked ear. At the intensities at which the tone was centered, the masked tone was softer than the unmasked tone according to alternate loudness balances.

A number of reports suggest that hard-of-hearing persons, even those with distinct interaural differences in sensitivity, localize sounds reasonably well (e.g., Nordlund, 1964; Dieroff, 1976). No systematic study, however, seems to be available that compares loudness matches to centering.

The hard-of-hearing person's ability to localize a sound in the median plane despite a large loudness difference between the ears probably results from long experience with environmental sounds. Florentine (1976) has nicely demonstrated this by wearing an earplug in one ear continuously for over 3 months. At first, she and other less heroic observers, who wore an earplug for only 5 to 27 days, judged 500- and 1000-Hz pure tones as centered when they were presented at earphone levels corresponding to equal loudness. These levels differed by as much as 30 dB. It was known that the tones were equally loud because the observers made alternate loudness balances between the two ears. Presumably, the earphone levels that yielded equal loudness resulted in equal levels at the eardrum, after attenuation by the monaural plug. After a few days of wearing earplugs, the observers set the earphone outputs close to equal intensity rather than to equal loudness in order to center the sound image. With constant, all-day exposure to environmental sounds, observers "learned" that a sound in the median plane meant unequal loudness at the two ears. This learning is wholly unconscious but recognizable as the observer gradually became more comfortable with environmental sounds and better able to localize them. Clearly, equal loudness at the two ears is not required for median-plane localization either in a sound field or through earphones (see also Jerger and Harford, 1960; Bauer *et al.*, 1966). The following results from prolonged exposure to a monaural sound buttress this conclusion.

2. Comparison of Changes in Loudness and Lateralization under Prolonged Listening

We have seen that an intermittent sound to one ear causes a progressive reduction in the loudness of a continuous sound in the other ear. Is this loudness reduction accompanied by a change in the locus of the sound image? If so, does the change in locus follow the same time course as the loudness change? Is it of comparable magnitude? Only Stokinger and Studebaker (1968) appear to have sought experimental answers to these questions, by asking 10 observers to judge alternately the loudness of a steady 1000-Hz tone and the locus of the tonal image. By a method of limits, the experimenter increased and decreased the level of the intermittent tone until either it was judged equal in loudness to the steady tone or the tonal image was centered, depending upon which instruction was in force. The matches were made before and after a 5-min exposure to the steady tone. To equal an 80-dB steady tone in loudness, the intermittent tone was set to 54 dB but to move the tonal image to center it was set to 27 dB. With a 50-dB steady tone, the levels were 32 and 22 dB. Under these conditions—1-sec tone bursts repeated every 3 sec—loudness is a great deal lower in the intermittent ear than in the steady ear when the sound is judged to be in the median plane. Here is additional evidence against the assumption that centering requires equal loudness at the two ears. Thus it is misleading to measure any kind of loudness adaptation from median-plane localization, and wholly wrong to infer monaural, simple, loudness adaptation from such measures.

Although Stokinger and Studebaker were the only ones to compare directly interactive adaptation for loudness and for lateralization, a number of other authors have explicitly asked observers to localize a sound image when exposed to a steady sound in one ear and an intermittent sound in the other (Carterette, 1955; Jerger, 1957; Tsuiki, 1965; Weiler, 1972; Wittich, 1966; Wright, 1959, 1960). The phenomenon itself had already been mentioned in 1859 by Dove who noted that when the output of a tuning fork was led first to one ear for some time and then to both ears, the sound was heard toward the previously unstimulated ear. Urbantschitsch (1881) and Sewall (1907) made similar observations.

The modern studies generally agree in showing more adaptation for lateralization at 2000 Hz and above than at lower frequencies, with the amount of adaptation increasing with level. Where quantitative data are given (Carterette, 1955; Jerger, 1957; Weiler, 1972; Wittich, 1966; Wright, 1959), the maximum amount of adaptation, i.e., the decrease in the level of the intermittent sound required for centering, is of the order of 25 dB after *approximately* 7 min of exposure to a steady sound. These studies measured much smaller amounts of adaptation than did Stokinger and Studebaker (1968), who correctly ascribed the difference to the shorter duration of their intermittent stimuli, 1 sec as compared to 15 sec used by the other authors. Wright in 1960 had found that he could obtain as much as 50-dB adaptation by reducing the duration of his intermittent stimuli from 15 sec used in his 1959 study, to 1 sec.

The large difference in adaptation based on loudness judgments and that based on lateralization judgments with brief, intermittent stimuli does not hold for the longer stimuli so often used. Hood (1950), using 10-sec stimuli repeated every 30 sec, obtained somewhat more adaptation, of the order of 35 dB, for loudness judgments than others obtained later for lateralization judgments. However, the repetition rate and other experimental details were different.

As to the time course of adaptation, it appears to be faster for lateralization, although few data are available that allow a direct comparison. Hood's (1950) figures suggest that loudness decreases primarily between the first and third minutes of exposure, whereas some of Wright's (1959) data suggest that a 15-dB lateralization shift occurs during the first minute of exposure.

One other type of experiment illustrates that equal loudness need not mean a centered image. Bartlett and Mark (1922) set the phase relation of a 157-Hz tone at the left and right ears so that a listener heard the tone in one ear only. After prolonged listening the phase was set to 0° and the image moved distinctly to the ear that had been "silent." Although loudness in the silent ear was not measured, it is unlikely that under equal stimulation to the two ears the loudness in one ear would have declined more than in the other. Moreover, Bartlett and Marks report no change in binaural loudness during the prolonged exposure.

From all this, we may conclude that adaptation of the lateralization mechanism, like induced loudness adaptation, occurs when a steady tone to one ear is accompanied by an intermittent tone to the other ear. The two phenomena have enough in common to suggest that they depend on a common mechanism, but they do diverge strongly when the duration of the intermittent tone is shortened. There can be no doubt that a centered sound need not be represented by equal loudness at the two ears, although such may be the usual condition.

The two types of adaptation also differ in that adaptation in lateralization normally occurs also when the steady sound is *not* accompanied by an intermittent sound in the contralateral ear. Thus, after monaural exposure to a continuous sound, the adaptation measured by "loudness balances" between that sound and a continuous sound of the same frequency introduced to the other ear almost certainly reflects adaptation of the lateralization mechanism; the postexposure tone is binaural and fuses to a single image that can be centered but for which interaural loudness balances are not possible. Accordingly, in those experiments, such as some of Hood's (1950), that were based on judgments of a postexposure binaural tone, the reported loudness balances must have been centering judgments. But let us return to induced loudness adaptation and its relation to lateralization.

3. Possible Basis for Induced Adaptation

In the presence of an intermittent sound in the contralateral ear, a steady sound declines in loudness and its apparent locus shifts toward the contralateral ear. Both changes require time to reach maximum value and, in that sense, may be considered forms of adaptation. Besides resembling each other with respect to the basic stimulus paradigm—a steady tone to one ear and an intermittent tone to the other—both changes increase with the level of the steady tone and are greater at frequencies above 1000 Hz than below. They differ in their magnitude; under similar stimulus conditions, centering judgments reveal much greater adaptation than loudness judgments. Also lateralization shifts decrease as the duration of the intermittent sound lengthens whereas loudness adaptation appears to increase.

We know enough about these processes to guess at the basic underlying mechanism which in turn leads to specific testable predictions. First let us recall what happens in the normal situation, when a brief, high-frequency sound arrives from a source off to one side of a listener. The sound arrives at the near ear sooner and with greater intensity than at the far ear. The interaural differences give rise to the impression of a sound coming from one side, the side from which it in fact originates. If the stimulus is mimicked with earphones then the listener hears only a tone at the ear receiving the more intense input sooner. The other ear is "silent." Békésy (1958) ascribes this effect to neural inhibition of a special kind which he calls *funneling*. Although the locus of the lagging, softer sound may go unperceived, it contributes to the overall loudness of the percept. This binaural funneling appears to take place whenever there is a sudden and rapid increase in intensity in one ear (or both), as if a sound had just arrived there. My hypothesis is that this sudden onset is at the root of induced adaptation both for lateralization and for loudness. Neural funneling takes place even in the absence of a sound at the other ear. The funneling hypothesis agrees with the finding that adaptation for lateralization is much more potent for short-duration than for longer duration intermittent stimuli. The funneling occurs immediately at stimulus onset (since it applies to interaural time differences well below 1 msec). A sound that continues as a steady sound for 10 or 15 sec loses its inhibitory potency, and the sound image moves toward the center. From the funneling hypothesis we should expect that the loudness of the intermittent sound is enhanced by the inhibited steady tone. [Botte *et al.* (1982) show that, in fact, the loudness of an intermittent sound nearly doubles when accompanied by a steady sound in the contralateral ear.]

What remains unclear is why the funneling effect increases with time (or perhaps with number of repetitions, since with only a single repetition as in many simultaneous dichotic loudness balances, one finds minimal decrease in loudness), which qualifies the effect as a form of adaptation. The best clue we have is that constant stimulation of one ear [or even of both ears (Bartlett and Mark, 1922) with lateralization to one side] results in subsequent lateralization or localization away from the "adapted" ear. Fatigued or adapted, the lateralization mechanism on one side is weakened and funneling occurs more readily toward the other unexposed side—thus the important role of duration of exposure.

Perhaps it is too soon to seek an answer to this question. First we must ascertain the limits of adaptation. A basic question is whether an intermittent sound in the ipsilateral ear can induce loudness adaptation and, if so, whether it is like adaptation induced contralaterally. Other questions concern temporal parameters. How long a time interval between the intermittent bursts suffices to unleash the adaptation process? Is it necessary to have the steady tone on during the intervals between intermittent sounds or would it suffice to turn it on 1 or 2 sec before the intermittent sound? Such a powerful effect probably can bridge gaps of at least a minute in a binaural system designed to handle time differences in the microsecond range. We should also expect it to be related to some useful property of the auditory system.

IV. CURRENT RESEARCH

The experiments reported below were carried out mostly at the Auditory Perception Laboratory at Northeastern University from 1976 to 1980. They concern primarily simple loudness adaptation, measured without recourse to interaural comparisons. A few experiments on induced loudness adaptation are considered separately. It was during the initial work on induced adaptation that we discovered that loudness adapts markedly at low levels even in the absence of an intermittent sound. Given all the negative outcomes in the recent literature whereby avoiding interaural interaction seemed to preclude loudness adaptation, we were indeed surprised to encounter potent adaptation at any level or frequency. Since simple loudness adaptation is the exception, we undertook to determine under what stimulus conditions it occurs. Knowing when loudness does adapt should help clarify why under most circumstances loudness does not adapt, why it is so unlike most other sensory atrributes in this respect. That understanding should in turn move us closer to unraveling the code for loudness in the auditory system.

Almost all the data have been collected by the method of successive magnitude estimation whereby the observer assigns numbers to express the loudness of a sound at successive time intervals.[3] Typical instructions to the observer are as follows:

You are to judge the loudness of a sound by choosing a number whose magnitude corresponds to the loudness. You may use any positive number no matter how small—including fractions or

---

[3]Meiselman (1968) appears to have been the first to use this procedure, to measure taste adaptation.

decimals—or how large. Do not, however, use negative numbers, but you may use zero if you do not hear the sound. The important point is that you choose a number that corresponds to the loudness you experience. First you will hear a brief sound repeated twice. Write the number you choose on the slip of paper provided.[4] After that you will hear a continuous sound. Whenever the light in front of you comes on you are to match a number to the loudness of the sound as you hear it during the 2 sec the light is on. Write each number down in its appropriate space. You will be asked to make X judgments; the light will come on every 10 to 30 sec. Please keep your head still while the sound is on, and do not touch the earphones.

The number of judgments, the intervals separating them, and the duration of the steady tone varied from experiment to experiment; duration was never less than 30 sec nor more than 4 min. The experimental values will be apparent from the figures and tables. Unless otherwise indicated, monaural stimuli were always presented to the observer's right ear. Each observer usually judged the same stimulus twice, with other stimuli normally separating the two sets of judgments. Stimulus variables other than duration were level, spectral characteristics, temporal characteristics, and mode of presentation (monaural vs binaural and earphone vs loudspeaker). The effect of observer variables such as age and absolute threshold is also considered. Finally, data are presented on loudness adaptation induced by an intermittent tone in the contralateral ear.

A. Stimulus Conditions Required for Simple Loudness Adaptation

1. Level

Neither those measures of loudness adaptation based on interaural loudness matches that avoid interaural interaction nor those based on monaural paradigms (such as tracking and cross-modality matching) have revealed any significant decrease in loudness as a function of stimulus duration, except sometimes at low levels. Given that the threshold for pure tones increases with prolonged, continuous stimulation ("tone decay"), the loudness of near-threshold tones ought to decrease over time. The method of successive magnitude estimation shows that the loudness of soft sounds does indeed decline as a function of time, and that the softer the signal the greater the decline.

Figure 4 presents results for 12 to 16 observers who judged the loudness of a steady 4000-Hz tone at successive intervals as indicated on the abscissa. In this early series, the tone was presented at the same three sound pressure levels to all observers without regard to individual thresholds. Accordingly, sensation level differed from observer to observer. Mean sensation levels are shown in the figure. On half the trials the tone was presented monaurally to the right ear and

---

[4]In later experiments and in all those in the free field, observers entered their numerical judgments into the memory bank of a calculator.

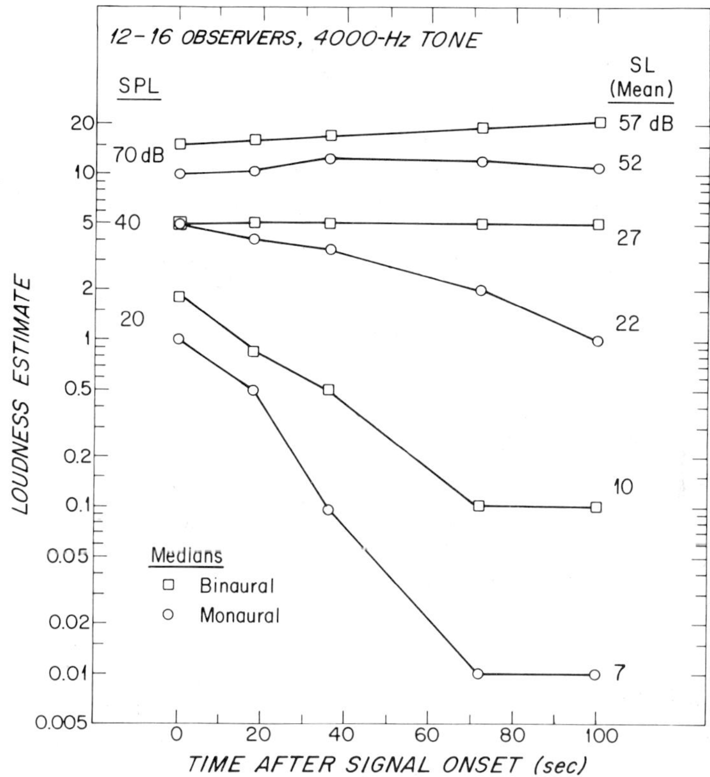

Figure 4   Median estimates of the loudness of a 4000-Hz tone as a function of signal duration. (Parameters on the curves are the sound pressure level of the tone and its corresponding mean sensation level.)

on the other half binaurally. The median loudness estimations are shown on the ordinate; each point stands for 32 judgments (except at 20 dB where only 12 observers could hear the tone). These medians are for the original numbers given by the observers who were always free to choose any number they desired. The overall picture is clear. At 70 dB SPL, loudness does not decrease over the 100-sec stimulus period; at 40 dB only monaural loudness decreases; at 20 dB both binaural and monaural loudness decrease dramatically, apparently reaching an asymptote by 70 sec. (The interaction between level and adaptation is significant at better than the 0.01 level as shown by a repeated-measures analysis of variance.) Similar results were obtained for a 1000-Hz tone, with the notable difference that at 20 dB SPL the loudness decrease was considerably less than for the 4000-Hz tone and at 40 dB monaural (as well as binaural) loudness did not decrease.

The principal finding from this original experiment, that loudness adapts at low levels but not at moderate levels, has stood up well—as shown below in a number of subsequent studies. Nevertheless, this early study suffers from two flaws. First, the tone was delivered at fixed sound pressure levels instead of being adjusted relative to each observer's threshold so as to be at a constant sensation level. It turns out that with respect to level, it is largely the sensation level that determines how much loudness adapts. (Moreover, at low sound pressure levels, some observers are unable to hear the sound. As noted above, four of the 16 observers in this first study could not hear the 4000-Hz tone at 20 dB SPL. In most of our subsequent studies, observers with high thresholds were excluded.) Second, termination of the tone coincided with the final light signal so that the observer judged the loudness of the sound just before it went off. These judgments at 100 sec were probably inflated owing to an "off-effect." At termination, soft sounds may often seem louder than earlier, and a steady tone that had become inaudible may be heard to go off (Dunlap, 1904). In our subsequent studies the steady tone continued for 2 or 3 sec after the light signal calling for a final magnitude estimation. These later studies suggest that adaptation continues beyond 70 sec, and does not stop there as in Fig. 4.

Although at least one previous report had suggested that loudness adapts at low levels (Lawrence *et al.*, 1949), a careful study by Margolis and Wiley (1976) uncovered no adaptation at 15 or 25 dB SL after 60 sec of continuous exposure to a 4000-Hz tone. Since their method, a delayed dichotic loudness balance, differed radically from our monaural (and binaural) method of magnitude estimation, we replicated part of their experiment. We used their method and stimulus configurations to measure the loudness of a 4000-Hz tone at 25 dB SL after 1 sec and after 30 sec. The observer judged whether a 1-sec tone in the left ear was louder or softer than a tone in the right ear that ended 400 msec earlier and that had lasted either 1 or 30 sec. The tone in the right ear was set at 25 dB SL. Figure 5 shows the SL in the left ear at which the tone was judged equal in loudness, by a method of constant stimuli, to the 25-dB SL tone in the right ear. Black dots are for 15 individual observers and the squares are the arithmetic means of those data. At the end of 30 sec the mean level in the left ear was nearly 10 dB lower than in the right ear. The corresponding means for the four observers of Margolis and Wiley, shown by the open circles, did not change over 30 sec. The large discrepancy between these two outcomes remains unexplained. Although four of our observers gave data similar to the four observers of Margolis and Wiley, it is highly unlikely that their observers represented an extreme sample unless they had been selectively chosen. Our own matches, however, show more adaptation than do our magnitude estimates. A 10-dB drop from 25 to 15 dB SL represents nearly a 3 : 1 change in loudness (Scharf, 1978). At 22 dB SL the magnitude estimates revealed only a 1.4 : 1 change in monaural loudness after 30 sec. Clarification of this discrepancy requires further exploration. However, it is clear

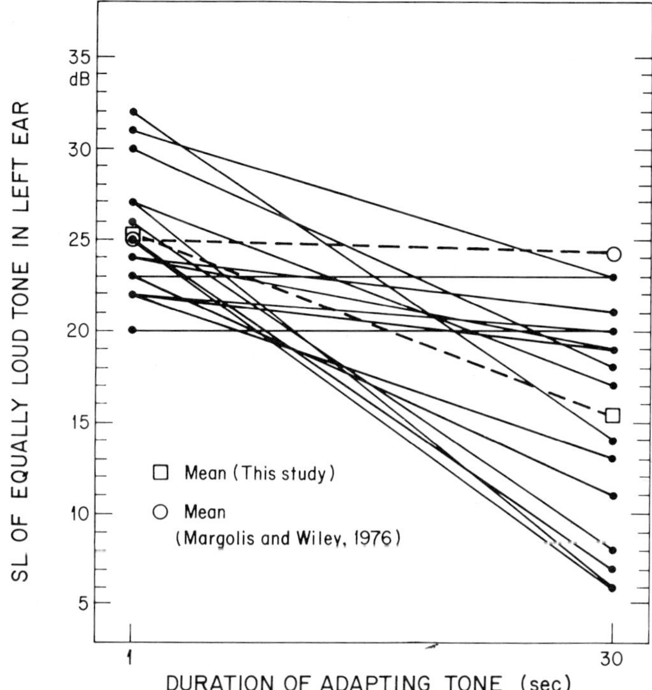

Figure 5 Sensation level at which a brief 4000-Hz tone burst to the left ear sounded as loud as the last part of a 25-dB tone to the right ear, plotted as a function of the duration of the right-ear tone. [Each solid line is for an individual observer. Circles are based on data from Margolis and Wiley (1976). Measurements were made by the method of constant stimuli.]

that adaptation can be demonstrated at low levels by delayed dichotic balances as well as by successive magnitude estimations. Magnitude estimation is the preferred method because it is far less time consuming than loudness balancing, and because it provides a snapshot of the dynamics of sensation, which is the essence of adaptation.

The data in Fig. 5 point up the large individual differences in loudness adaptation. Similar variability was true of the magnitude estimations at low levels presented in Fig. 4 but that variability was exaggerated by the large differences in sensation levels from observer to observer. Nevertheless, the variability at 70 dB SPL was small in comparison to that at 20 dB. No observer showed consistent adaptation at the higher level. Whereas loudness adaptation seems to be almost universally absent at high levels, it is not universally present at low levels; some observers show no adaptation at levels as low as 10 dB above threshold. Section IV,B treats extensively the question of differences among individuals. The next set of experiments eliminates interindividual variation caused by the use of different sensation levels for each subject; all stimuli were presented at levels relative to each observer's threshold.

Measurements were made with a 4000-Hz tone at sensation levels from 5 to 30 dB on 8 observers. An adaptive two-interval, forced-choice procedure provided an accurate, criterion-free threshold measure in the same session that successive magnitude estimations were made. On three separate days, each observer estimated the loudness of the tone presented at all five levels either monaurally—1 day to the left ear, 1 day to the right ear—or binaurally. To facilitate comparison among the data, only the first and final estimates are considered. The estimate, E_t, at time, t (usually the final estimate), is subtracted from the initial estimate, E_0. Dividing the difference by the initial estimate yields an *adaptation quotient*, AQ, according to the equation, $AQ = (E_0 - E_t)/E_0$. The AQ may be specified by the value of t as AQ_t. (The subscript, t, will be usually omitted when the AQ is computed from the final estimate.) The larger the AQ, the more adaptation. A quotient of 1 means complete adaptation: the tone became inaudible. A quotient of 0 means no adaptation: loudness was the same at the end as at the beginning of the adaptation period.

Figure 6 plots the mean AQ as a function of sensation level. (Mean sound pressure level at threshold is shown on the graph; the binaural value is the average of -1.5 dB in the right ears and 3.5 dB in the left ears of the eight

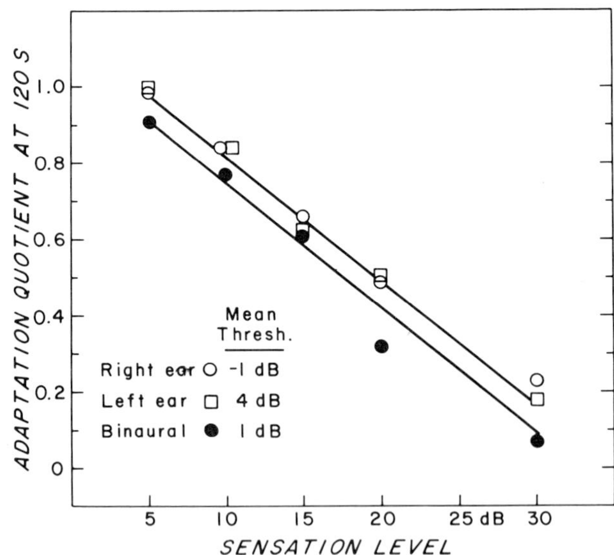

Figure 6   Adaptation quotient for a 4000-Hz tone presented either monaurally or binaurally as a function of sensation level. (Each point is the mean of 16 AQs from eight observers.)

observers.) Loudness adaptation depends heavily on level. With increasing sensation level, AQ decreases monotonically from over 0.9 at 5 dB to 0.2 and less at 30 dB. The binaural quotient is 0.07 and the monaural quotients are around 0.2 at 30 dB, indicating average decreases in loudness over a 2-min listening period of only 7 and 20%. (Section IV,A,4 treats the apparent differences between monaural and binaural modes of signal presentation.) The monaural quotients of nearly 1.0 at 5 dB mean that adaptation was nearly complete at 120 sec. Indeed, on only 6 of the 32 trials could the monaural tone be heard for the full 120 sec; on the other 26 trials the tone disappeared.

2. Spectral Characteristics

Our first near-threshold measurements suggested that loudness adapts more at 4000 Hz than at 1000 Hz. Hints can also be found in the literature that high frequencies adapt more than low (e.g., Rayleigh, 1882; Snyder, 1973). To determine just how adaptation depends on spectral characteristics, we used tones with frequencies from 250 to 15,000 Hz as well as filtered noise and two-tone complexes. First the results for pure tones at various frequencies are presented and then the results for sounds of varying spectral complexity.

a. Frequency. The method of successive magnitude estimation was applied throughout, with sensation level set to the same value for every observer. Thresholds were again measured at the beginning of each session by a 2IFC procedure. Seven observers estimated the loudness of monaural tones set to four frequencies at five sensation levels. Figure 7 presents the mean AQ at 120 sec as a function of sensation level. Parameter on the curves is the frequency of the tone. Each mean is based on 14 values, two for each of the seven observers. The major effect of level is evident at all frequencies. The effect of frequency is small and statistically insignificant ($p > 0.05$ by ANOVA). But at 10 and 15 dB SL, adaptation at 4000 Hz does seem to exceed adaptation at the lower frequencies. At 20 dB SL adaptation is small at all four frequencies, and at 30 dB SL adaptation is negative at all frequencies, meaning that observers reported a small increase in loudness over the 2-min listening period. Thus, a clear effect of frequency on adaptation may be measurable most easily in the neighborhood of 10 dB SL.

Several other series of measurements honed in on the frequency effect. In one series, 11 observers made magnitude estimations of tones at 250, 1000, 2000, and 4000 Hz over intervals of 100 sec. In a second series, another 12 observers made estimations of tones at 1000, 1500, 4000, and 6000 Hz over intervals of 120 sec. In a third series, 16 observers made estimations at 4000, 6000, 8000 Hz and 14 observers at 10,000 Hz over intervals of 110 sec. Finally, in a fourth series, 15 observers made estimations at 2000 and 4000 Hz over intervals of 100 sec. All measurements were at 10 dB SL, with the threshold determined rapidly

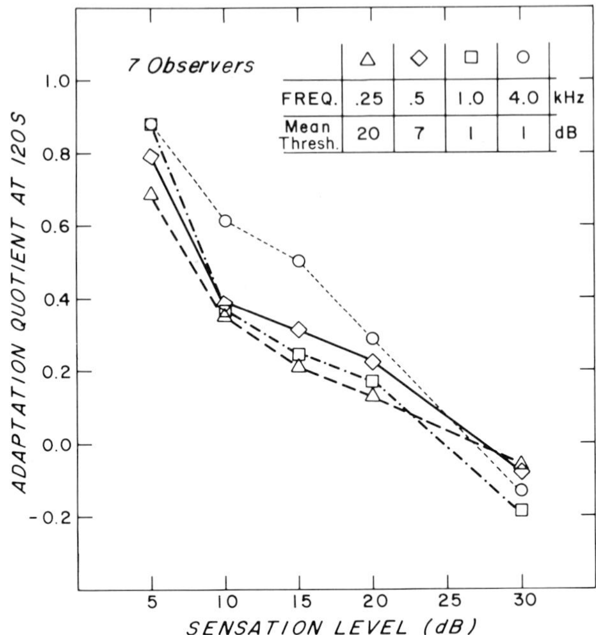

Figure 7 Mean adaptation quotient for four different frequencies as a function of sensation level.

by a method of limits comprising three descending and three ascending series. Figure 8 gives the obtained AQs as a function of frequency. Means are based on the combined results from one to three groups of observers; groups were combined whenever the signal frequency was the same. Thus the number of observers varies from a minimum of 11 at 250 Hz to a maximum of 54 at 4000 Hz, as shown at the top of the figure. Every observer made two estimations at each duration so that each mean AQ is based on four judgments by each observer, two for the initial estimation and two for the estimation at time, t, which was between 100 and 120 sec.

At 250 and 1000 Hz, adaptation is less than 40% after about 120 sec. It increases to approximately 50% at 1500 and 2000 Hz, and then hovers above 60% at frequencies between 4000 and 10,000 Hz. Data collected in a free field (see below) suggest that adaptation remains approximately constant at still higher frequencies, up to 15,000 Hz. We, like other investigators (see Ward, 1973, p. 304), have thus been unable to confirm Rayleigh's report (1882) that a 10,000-Hz tone at "moderate intensity" becomes inaudible in 3 to 4 sec. Of the 14 observers who listened in the free field, only one reported that the 10,000-Hz tone disappeared and only after 2 min of exposure. Of the 14 other observers who

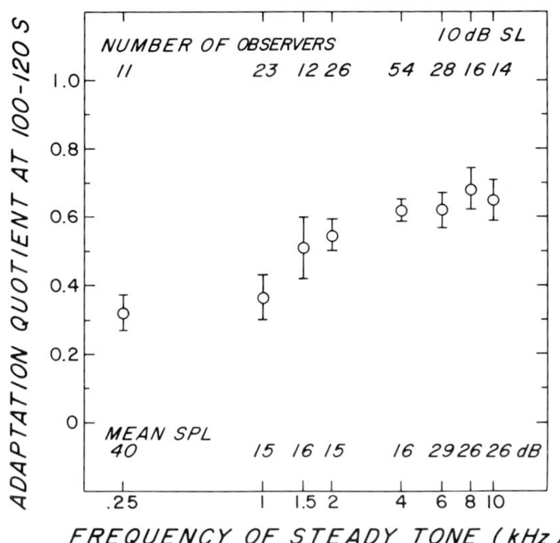

Figure 8 Mean adaptation quotient at 10 dB SL as a function of frequency. Number of observers who judged each frequency and the mean sound pressure level at 10 dB SL are shown above the corresponding frequency. Each observer contributed two AQs at each data point. Vertical lines are two standard errors of the mean.)

judged under earphone listening, four reported that the tone disappeared, after 20 to 80 sec of exposure. Perhaps Rayleigh listened to a tone less than 10 dB above his threshold; according to the data collected at 5 dB SL (see Fig. 6), a 4000-Hz tone disappears for many listeners when so close to threshold, and no doubt so does a 10,000-Hz tone.

Figure 8 gives the mean sound pressure level at which each frequency was presented in order to be at 10 dB SL. Differences in adaptation at low and high frequencies cannot be ascribed to differences in physical intensity. Although the 250-Hz tone was about 25 dB more intense than the 4000-Hz tone, the 1000-Hz tone was 1 dB *less* intense. Similarly, initial loudness was approximately 0.25 sones for the 250-Hz tone but about the same—0.06 sones—for the 1000- and 4000-Hz tones (from Scharf, 1978). Thus loudness apparently adapts less at the lower frequencies because the frequency is lower and not because some other stimulus attribute such as intensity or some subjective attribute such as loudness changes with frequency.

Figure 9 illustrates the similarity of the adaptation curves for frequencies from 4000 to 10,000 Hz. Median loudness estimates by 16 observers are plotted as a function of stimulus duration. (At 10,000 Hz, 14 observers participated.) Filled symbols are for the four different frequencies; open symbols are for noises that are discussed below. This group of observers comprised either a part of or the entire group of observers whose AQs are given in Fig. 8. All measurements were

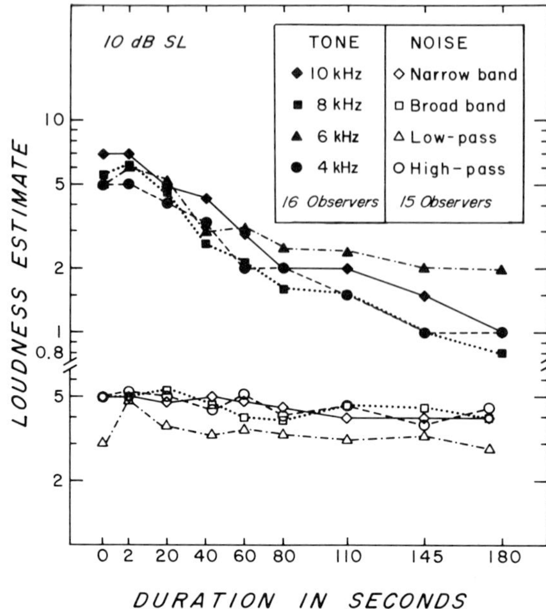

Figure 9   Loudness estimate of tones at four different frequencies and of four different kinds of continuous-spectrum noise, plotted as a function of the duration of the sound. (Each point is the median of 32 judgments of the tones and of 30 judgments of the noises.)

made at 10 dB SL. The course of loudness over the 3-min listening period is similar at three of the four frequencies; at 6000 Hz, loudness seems to adapt least. However, the data from these 16 observers, when combined with those of 12 other observers run earlier, yielded an average AQ close to that at the other three frequencies (as seen in Fig. 8). Moreover, a repeated-measures ANOVA showed that the interaction between frequency and duration of the signal was not significant so that adaptation was the same at all four frequencies. (The ANOVA was performed on the adaptation quotients in order to eliminate differences among observers and frequencies caused by the use of different initial numbers in the magnitude estimations.)

b. Spectral Complexity. In the next two series of measurements, the effect of spectral complexity on adaptation was investigated, first for continuous-spectrum noise and then for two-tone complexes.

The noise data appear in Fig. 9 which presents median loudness estimates as a function of listening duration. Fifteen observers judged the loudness of various configurations of noise at 10 dB SL. The low-pass and high-pass noises had cut-off frequencies in the vicinity of 2000 Hz. The slopes from the two ganged

Allison-2B filters were 70 dB per octave. The broad-band noise was white noise that went through a low-pass filter set to a cut-off at 7000 Hz. The narrow band had a width from 3800 to 4200 Hz with slopes steeper than 200 dB per octave. Each observer judged the four noises twice each in a single 1-hour session. Thresholds were measured by a rapid method of limits immediately before the loudness judgments.

The contrast between the high-frequency data in Fig. 9 and the noise data is striking. Whereas the loudness of the high-frequency tones decreases dramatically with time, the loudness of the noises decreases only slightly. The mean AQ for each of the four noises at 110 sec is under 0.3. The mean AQ for pure tones above 2000 Hz exceeds 0.6. These differences between adaptation for the noises and for the tones are highly significant by ANOVA. (An earlier study with a different group of 13 observers yielded an AQ_{120} of 0.18 for a broad-band noise at 15 dB SL, as compared to 0.61 for a 4000-Hz tone at the same level.)

Since the high-pass noise shows as little adaptation as the low-pass or broad-band noise, the decrease in adaptation cannot be ascribed to the presence of low-frequency components which adapt less than high-frequency components. Nor does greater bandwidth account for the decrease in adaptation, since the narrow-band noise adapted weakly although it was centered on 4000 Hz (where a pure tone adapts strongly) and its energy was confined to less than a critical band (see Scharf, 1970). Accordingly, neither frequency nor bandwidth per se provides a likely explanation for the reduced adaptation of continuous-spectrum noise. A likely candidate is the presence of fluctuations of amplitude within the component critical bands of a continuous-spectrum noise. Amplitude may fluctuate slowly enough to prevent or at least reduce adaptation. Thus, it would appear that amplitude modulation—or its equivalent—over a restricted range of frequencies is sufficient to reduce and perhaps eliminate loudness adaptation. Before considering the effect of modulating a pure tone, we examine the results of spreading excitation within the auditory system by increasing the frequency separation between two pure tones.

Figure 10 presents the mean AQ at 120 sec as a function of a frequency separation, ΔF, between two tones centered on 4000 Hz. Four series of measurements were run at 10 dB SL with different groups of observers; of the 18 observers who participated in the four series, two participated in all four series and one in three series. The AQ for a single tone at 4000 Hz (ΔF equals 0 Hz) is more than 0.6. For two tones with a ΔF of only 2 Hz, adaptation plummets to nearly 0 and only gradually increases with ΔF until beyond a ΔF of 700 Hz, adaptation is nearly as great as that for the single tone. The disappearance of adaptation at the narrowest ΔFs is surely due to beating between the two tones which causes the overall amplitude to fluctuate widely, going from a maximum to a null two times per second when ΔF is 2 Hz, four times per second when ΔF is 4 Hz, and so forth. Even when one tone is weaker than the other so that the

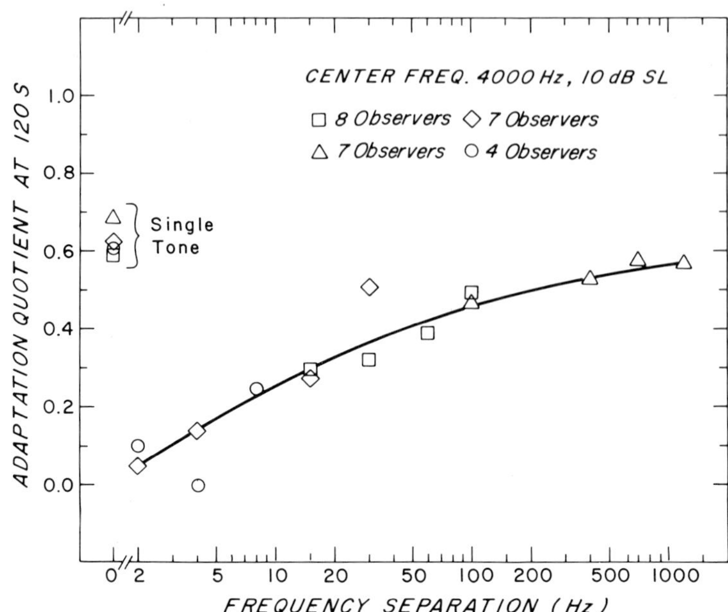

Figure 10   Mean adaptation quotient for a two-tone complex at 10 dB SL, plotted as a function of the frequency difference between the two components of the complex. (Each symbol is for a different series of measurements with varying numbers of observers.)

depth of modulation is less than 100%, adaptation for a two-tone complex with a ΔF of 100 Hz is half what it is for a single tone. Just how adaptation depends upon depth of modulation remains to be investigated. It is clear that the amplitude fluctuations in a two-tone complex, like those in the continuous-spectrum noises, sharply reduce adaptation. As ΔF increases, the fluctuations speed up and become too rapid to prevent adaptation which then increases. At the widest ΔFs, the tones are so far apart that they fail to interact significantly. Since both tones are at high frequencies, adaptation approaches that of a single high-frequency tone.[5]

The frequency separation at which adaptation appears to reach maximum in Fig. 10 is close to the critical band, which is 700 Hz at a center frequency of 4000 Hz. Similar data were collected at a center frequency of 2000 Hz, where adaptation also increased with ΔF, reaching a maximum in the vicinity of 300 Hz which is the critical band at 2000 Hz. Although these data must be considered

---

[5]Békésy (1960) also reported a decrease in loudness adaptation for two beating tones. However, he used a dichotic loudness balance to measure the adaptation of a 1000-Hz tone at 80 dB SPL. Since at such a high level, monaural measures reveal no adaptation, it is likely that Békésy demonstrated a decrease in induced loudness adaptation by introducing beats.

highly tentative with respect to the precise relation between adaptation and ΔF, adaptation ought to be reduced when tones interact to produce significant amplitude variations that are not too rapid. Moreover, since interaction between two tones is greatest when they are within the same critical band (particularly at low levels), a critical-band effect is to be expected. From this point of view, the hypothesis that loudness adaptation requires a restricted spread of excitation cannot be rejected. At 10 dB SL the spread of excitation around each component tone is so limited that little additional spread is obtained when the frequency separation is increased. On the other hand, the near disappearance of adaptation at narrow ΔFs suggests an important role for temporal variables. Loudness adaptation may require a steady stimulus, one that varies little over time. Owing to audible beating, two tones close in frequency are heard as varying strongly over time.

3. Temporal Characteristics

The importance of temporal variation in loudness adaptation is evident not only in these new measures of loudness adaptation of complex sounds, but also in old measures of tone decay (Carhart, 1957). Patients with acoustic neuromas continue to hear an intermittent tone over prolonged exposures; a steady tone quickly disappears. Pathological tone decay and normal loudness adaptation may have some elements in common.

The tone-decay data plus the results described above lead to the prediction that the loudness of an intermittent tone, even close to threshold, would not decrease over time. Surprisingly, this prediction is only partly correct. A 4000-Hz tone at 10 dB SL was turned on and off in nine different ways by means of a Grason-Stadler electronic switch (829E); the envelope was Gaussian and the rise–fall time was 25 msec. The period was 250, 500, or 1000 msec and the on time varied from 100% (steady tone) to 50% of the period. Table I gives the mean

TABLE I

MEAN AQ_{110} FOR A 4000-Hz TONE AT 10 dB SL[a]

Period (msec)	Duty Cycle (% Time Signal On)				
	50	80	90	95	100
1000	0.36	0.33	0.63	—	—
500	0.31	0.24	—	0.62	—
250	0.25	—	0.50	—	0.58

[a] Each of 15 observers judged six of the nine signals over one listening interval, so that each mean is based on 10 AQs.

AQs at 110 sec. Most striking is that even with a 50% duty cycle, adaptation was significantly greater than 0; loudness decreased by about one-third even when the off period was as long as 500 msec. Adaptation increased with duty cycle so that by 90%, it was as great as for a steady tone. Results for the shortest period of 250 msec suggest somewhat less adaptation than for longer periods.

The amount of adaptation depends on the length of both the on and off periods. Therefore, it is difficult to state what the longest off period is at which adaptation vanishes. Clearly, adaptation is measurable even for off periods as long as 500 msec. (Preliminary data on recovery suggest the required off period varies greatly from person to person, and may be as long as 10 sec.)

The resistance of adaptation to intermittency seemed especially surprising in light of the failure of a two-tone complex beating two times a second to adapt (Fig. 10). Such a stimulus follows a temporal course like that of a tone turned on and off twice a second. However, differences in the details of the envelope are sufficient to produce a large difference in AQ between the 8 observers who judged the two-tone complex and the 10 observers who judged the intermittent tone. One AQ is 0.31 and the other is 0.08. Although not statistically significant ($t=1.9$, $p<0.1$) when considered alone, a comparison of all the data at narrow ΔFs in Fig. 10 with the AQs in Table I suggests that this difference is meaningful. But why should a soft intermittent tone adapt more than a soft beating, two-tone complex? First it is to be noted that a complex with a ΔF of 2 Hz is effectively off just as long as an intermittent tone with a 500-msec period and a 50% duty cycle. That is so because during the troughs in the envelope of the beating tones, the instantaneous sound pressure may well fall below threshold for intervals as long as 250 msec. The important difference is that during each ''on'' period of beating tones, amplitude first increases and then decreases, reaching maximum only briefly, whereas an intermittent tone remains at maximum amplitude throughout most of its on period. The general rule may be that a continually changing stimulus, such as a two-tone complex, adapts least of all. It adapts less than an intermittent stimulus with alternating on and off periods, provided that the intermittent stimulus maintains a fairly constant level during the on periods and that its off periods are not too long.

An investigation of the effects of frequency modulation (FM) on adaptation lends further support to the notion that variation in level (probably in excitation level) is required to reduce or eliminate adaptation. Frequency modulation had no discernible effect on loudness adaptation. Varied sinusoidally over a range from 3900 to 4084 Hz at a rate of 50 Hz, a modulated tone showed as much adaptation as did an unmodulated, 4000-Hz tone. For the FM tone, the mean AQ was 0.62; for the pure tone, it was 0.61. Over this range and rate of modulation, the FM stimulus has almost all its energy confined to a single critical band. A more precise statement may be that a change in excitation level, over time, is required *within a critical band* in order to reduce adaptation. The amplitude of an

FM tone remains constant over time. Successive changes in the level of excitation over neural elements within a critical band is not the same as a simultaneous change in excitation over all the involved neural elements. If this preliminary finding and its interpretation hold up, they would suggest that loudness adaptation takes place beyond the point of integration of excitatory inputs from within a single critical band.

4. Mode of Stimulus Presentation

Before examining data that bear directly on the basis for loudness adaptation, we return to the question of whether adaptation is the same for binaural as for monaural sounds. Also is adaptation the same when listening through earphones as when listening in a sound field?

Figure 4 did suggest greater adaptation for a monaural 4000-Hz tone than for a binaural tone, but the binaural tones were presented at higher sensation levels. Yet, when set to the same sensation levels, monaural tones yielded higher AQs as Fig. 6 showed. Although an analysis of variance did not yield a significant ear effect for those data (binaural versus left ear versus right ear) because the left- and right-ear quotients were so similar, as they were expected to be, the monaural AQs were higher at all five levels than the binaural AQs. The reason for this difference appears to be that the loudness of the binaural signal adapted no more than the *less* adapting of the two ears. The binaural adaptation quotient was only slightly lower than the mean of the smaller of the two monaural quotients from each observer. A later experiment on 12 observers showed that "binaural" adaptation was nil when one ear was stimulated at 40 dB SL while the other ear was stimulated at 10 dB SL. Clearly, the less adapting ear determines the amount of loudness adaptation under binaural stimulation. (For the eight observers whose data are shown in Fig. 6, differences in adaptation between the ears of a given observer were small. Moreover, mean AQs for the left and right ears were about the same. In a later experiment with another 10 observers, mean adaptation to a 4000-Hz tone at 10 dB SL was also about the same in the left and right ears.)

Two direct studies of possible interaural and binaural effects in simple adaptation were undertaken. A 4000-Hz tone at 10 dB SL was presented for 90 sec to the right ears of 12 observers. Its loudness declined by 77% (AQ = 0.77). At the end of 90 sec, the tone was switched to the left ear for another 90 sec. The observers assigned an initial value to the tone in the unadapted left ear that was much higher than the terminal value they had just assigned, after 90 sec, to the tone in the right ear. However, the value was not as high as that assigned initially in the right ear, owing to the switch from listening to one ear to the other ear, as a later experiment showed. (Using a light to warn the observer a few seconds beforehand of the impending switch in ears raised the initial estimate in the unadapted ear to its expected level.) At the end of 90 sec of stimulation of the left ear, the mean estimation dropped to the same value it had reached at the end of

90 sec of stimulation of the right ear. Clearly, strong adaptation of one ear over 90 sec results in little (probably no) adaptation in the other ear.

A second experiment, on the same 12 observers, further demonstrates the independence of the two ears with respect to simple loudness adaptation. A 4000-Hz tone was led for 90 sec to the left ear at a sensation level of 40 dB and to the right ear at a level of 10 dB. The large level difference meant that the tone was completely lateralized toward the left ear, where its loudness remained essentially unchanged (AQ = 0.18) over the 90-sec listening period. At the end of 90 sec the tone to the left ear terminated, while the weaker tone to the right ear continued for an additional 90 sec. Immediately after termination of the strong tone, the loudness of the weak tone, unheard until then, was nearly down to the value such a tone usually reaches after 90 sec of steady stimulation. Adaptation continued during the next 90 sec just as if the tone had been presented by itself all along. After 180 sec the AQ was 0.89. The nonadapting tone in one ear had no effect on the course of adaptation in the other ear.

These various results suggest that loudness adaptation depends on what is going on in each ear and is unaffected by binaural summation or interaural interaction. Perhaps then adaptation depends on neural events that precede the place in the auditory system where inputs from the two ears come together.

Adaptation is not restricted to earphone listening. Fifteen observers judged a 4000-Hz tone presented binaurally either through earphones or from a loud-speaker. The loudspeaker was about 2 m from the observer who sat in a sound-proof, semireverberant room with his chin in a chin rest to reduce head move-ments. The mean AQ_{120} at 15 dB SL was 0.49 for earphone listening and 0.45 for loudspeaker listening. Measurements in a large anechoic room yielded simi-lar results. (See Canévet *et al.*, 1981.) Thirty-nine observers listened at 10 dB SL to a 4000-Hz tone coming from a loudspeaker 3.7 m in front of them. The observer sat with the back of his head against a head rest. The AQ at 120 sec was 0.45; at 180 sec it was 0.59. The value of 0.45 is lower than that of 0.62 measured with 54 observers who listened with their right ear only through an earphone (Fig. 8). The reduced adaptation in the free-field condition must be due in part to a difference between binaural and monaural listening, with the less adapting ear determining the amount of adaptation. Another part of the difference must result from dif-ferences between the two groups of observers. When data for the same observers who were run under earphone and sound-field conditions are compared, dif-ferences between the two conditions are minimal. Nor are there differences at higher levels where loudness does not adapt. Twelve observers who listened to a 4000-Hz tone at 50 dB SL in a free field showed no loudness adaptation whatsoever.

At low sensation levels, adaptation depends on frequency in the free field much the same way as in monaural earphone listening. At 400 Hz adaptation was considerably less than at frequencies between 4,000 and 15,000 Hz. At the higher frequencies, adaptation was relatively constant except for a 20% jump at 15,000 Hz.

A difference between earphone and sound-field listening that is not evident in the data is a waxing and waning of the loudness of a steady tone presented in a sound field. Many observers report that loudness does not remain steady when the sound from a loudspeaker is a low-level 4000-Hz tone. Rather the loudness tends to increase and decrease during the adaptation period. Some observers also reported a waxing and waning for earphone listening, but no attempt has yet been made to determine the incidence of this phenomenon or its relation to the degree of adaptation.

On the whole, however, loudness adaptation seems about the same whether low-level tones are present monaurally or binaurally through earphones or in a sound field, whether semireverberant or anechoic.

5. *Adaptation under Partial Masking*

Near threshold, the loudness of a steady pure tone usually adapts. The adaptation can be reduced by lowering the frequency of the tone, modulating its amplitude, or replacing it by a continuous-spectrum noise. The adaptation can be almost entirely eliminated by adding a tone at a nearby frequency to produce audible beats. These data suggest that in order for loudness adaptation to occur, a sound must be steady (or be changing so rapidly as to be effectively steady). Since loudness does not adapt above 30 dB SL, the question poses itself: Does an intense tone or the response it evokes in the auditory system show temporal variations in level? If such temporal variations exist, they are not obvious. What is obvious about the way the response to a pure tone changes in level, obvious both from psychoacoustical data and from physiological data, is that the spread of excitation in the auditory system increases with level. Perhaps this spread engenders an effective fluctuation within the auditory nervous system. Whatever the mechanism, if spread of excitation plays a role in preventing adaptation at high levels, then reducing that spread could cause the loudness of even an intense sound to adapt.

An effective means for limiting the spread of activity is to introduce a high-pass noise which masks those parts of the auditory system that normally respond to the high-frequency tail produced by a sound. Accordingly, we measured adaptation at 4000 Hz with and without such a noise. The noise was white noise passed through a Krohn-Hite (310A) filter whose low-frequency rolloff was 18 dB/octave measured from the 3-dB-down point at 4000 Hz. The tone was set to 15 dB above its masked threshold in the presence of three levels of noise, and also to 15 dB SL in the quiet. The open symbols in Fig. 11 are the geometric means for 10 observers who listened monaurally for 120 sec. Even a tone whose mean SPL was 73 dB showed considerable adaptation (mean $AQ_{120} = 0.52$)

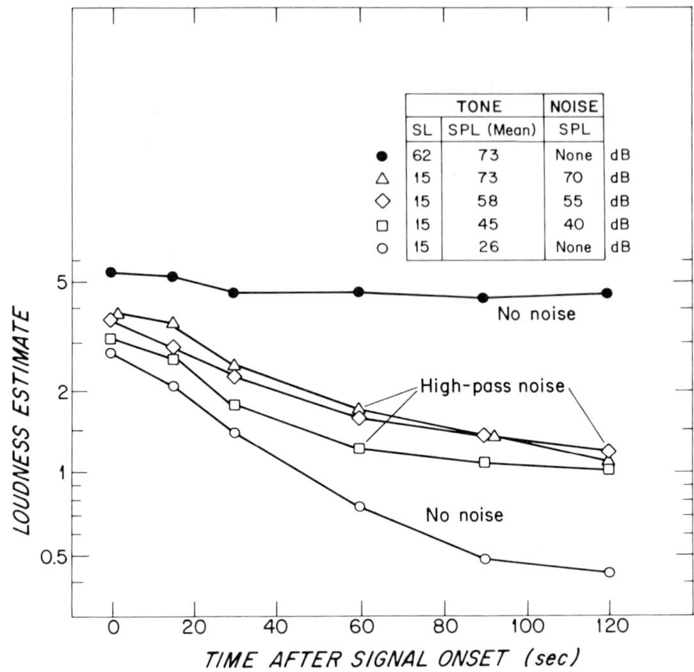

Figure 11   Median estimate of the loudness of a 4000-Hz tone as a function of the duration of the tone. (Open symbols mean the tone was presented at 15 dB SL either in the quiet or against a high-pass noise whose level is shown in the inset. Filled circles are for the tone set at 62 dB SL and presented in the quiet. Each point is based on two judgments by each of 10 observers.)

when partially masked by a 70-dB noise. Adaptation, as indexed by AQ_t, did not differ significantly among these conditions. The same 73-dB tone presented in the quiet showed almost no adaptation as indicated by the filled circles. The results lend tentative support to the hypothesis that for loudness to adapt, the spread of activity in the auditory system must be restricted.[6]

A restricted spread of activity may be a necessity but it is not a sufficient condition for loudness adaptation. Several stimuli, whose spread is naturally limited by their weak intensity, have been shown to adapt little or not at all at 10 dB SL. These include a beating two-tone complex, a narrow-band noise (centered on 4000 Hz), and a 250-Hz tone. Moreover, a 250-Hz tone shows no more

[6]Dirks *et al.* (1974) reported similar results, using a heterophonic simultaneous matching procedure (steady 4000-Hz tone in one ear matched in loudness to an intermittent 2000-Hz tone in the other ear), which seemed immune to interaural effects. The loudness of a 4000-Hz tone adapted when presented at 70 dB SPL in the presence of an octave band of noise but not when presented in the quiet at the same sound pressure level.

adaptation at 15 dB SL (mean SPL = 51 dB) in the presence of a 70-dB high-pass noise than it does at 15 dB SL (mean SPL = 33 dB) in the quiet.

These results along with the data on low-level loudness adaptation are considered below in an attempt to uncover the basis for the failure of loudness adaptation at most stimulus levels. First, however, other aspects of loudness adaptation are examined.

B. Individual Differences and Relation of Adaptation to Other Variables

This section looks at individual differences in loudness adaptation, and then considers the relationship between adaptation and individual characteristics such as threshold, age, and sex for which relevant measures or information were obtained. Possible connections between adaptation and auditory pathology are also discussed.

1. Individual Differences

Throughout these studies of simple loudness adaptation, differences among individual listeners have been large. One listener may report no change in the loudness of a low-level tone whereas another listener reports that the loudness decreased until the tone became inaudible. From experience with a small number of laboratory personnel who served as observers over a period of months or years, sometimes in trial runs, sometimes in final runs, it appears that most observers are consistent adaptors—to varying degrees. Others are consistent nonadaptors or poor adaptors. Too few data are available on consistency across sessions to buttress this impression statistically. However, within-session data reveal a high correlation between the AQ from an observer's first set of judgments and that from a second set. For 48 observers who judged a 4000-Hz tone over 110 sec, the correlation coefficient was 0.71 between first and second AQs. Increasing the number of observers to 63 by including observers who also judged a broad-band noise increased the correlation coefficient to 0.75. The correlation was also high between the AQ_{110} for a 4000-Hz tone and for a 6000-Hz tone, equalling 0.63 for 28 observers.

To give a better picture of the variability among observers, Table II provides a breakdown of AQs for 54 observers (two AQs each) who judged a 4000-Hz tone presented through a single earphone at 10 dB SL. Table II also gives the AQs for 39 observers who judged a 4000-Hz tone in an anechoic room. Under both listening conditions entries appear in all the cells of the table. More than half the observers had an AQ of 0.6 or greater, but few reported that the tone disappeared completely (AQ = 1.0). Under earphone listening only 16% of the observers experienced essentially no adaptation (AQ under 0.2) whereas in free-field lis-

TABLE II

Distribution of AQs[a]

			AQ			
	<0.2	0.2–0.39	0.4–0.59	0.6–0.79	0.8–0.99	1.0
Earphone[b]	16	5	22	17	32	8
Free field[c]	28	8	8	23	28	5

[a] 4000-Hz tone at 10 dB SL (percentages).
[b] Fifty-four observers contributed two AQs_{110} each.
[c] Thirty-nine observers contributed one AQ_{120} each.

tening 28% experienced little or no adaptation. As suggested by the within-session correlations these differences among listeners are probably stable individual characteristics.

Another way of looking at interindividual variability is to examine the time it took before the observer reported that the loudness had decreased to half its original value. Table III gives the distribution for the same observers whose AQs are given in Table II. Under both earphone and free-field listening conditions, about 38% of the half-loudness judgments occurred within 40 sec of stimulus onset. At the other end about 30% of the judgments did not decline to half within a 120-sec listening period.

The large variability in AQ values makes it meaningful to evaluate the correlation between AQ and individual characteristics such as threshold, age, and sex.

TABLE III

DISTRIBUTION OF DURATIONS REQUIRED FOR A 4000-Hz TONE
AT 10 dB SL TO REACH HALF LOUDNESS[a]

	Duration (sec)			
	0–40	41–80	81–120	>120
Earphone (54 observers)[b]	37	29	8	26
Free field (39 observers)[c]	38	10	18	33

[a] Percentages.
[b] Two runs each.
[c] One run each.

2. Threshold and Adaptation

Three different hypotheses about the relation between adaptation and absolute threshold seem plausible. (1) Adaptation is negatively correlated with threshold. This hypothesis assumes that adaptation becomes greater, the lower the sound pressure reaching the cochlea. Persons with lower thresholds may receive lower sound pressures at the cochlea and therefore may experience more adaptation at a given sensation level than persons with high thresholds. (2) Adaptation is uncorrelated with threshold. This hypothesis also assumes that adaptation depends on the sound pressure at the cochlea. However, differences in threshold at 4000 Hz are assumed to be due largely to differences in the ear's transmission characteristics. Thus sound pressure at the cochlea would be similar even for persons with different thresholds. (3) Adaptation is positively correlated with threshold. This hypothesis assumes that adaptation is smaller for healthier auditory systems, and that low thresholds are associated with healthier systems.

To test these hypotheses, correlations are needed between threshold and AQ. Attention, however, must be paid to the range and variability of the thresholds for the groups of observers studied. The 54 observers whose data are given in Table II had thresholds that varied from -3 to 27 dB SPL. However, 80% of the thresholds fell between 2 and 15 dB. This narrow range may be why the correlation coefficient between threshold and AQ is low, 0.36, although statistically significant at the 0.01 level. To overcome the heavy weighting toward low thresholds—a natural outcome of the selection of normal-hearing observers from a college population—I averaged separately the AQs for the six observers with thresholds below 0 dB and for the five observers with thresholds above 15 dB. The AQ for the low-threshold group is 0.37; the AQ for the high-threshold group is 0.82. This comparison, together with the positive correlation between threshold and AQ, lends some support to the hypothesis that adaptation is stronger near high thresholds than near low thresholds.

The 39 observers who listened in the free field had a larger dispersion of thresholds at 4000 Hz (owing to the inclusion of many older persons) than did the 54 observers who listened through earphones. Accordingly, a correlation between adaptation and threshold may be more apparent for this group. In the free field as under earphone listening, threshold was measured by a rapid method of limits. The sound pressure level was measured in a microphone positioned at the locus of an observer's head, in the absence of the listeer. [Owing to diffraction effects for the head, the level at the entrance to the ear canal would be about 6 dB higher (Békésy, 1960, p. 269).] Threshold varied from -14 to 42 dB with the mean equal to 7 dB and the standard deviation equal to 14 dB. Correlation between AQ_{180} (mean $= 0.59$, standard deviation $= 0.45$) and threshold is 0.0. Other, unknown factors apparently swamped the small effect of threshold.

3. Age and Adaptation

The present data provide no evidence for a relation between age and loudness adaptation. The correlation between age and AQ for the 39 observers tested in an anechoic room is close to 0, despite the wide range of ages—from 22 to 64 years. Moreover, whereas the group of 54 observers who were nearly all in their early 20s had an AQ at 120 sec of 0.62, the older group (mean age of 38 years) had an AQ of 0.45. As noted earlier, this difference is due only in part to the difference in adaptation under monaural earphone and sound-field listening. Most of the difference is probably due to differences between the two groups other than age, since age is not correlated with AQ.

Even if not correlated with age among adults, there may be a difference between adults and children. Adaptation was measured in 14 children whose ages ranged from 9 to 16 years with the mean at 12.4 and the standard deviation equal to 1.0. The children were all run in the anechoic room and judged a 4000-Hz tone at 10 dB SL for 180 sec. Their mean AQ_{120} was 0.33 and their mean AQ_{180} was 0.34, compared to 0.45 and 0.59 for the 39 adults. Moreover, whereas of the 14 children, 6 (43%) showed no adaptation over 3 min (AQ $\leq$ 0.0), of the 39 adults, only 7 (18%) showed no adaptation. These differences between mean AQs and proportions, however, reach only borderline significance ($p<0.10$). A larger sample of children is needed. The eight children who did adapt seemed to do so more slowly than the adults; the AQ at 60 sec was only 0.06 for the children and was already up to 0.33 for the adults. These tentative results are reminiscent of Kärjä's (1968) report of no interaurally induced loudness adaptation for a 4000-Hz tone at 60 dB SL for children under 15 years compared to an average of nearly 30 dB of adaptation after 3 min for an adult group.

4. Adaptation and Sex

A major known difference between the auditory abilities of men and women is the greater sensitivity of women to higher frequencies, a difference that increases with age (Hinchcliffe, 1959). Given the small positive correlation between adaptation and threshold, somewhat greater adaptation would be expected for men than for women at 4000 Hz. Of the 54 observers in the earphone-listening group, 29 were men and their mean AQ was slightly higher than that of the 25 women. The difference was not statistically significant. Moreover, of the 39 observers in the free-field group, 26 were men and their mean AQ was slightly lower than that of the 13 women. Adaptation and sex seem to be unrelated.

5. Adaptation and Use of Numbers in Magnitude Estimation

Magnitude estimation requires that observer assign numbers to the loudness of a sound. In the studies described above observers were always free to choose the number that seemed best to match the loudness of the two sound bursts presented prior to the beginning of the adaptation period. Many observers chose small numbers since the sounds were so soft. As loudness adapted and the sound became still softer, observers used very small numbers to express the reduced loudness. I doubt that the ratio between numbers like 0.01 and 0.001 has the same meaning for an observer as the ratio between 10 and 1. Often an observer meant only that a sound became softer when he went from 0.01 to 0.001, and not that the loudness went down tenfold. To keep the observer from using very small numbers and exaggerating the degree of loudness adaptation, it would be necessary to assign the initial sound a large number which the observer is to use as his standard. But forcing the observer to use large numbers for soft sounds would probably result in his assigning smaller numbers to subsequent sounds simply because they are so soft to begin with and not only because their loudness has diminished over time. The result would again be to exaggerate the degree of adaptation.

In a study with 12 observers it turned out that the free choice of the initial numbers exaggerated adaptation no more than did forcing the observer to begin with a larger number. At 10 dB SL, AQ_{180} was 0.88 when observers chose freely the initial value (which was 4.6 on the average) and it was 0.77 when the assigned initial value was 10. On the other hand, at 40 dB SL, AQ_{180} was 0.10 when observers chose freely (initial value was 9.4) and rose to 0.25 when the assigned value was 100. Although neither of the differences between the AQs was statistically significant, their being in opposite directions is reasonable. At 40 dB, where there is no true adaptation, forcing observers to start with a number 10 times greater than their free choice resulted in a larger AQ. At 10 dB, where true adaptation is strong, observers who started with lower, freely chosen initial values ended up with very small numbers that slightly exaggerated the already strong adaptation. The resulting individual AQs, some of which are inflated, have a minimal effect on the mean AQ. The effect is small because the arithmetic mean gives little weight to small differences among AQs above 0.99 which usually correspond to the assignment of tiny fractions at the end of a listening period. Accordingly, the averaging procedure attenuates exaggerated ratios in the observer's estimations, and the mean AQ values provide a fair representation of the degree of adaptation.

The drift away from the assigned standard at 40 dB SL is in accord with the results of Zwislocki and Goodman (1980) who measured loudness as a function of level rather than of exposure duration. They showed that, on the average, observers gravitate toward a standard set of numbers, almost regardless of the initial number assigned by the experimenter. The farther away in level or time from the initial judgment, the stronger the influence of the observer's own absolute scale and the weaker the influence of the initially assigned number. In studies of loudness adaptation at low levels, assigning a number for the observer will probably have minimal adverse effects on the judgments provided the assigned value is near the average value that observers usually choose; it may have the advantage of keeping some observers who would have chosen a small initial value from ending up with double and triple decimals.

This advantage is negligible, when interest focuses on the overall amount of adaptation as measured by the AQ. Thus, in the current studies, where the observer chose the initial value freely, there was no relation between the size of the initial magnitude estimate and AQ. At 10 dB SL, correlation coefficients are small and statistically insignificant for both the earphone and free-field groups.

6. Pathology and Auditory Fatigue

All observers in the series of studies reported above had normal hearing for their age. Therefore, these data provide no information about possible effects of pathology on loudness adaptation. Since, however, persons with acoustic neuroma often show marked tone decay, could it be that the large differences in loudness adaptation among normally hearing persons are related to differences in incipient pathology or to susceptibility to pathology? Are these differences related to differences in auditory fatigability? Do persons with auditory pathology adapt differently from normally hearing persons, and does the course of adaptation differ among the various kinds of pathology? Answers are difficult to come by from the data available in the literature. Many of the data have to do with induced loudness adaptation rather than simple loudness adaptation.

Of those studies that have attempted to measure simple adaptation in pathological ears, two revealed little loudness adaptation in listeners with cochlear impairment and one revealed sizable adaptation. Using a monaural procedure, Wiley *et al.* (1976) found adaptation in only three of six patients with noise-induced hearing loss, and that only for a 4000-Hz tone at 10 dB SL. Using a dichotic delayed balance, Margolis and Wiley (1976) found only small amounts of loudness adaptation at 15 and 25 dB SL in four persons with cochlear impairment (but they also found no adaptation in four normally hearing observers as noted above in Section III,A). Dirks *et al.* (1974) did measure a 10-dB drop in loudness level for two listeners with a cochlear hearing impairment over 3 min of listening to a 4000-Hz tone at 70 dB SPL. The corresponding sensation levels were about 25 dB. A third impaired listener showed a 7-dB drop in loudness level at approximately 20 dB SL; a fourth showed no adaptation at 20 dB SL. Dirks *et al.* used a simultaneous loudness matching procedure with a steady tone in one ear and an intermittent tone at a different frequency in the other ear. At most levels and frequencies they found no adaptation for the steady tone, which suggests that induced adaptation was avoided. These four hearing-impaired observers gave results similar to those for normally hearing listeners with respect to the amount and variability of adaptation.

On the whole, these three studies suggest that persons with cochlear impairment adapt at low sensation levels about as much as normally hearing persons. The literature on induced loudness adaptation leads to a similar conclusion, although the results differ greatly from one study to another. For example, Hood (1950) measured more adaptation in persons with Menière's disease than in normals whereas Kärjä (1974) measured less. Except for acoustic neuroma, other more peripheral insults to the auditory system seem not to provoke notable changes in adaptation, whether simple or induced. But this conclusion rests on a weak data base—too few data on simple loudness adaptation and procedurally weak data on induced adaptation.

Schubert (1944) long ago speculated that loudness adaptation might be related to susceptibility to noise-induced hearing loss. No one seems to have tested this possibility although Hood (1969) has reiterated Schubert's speculation. Schubert wrote about simple, near-threshold adaptation which he had measured by determining how long it took a tone to disappear. Finding large differences among normally hearing persons, he suggested that the inability to hear a soft sound over long durations may be related to an inability to withstand damage from noise. An obvious if weak test of this hypothesis would be to measure the correlation between temporary threshold shift (TTS) and simple loudness adaptation. This test is weak because TTS does not seem to predict susceptibility to permanent hearing loss. Nevertheless, both TTS and adaptation vary so much from person to person that the possibility of a significant correlation exists. Indeed, should there be a strong correlation, it would become reasonable to consider a longitudinal study to answer the question of whether adaptation is related to incipient auditory pathology or to susceptibility to such pathology. Perhaps even without a strong correlation between TTS and adaptation, some attempt should be made to determine whether the ability of the auditory system to maintain loudness and audibility over long durations is related to the system's vulnerability.

C. Effect of Adaptation on Other Auditory Functions

1. Loudness Function

Loudness adaptation decreases rapidly as a function of level as Figs. 6 and 7 show so clearly. This change in AQ means that the function relating loudness to level must vary as a function of signal duration. The loudness of signals lasting less than 2 sec or so would follow the standard function which has a slope of 0.6 above about 30 dB SL and an increasingly steep slope at lower levels. Generally, loudness grows more rapidly as a function of level near threshold than at higher levels (Scharf, 1978; Scharf and Stevens, 1961). This increase in slope is exaggerated for longer duration tones, especially those above 2000 Hz, because the closer a tone is to threshold the more its loudness declines with duration. The inevitable result of this is loudness recruitment—a more-rapid-than-normal increase in loudness as a function of level. In part, recruitment is caused by an increase in the effective threshold for a pure tone at longer durations. An increased threshold means that loudness reaches normal values over a shorter span of intensities. The term "effective threshold" seems especially appropriate because the detection threshold would be difficult to measure for a steady tone after 2 min of stimulation and because detection is probably irrelevant to determining the point at which loudness begins to increase with level. The shift in the effective threshold at long durations may be much larger than the shift in the "true" detection threshold. Measurements of the loudness of short- and long-duration tones as a function of level should clarify these issues.

2. Intensity Discrimination

Some authors (Teghtsoonian, 1971) have argued that the ability to discriminate an increment in intensity should be greater when loudness changes more rapidly as a function of level. The reasoning is that the just discriminable change in intensity, ΔI, gives rise to a subjective change in loudness, ΔL, that is proportional to the slope of the loudness function. The steeper that function the smaller the ΔL and the better discrimination ought to be. Accordingly, discrimination at low levels should improve with sound duration since the loudness function steepens with duration near threshold. The only report that seems to address this issue for normal listeners indicated no increase in discrimination over time (Bartholemeus and Swisher, 1971). However, Bartholemeus and Swisher used the SISI test to measure discrimination, incrementing the level of a continuous tone every 6 sec. This modulation of the tone may have reduced or eliminated adaptation so it does not provide a fair test of the hypothesis. Since, however, intensity discrimination for short-duration tones is worse near threshold (Jesteadt *et al.*, 1977), where the loudness function is steeper anyway, than at higher levels, it is difficult to believe that discrimination would improve with duration owing to a further steepening of the loudness function (although it might improve for other reasons).

Fechner (1860) predicted that adaptation should have no effect on discrimination since the standard stimulus and the stimulus to be discriminated would both decrease in subjective intensity. Thus the relative change required for discrimination should remain the same. Fechner believed that the subjective jnd is a constant and would not change under adaptation in any case.

To complete the circle, one could also argue that discrimination of a tone at a constant low level ought to worsen as duration increases. The reasoning is simple. Discrimination becomes poorer at low levels. Therefore, as the loudness of a sound decreases, discrimination should worsen because the system deals with a stimulus that is effectively weaker.

The effect of adaptation on intensity discrimination is wholly unknown. Theoretically, it may be argued that the discrimination improves, worsens, or remains the same when loudness adapts. Data are needed.

3. Pitch

Many observers who estimated the loudness of weak tones over time reported, often spontaneously, that the pitch of a pure tone became unclear as the loudness decreased, that the tone became noisy and fuzzy. The literature contains numerous reports of this phenomenon (e.g., Green, 1963; Harbert *et al.*, 1966; Schubert, 1944; Snyder, 1973). It is as if the tone descends into the "atonal interval," that narrow range of levels from threshold up to 5 dB or so above threshold where most listeners show increased variability in pitch matching (Harris and Myers, 1949; Pollack, 1948). Harris and Myers showed how the region of uncertainty—measured in Hertz—widens as the level of a pure tone is reduced from 10 dB SL down to threshold. Thus, the loss of pitch at low levels that accompanies prolonged stimulation and the loss induced by decreasing the level of a brief tone may have a common underlying cause. In both cases, changes in the quality of the tone may reflect a decrease in those neural processes that seem to lead to a sharpening of the excitation evoked by a tone. Lacking any systematic studies of the psychophysical phenomenon, one is free to speculate but the notion of an increased spread of excitation may prove useful in theorizing about the source of adaptation.

D. Induced Loudness Adaptation

The evidence is overwhelming that under simple monaural or binaural conditions, loudness adapts only near threshold. Yet in the presence of an intermittent sound in the contralateral ear, the loudness of a steady sound at high levels also decreases over time (see Fig. 3).[7] The intermittent sound may also provoke some decline in loudness when presented to the same ear as the steady sound. Accordingly, an appropriately neutral name for this phenomenon is induced loudness adaptation.

In most previous measurements of induced adaptation, the intermittent tone served as the comparison sound, whose level was varied and whose loudness was matched to that of the steady tone. Since, as it turns out, the intermittent tone induces the loudness loss of the steady tone, it is methodologically clearer to

---

[7]A continuous sound in one ear may also cause the loudness of a continuous sound in the other ear to decrease. We have only just begun to investigate this phenomenon. Our first results show that a steady 1640-Hz tone to one ear induces loudness adaptation of a steady 1000-Hz tone to the other ear. Both tones were at 60 dB SPL; the 1640-Hz tone came on 20 sec after the 1000-Hz tone. We do not yet know what temporal, spectral, and intensive relations must obtain between dichotic sounds in order to demonstrate such adaptation.

leave unchanged the intermittent tone as well as the steady tone. Successive magnitude estimation permits this methodological clarification. Some early results are described to show the efficacy of the method and the magnitude of the adaptation.

A steady 4000-Hz tone was presented at 50, 60, 70, or 80 dB SPL to the right ear, and an intermittent tone at the same level to the left ear. The observer was told to ignore the intermittent tone and estimate only the loudness of the sound in his right ear. A light came on at 3, 6, 12, 18, 24, and 30 sec; the observer

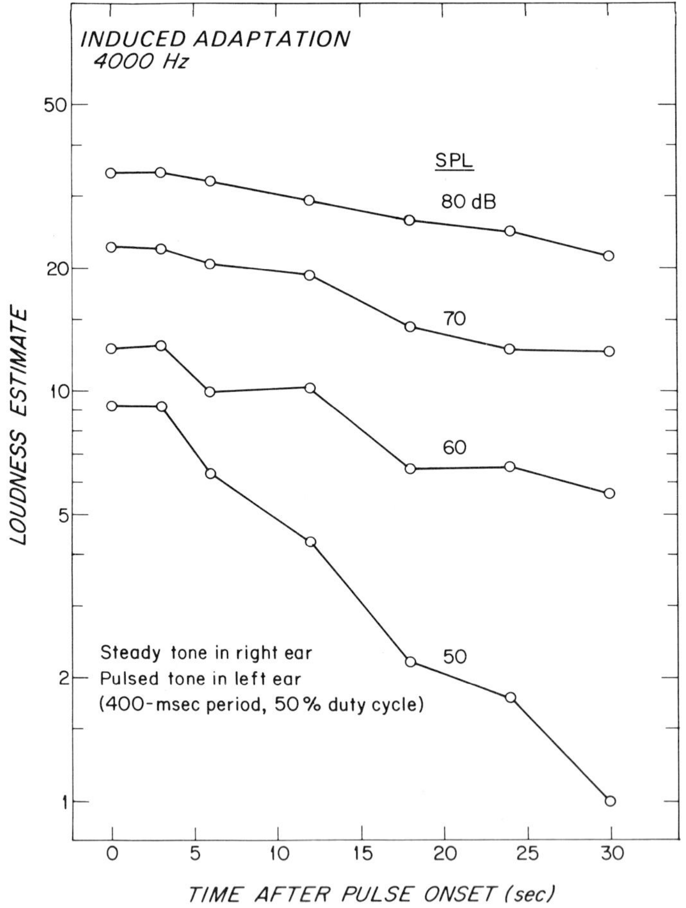

Figure 12 Loudness estimation of a steady 4000-Hz tone plotted as a function of the duration was heard in the presence of a pulsed tone in the contralateral ear. (Parameter on the curves is the sound pressure level of the steady tone and also of the pulsed tone, which was on for 200 msec and off for 200 msec during the 30-sec period.)

estimated the loudness of the tone at that moment and wrote down the number corresponding to the loudness. Both tones had rise–fall times of 10 msec. Figure 12 gives the geometric means of the loudness estimations by five observers (two judgments by each observer) as a function of the duration after the onset of the intermittent tone. Those data are for a 4000-Hz steady tone in the right ear and a 200-msec tone that came on every 400 msec in the left ear. Parameter on the curves is the sound pressure level of the steady tone and of the intermittent tone. Loudness decreased over the 30-sec interval at all levels, but more so the lower the level. Differences among the four levels in the amount of adaptation was highly significant as shown by a repeated-measures ANOVA performed on the adaptation quotients. Measurements were also made with longer intermittent tone bursts (500 msec on, 500 msec off) set 20 dB lower than the continuous tone instead of to the same level. Both lengthening the period and lowering the level of the intermittent tone reduced but did not eliminate adaptation.

The most striking result in Fig. 12 is that loudness adaptation increases markedly as the level of the continuous and intermittent tone goes down. Hood (1950) and Kärjä (1968) had found that adaptation *decreases* as the level goes down. However, Hood and Kärjä were referring to adaptation over a 3-min period. A close look at Kärjä's data for the same stimulus conditions as represented in Fig. 12 reveals that after 30 sec the loudness of the steady tone declined by 37% at 80 dB SPL and by nearly 60% at 60, 40, and 20 dB SL. The discrepancy then is mainly at 50 dB where we measured a 90% decrease in loudness. I believe that the difference is caused mainly by our use of magnitude estimation with a pulsed tone at a constant level and by Kärjä's use of a tracking procedure with a pulsed tone decreasing in level. Especially at lower levels, making a soft intermittent tone still softer could very well reduce its ability to induce loudness adaptation in the contralateral ear.

Besides level, other stimulus variables that seem to affect the amount of induced loudness adaptation are frequency of the steady sound, frequency difference between the steady and intermittent tones, and level and temporal characteristics of the intermittent sound. There remains the question of observer characteristics such as auditory pathology, individual differences, and age. For example, using his tracking procedure, Kärjä (1968) found that observers under 15 years of age almost never adapted. The method of successive magnitude estimation makes feasible the study of these many variables. An additional example of some relevant results is given in Fig. 13.

Figure 13 gives the mean AQ as a function of the duration of a continuous 1000-Hz tone at 60 dB SPL in the right ear. The variables of interest are the frequency of the intermittent tone in the left ear (1000 or 1100 Hz) and its on–off cycle (200/800 or 200/200 msec). In a control condition, the observer judged the loudness of the continuous tone presented alone. The dashed vertical lines indicate the start and finish of the intermittent tone. Although loudness for this group

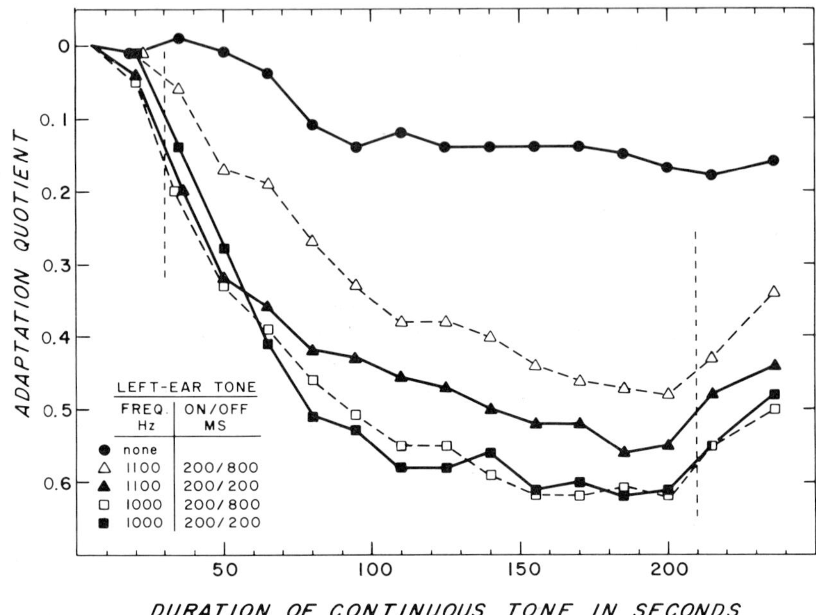

Figure 13   Mean AQ for 10 observers as a function of the duration of a continuous 1000-Hz tone at 60 dB SPL presented to the right ear. [In a control condition (filled circles), the continuous tone was presented alone. In four other conditions, an intermittent tone at either 1000 Hz (squares) or 1100 Hz (triangles) went to the left ear. The on–off cycle was either 200 and 800 msec (filled triangles and squares) or 200 and 200 msec (open symbols). Dashed vertical lines indicate the beginning and end of the intermittent tone.]

of 10 observers decreased on the average by over 15% in the control condition, this decrease was not significantly different from no decrease. More important, the decreases were as much as 60% in the presence of the intermittent tone in the contralateral ear. Loudness decreased most rapidly during the first minute of the intermittent tone and quite slowly after 2 min. It appears that asymptote had been reached after 150 sec in three of the four intermittent stimulus conditions. An analysis of variance combined with Dunnett's test for comparisons involving a control mean (Kirk, 1968) showed that the control condition differed significantly from each of the four experimental conditions, i.e., adding an intermittent tone to the contralateral ear induced a significant decrease in the loudness of a continuous tone. However, although the 1100-Hz intermittent tone appears to have caused less adaptation than the 1000-Hz tone, the difference is not statistically significant. Also, the interaction between the rate of intermittency and the frequency was not significant. Both these variables are currently being studied more intensively.

Induced adaptation is a powerful effect. It is not simply the result of lateralization; a much weaker intermittent tone readily induces adaptation of a 20- or 30-dB more intense continuous tone in the contralateral ear. The observers had no difficulty judging the loudness of the continuous tone even though it sometimes disappeared each time the intermittent tone came on. When the intermittent tone was off, the continuous tone was heard in its own ear and its loudness could be judged without difficulty. Moreover, not only did loudness decrease steadily as a function of time, but it did not return to its original value even after the intermittent tone stopped. Indeed, later experiments show that loudness remains reduced for at least 80 sec after cessation of the intermittent tone. It may be that loudness does not return to normal unless the continuous tone is first turned off and then, after some interval, on again.

Many other data have been and continue to be collected at the Auditory Perception Laboratory on induced loudness adaptation. The results in Figs. 12 and 13 may be considered suggestive of the likely relations to be uncovered in induced loudness adaptation. (See Botte *et al.*, 1982.)

V. POSSIBLE BASIS FOR SIMPLE LOUDNESS ADAPTATION

First it is shown that simple adaptation is most unlikely to have a central nonsensory basis such as reduced attention. Next relevant neurophysiological data are discussed, and finally a highly tentative basis for loudness adaptation is suggested, a basis that could also apply to induced loudness adaptation.

A. Central Mechanisms

Could it be that listeners assign smaller and smaller numbers to soft sounds as a function of time because they are unable to maintain a constant level of attention? Reduced attention would seem plausible at low levels owing to the weakness of the sensory experience. At higher levels where magnitude estimations do not decline over time, the sensations are strong enough to keep the observer listening. Several lines of evidence speak against this interpretation. Most important, not all soft sounds show adaptation. A beating two-tone complex does not decline in loudness even though it is at only 10 dB SL. Noises and low-frequency tones adapt much less than high-frequency tones. Since neither a low-frequency tone nor broad-band noise has perceptible fluctuations, we cannot attribute their reduced adaptation to greater attention-getting properties that stem from fluctuations over time as in beating tones or narrow-band noises. It seems far-fetched to ascribe adaptation to an attention mechanism that depends so strongly on spectral and temporal, as well as intensive, characteristics of the signal.

A second argument against an attention hypothesis is that experienced observers report that they cannot prevent the loudness of a soft tone from diminishing by, for example, concentrating on it nor can they bring loudness back to its initial value by any kind of subjective effort. To the adapting listener, it is very much as if the stimulus level had been reduced.

B. Physiological Changes in the Auditory Nervous System over Time

Few data are available on how neural responses within the auditory system depend on time beyond durations of 1 or 2 sec. It has often been demonstrated that a sound evokes an initial burst of rapid firing in a single eighth-nerve fiber, and that within the first 50 msec the rate decreases to a more or less steady value. But just how steady that value remains over the next several minutes is not clear. Kiang (1965, p. 78) published two figures showing how the firing rate of two different units in a cat's auditory nerve decreased continuously over a 13-min period. Most of the approximately 30% decrease in absolute spike rate took place during the first 5 min or so. One unit was driven by an 1800-Hz tone at a level 66 dB above the unit's threshold; the other unit was driven by an 8900-Hz tone at a level 38 dB above threshold. These levels are higher than those at which simple loudness adaptation has been demonstrated psychophysically in humans. No neurophysiological data were furnished for weaker stimuli.

Young and Sachs (1973) did show, also for two different cat fibers, how discharge rate changes as a function of time at low as well as at high stimulus levels. At sound pressure levels from 28 to 89 dB, the response to a 60-sec tone near 2000 Hz decreased rapidly during the first few seconds of stimulation and then slowly throughout the remainder of the 60-sec period. The rate of long-term decline was approximately the same at all levels, with only a hint of a slightly larger decline at the lowest level.

The effect of level on neurophysiological responses in the cochlear nucleus is seen in a report by ten Kate *et al.* (1977). They showed how spike rate in units of the dorsal cochlear nucleus of the cat decreases with duration in response to a steady 100-sec tone or white noise. For both kinds of stimulus, the decline in firing rate as a function of duration increased with stimulus level. Indeed, whereas the initial spike rate increased with level, the firing rate after 100 sec was faster to a low-level tone than to a tone 80 dB more intense. These findings are just the reverse of the psychophysical data from humans who show a decrease in adaptation with increasing level until, by 30 dB SL, simple loudness adaptation is hardly measurable. The rather sparse neurophysiological data suggest that either loudness adaptation is not reflected in spike rate or it is based on neural events at levels beyond the cochlear nucleus.

C. Possible Basis for Loudness Adaptation

Taken all together, the data on simple and induced loudness adaptation suggest that adaptation is avoided where stimuli continue to evoke on-responses in units of the auditory system at some level beyond the cochlear nucleus. Let us assume that on-responses occur when the level of excitation increases sufficiently either because of an increase in stimulus intensity over a small group of fibers or because of variations in the pattern of excitation across fibers. Changes in stimulus intensity at low levels are needed to evoke on-responses—otherwise the excitation remains relatively fixed over a small group of units. Variation in excitation patterns occurs at higher levels where the pattern evoked by a tone is widespread and unstable as a large number of fibers fire out of phase. This variation which prevents adaptation at higher levels is overridden when a more strongly varying stimulus accompanies the steady stimulus and induces loudness adaptation.

In vision and taste, fluctuations in the stimulus imposed at the receptor have been shown to reduce adaptation. Involuntary eye movements (nystagmus) prevent adaptation. When nystagmus is circumvented by stimulating the eye with light reflected from a mirror attached to the cornea, visual images disappear within a minute (Riggs *et al.*, 1953). Likewise, tongue movements reduce adaptation to taste stimuli (Abrahams *et al.*, 1937). When they are avoided by stimulating a portion of the tongue with filter paper soaked in a taste solution, adaptation is strong and often complete within a couple of minutes (Gent and McBurney, 1978). On the other hand, pulsing a taste stimulus eliminates adaptation altogether and enhances subjective magnitude (Meiselman and Halpern, 1973).

The general rule may be that sensory systems adapt to steady, prolonged stimulation that is concentrated on a constant set of receptor units. Fluctuations in the level of stimulation reduce or elminate adaptation. Fluctuations may be in the stimulus or in the sensory organ (as when the particular units exposed to a steady stimulus vary). If this rule is generally true, then, with respect to loudness, the question remains of just how and where in the auditory system temporal variations are imposed on the level of excitation so as to avoid adaptation under most listening conditions even to steady and prolonged stimulation.

VI. CONCLUSIONS

From the survey of the literature and from the new data offered, the following conclusions seem warranted. A sound presented alone adapts only if it is below 30 dB SL. High-frequency pure tones adapt more than low-frequency tones or than noises, whether broad-band or narrow-band. Steady sounds adapt more than modulated sounds, and if the sound amplitude is modulated sufficiently adaptation may disappear altogether as when two tones beat together. People differ widely with respect to the degree of adaptation they experience. Although most people hear the loudness of a high-frequency, low-level tone decline by at least half within 1 min, others report no change in loudness and still others report that the tone disappears. No relation has been found, however, between the degree to which a person adapts and individual characteristics such as threshold, age, and sex, although there is some evidence that children under 15 years adapt less than adults. Free-field listening may produce less adaptation than earphone listening.

Loudness adaptation may also be induced by presenting a steady sound in one ear and an intermittent sound in the other. The loudness of the steady sound decreases markedly over 2 or 3 min even at high levels where its loudness does not change when presented alone. This form of adaptation is ascribed to the overriding of the normal variation in excitatory inputs from a high-level steady sound by the much greater variation from the intermittent sound. The role of interaural interaction and of lateralization in this adaptation is obscure, especially since the intermittent sound may induce some adaptation when in the same ear as the steady sound.

Although attentional mechanisms can almost surely be excluded as a basis for low-level adaptation, a scarcity of relevant physiological data permits only vague speculation about the basis for loudness adaptation or, more generally, for the lack of adaptation under most conditions. It is clear, however, that adaptation to intense sounds would not be beneficial to the organism. Exposure to intense sounds damages the hearing organ, and even mildly intense sounds can produce damage over long enough exposures. Since loudness is a major component of sound annoyance (Scharf, 1974), a diminution of loudness over time would mean that loud sounds would generally become less aversive and the exposed organism would be less likely to leave areas of intense sound.

Acknowledgments

A number of people contributed to the collection and analysis of data presented in this article. David Fishken and Thomas Horton were especially active in planning and executing many of the experiments. Mary Johnson and Phillip Duncan as well as Elinor Arpino, Ronald Diamond, Janet Harr, and Mary Testa were undergraduate students who helped enormously. The free-field data have all been collected at the Laboratoire de Mécanique et d'Acoustique, CNRS, in Marseille with the collaboration of Georges Canévet, Roger Germain, and Alain Marchioni. People who offered helpful comments about an earlier draft of this article include W. Dix Ward, W. Hartmann, E. M. Weiler, J. D. Hood, J. D. Harris, D. N. Elliott, and D. Fishken. Some of these readers disagree strongly with some of my interpretations of the data, and I could not accept all their suggestions in revising the manuscript. I am grateful to all these people and to the many observers who participated in the many experiments.

Part of this research was supported by a grant (2R01NS07270) from the National Institute of Neurological and Communicative Disorders and Stroke, a grant (RR07143) under HEW's Biomedical Research Support Program, and by the Laboratoire de Mécanique et d'Acoustique of the Centre National de la Recherche Scientifique.

References

Abrahams, H., Krakauer, D., and Dallenbach, K. M. (1937). Gustatory adaptation to salt. *Am. J. Psychol.* **49**, 462–469.

Ahaus, W. A., Stokinger, T. E., and Wylde, M. A. (1975). Influence of duty cycle and off time of comparison-tone pulse trains on the measurement of perstimulatory adaptation. *Percept. Psychophys.* **18**, 287–292.

Bartholomeus, B., and Swisher, L. (1971). Tone decay and SISI scores. *Arch. Otolaryngol.* **93**, 451–455.

Bartlett, F. C., and Mark, H. (1922). A note on local fatigue in the auditory system. *Br. J. Psychol.* **13**, 215–218.

Bauer, R. W., Matuza, J. C., Blackmer, R. F., and Glucksberg, S. (1966). Noise lateralization after unilateral attenuation. *J. Acoust. Soc. Am.* **40**, 441–444.

Békésy, G., von (1929). Zur Theorie des Hörens; Über die Bestimmung des einem reinen Tonempfinden entsprechenden Erregungsgebietes der Basilarmembran vermittelst Ermüdungserscheinungen. *Phys. Z.* **30**, 115–125.

Békésy, G., von (1958). Funneling in the nervous system. *J. Acoust. Soc. Am.* **30**, 399–412.

Békésy, G., von (1960). "Experiments in Hearing." McGraw-Hill, New York.

Berglund, U., and Berglund, B. (1970). Adaptation and recovery in vibrotactile perception. *Percept. Motor Skills* **30**, 843–853.

Bocca, E., and Pestalozza, G. (1959). Auditory Adaptation: Theories and facts. *Acta Oto-Laryngol.* **50**, 349–353.

Botte, M.-C., Canévet, G., and Scharf, B. (1982). Loudness adaptation induced by an intermittent tone. *J. Acoust. Soc. Am.* **72**, 727–739.

Bray, D. A., Dirks, D. D., and Morgan, D. E. (1973). Perstimulatory loudness adaptation. *J. Acoust. Soc. Am.* **53**, 1544–1548.

Canévet, G., Germain, R., Marchioni, A., and Scharf, B. (1981). Adaptation de pomi. *Acustica* **49**, 239–244.

Carhart, R. (1957). Clinical determination of abnormal auditory adaptation. *Arch. Otolaryngol.* **65**, 32–39.

Carterette, E. C. (1955). Perstimulatory auditory fatigue for continuous and interrupted noise. *J. Acoust. Soc. Am.* **27**, 103–111.

Cocholle, R. (1946). Les temps de réaction absolus binauraux. *C. R. Séances Soc. Biol.* **140**, 496–497.

Davis, J. M., and Weiler, E. (1976). Monaural auditory adaptation as measured by simple reaction time. *Br. J. Audiol.* **10**, 102–106.

Dieroff, H. G. (1976). Possibilities of improving the diagnosis of noise-induced hearing damage by means of directional audiometry, the dichotic speech discrimination test, and the EEG. *Audiology* **15**, 152–162.

Dirks, D. E., Morgan, D. E., and Bray, D. A. (1974). Perstimulatory loudness adaptation in selected cochlear impaired and masked normal listeners. *J. Acoust. Soc. Am.* **56**, 554–561.

Dove, H. W. (1859). Beweiss, dass die Tartinischen Töne nicht subjectiv, sondern objectiv sind. *Ann. Phys.* **107**(Ser. 2), 652–654.

Dunlap, K. (1904). Some peculiarities of fluctuating and of inaudible sounds. *Psychol. Rev.* **11**, 308–318.

Egan, J. P. (1955). Perstimulatory fatigue as measured by heterophonic loudness balances. *J. Acoust. Soc. Am.* **27**, 111–120.

Egan, J. P., and Thwing, E. J. (1955). Further studies on perstimulatory fatigue. *J. Acoust.Soc. Am.* **27**, 1225–1226.

Ekman, G., Berglund, B., Berglund, U., and Lindvall, T. (1967). Perceived intensity of odor as a function of time adaptation. *Scand. J. Psychol.* **8**, 177–186.

Elliot, D. N., and Fraser, W. R. (1970). Fatigue and adaptation. *In* "Foundations of Modern Auditory Theory" (J. V. Tobias, ed.), pp. 157–202. Academic Press, New York.

Feaster, S. A., and Weiler, E. M. (1975). The effects of monaural auditory adaptation in the speech range. *Br. J. Audiol.* **9**, 81–83.

Fechner, G. T. (1860). "Elemente der Psychophysik," Vol. I. Breitkopf & Härtel, Leipzig.

Fishken, D., Arpino, E., Testa, M., and Scharf, B. (1977). Loudness may adapt, after all. *J. Acoust. Soc. Am.* **61**, S61 (A).

Florentine, M. (1976). Relation between lateralization and loudness in symmetrical hearing losses. *J. Am. Audiol. Soc.* **1**, 243–251.

Fraser, W. D., Petty, J. W., and Elliott, D. N. (1970). Adaptation: Central or peripheral? *J. Acoust. Soc. Am.* **47**, 1016–1021.

Gent, J. F., and McBurney, D. H. (1978). Time course of gustatory adaptation. *Percept. Psychophys.* **23**, 171–175.

Green, D. S. (1953). The modified tone decay test, as screenning procedure for 8th nerve lesions. *J. Speech Hear. Disord.* **28**, 31–36.

Gruber, J., and Braune, H. (1974). Auditory adaptation measured by cross-modality matching. *Int. Congr. Acoust. 8th* 130.

Gummlich, H. (1971). Veränderungen des Lautstärkeeindruckes bei langzeitiger Gerauscheinwirkung (Changes in the impression of sound intensity during protracted noise.) *Proc. Int. Congr. Acoust, 7th* **3.**

Harbert, F., Weiss, B., and Wilpizeski, C. R. (1966). Some effects of stimulus parameters on the measurement of suprathreshold auditory adaptation. *J. Audit. Res.* **6**, 409–418.

Harbert, F., Weiss, B. G., and Wilpizeski, C. R. (1968). Suprathreshold auditory adaptation in normal and pathological ears. *J. Speech Hear. Res.* **11**, 268–278.

Harris, J. D., and Myers, C. K. (1949). The emergence of a tonal sensation. *J. Exp. Psychol.* **39**, 228–237.

Harris, J. D., and Pikler, A. G. (1960). The stability of a standard loudness as measured by compensatory tracking. *Am. J. Psychol.* **73**, 573–580.

Hempstock, T. I., Bryan, M. E., and Tempest, W. (1964). A redetermination of quiet threshold as a function of stimulus duration. *J. Sound Vib.* **4**, 365–380.

Hinchcliffe, R. (1959). The threshold of hearing as a function of age. *Acustica* **9**, 303–308.

Hood, J. D. (1950). Studies in auditory fatigue and adaptation. *Acta Oto-Laryngol. S92.*

Hood, J. D. (1969). The role of deranged metabolism in susceptibility to noise induced hearing loss. *Sound* **3**, 58–60.

Jerger, J. E. (1957). Auditory Adaptation. *J. Acoust.Soc. Am.* **29**, 357–363.

Jerger, J. E., and Harford, E. R. (1960). Alternate and simultaneous binaural balancing of pure tones. *J. Speech Hear. Res.* **3**, 15–30.

Jesteadt, W., Wier, C. G., and Green, D. M. (1977). Intensity discrimination as a function of frequency and sensation level. *J. Acoust. Soc. Am.* **61**, 169–177.

Kärjä, J. (1968). Perstimulatory suprathreshold adaptation. I. Basic studies on normal-hearing persons. *Acta Oto-Laryngol.* **S241.**

Kärjä, J. (1974). Perstimulatory suprathreshold adaptation III. Sensorineural Deafness. *Acta Oto-Laryngol.* **78**, 73–80.

Kiang, N. Y.-S. (1965). "Discharge patterns of Single Fibers in the Cat's Auditory Nerve" (with the assistance of T. Watanabe, E. C. Thomas, and L. F. Clark). Research Monograph No. 35. MIT Press, Cambridge, Massachusetts.

Kirk, R. E. (1968). "Experimental Design: Procedures for the Behavioral Sciences." Brooks/Cole, Belmont, California.

Lawrence, M., Windsor, R. B., and Hegeman, J. S. (1949). Discrimination of a sound changing gradually in intensity. *J. Aviat. Med.* **20**, 211–220.

Maré, G., de (1939). Audiometrische Untersuchungen. Ueber das Verhalten des normalen und schwerhörigen Ohres bei funktioneller Belastung nebst Bemerkungen zur Theorie des Gehörs. *Acta Oto-Laryngol.* **S31**, 1–173.

Margolis, R. H., and Wiley, T. L. (1976). Monaural loudness adaptation at low sensation levels in normal and impaired ears. *J. Acoust. Soc. Am.* **59**, 222–224.

Marks, L. E. (1974). "Sensory Processes." Academic Press, New York.

Meiselman, H. L. (1968). Magnitude estimations of the course of gustatory adaptation. *Percept. Psychophys.* **4**, 193–196.

Meiselman, H. L., and Halpern, B. P. (1973). Enhancement of taste intensity through pulsatile stimulation. *Physiol. Behav.* **11**, 713–716.

Melnick, W. (1967). Comfort level and loudness matching for continuous and interrupted signals. *J. Speech Hear. Res.* **10**, 99–109.

Mirabella, A., Taug, H., and Teichner, W. H. (1967). Adaptation of loudness to monaural stimulation. *J. Gen. Psychol.* **76**, 251–273.

Morgan, D. E., and Dirks, D. D. (1973). Suprathreshold loudness adaptation. *J. Acoust. Soc. Am.* **53**, 1560–1564.

Nordlund, B. (1964). Directional Audiometry. *Acta Oto-Laryngol.* **57**, 1–18.

Palva, T., and Kärjä, J. (1969). Suprathreshold auditory adaptation. *J. Acoust. Soc. Am.* **45**, 1018–1021.

Palva, T., Kärjä, J., and Palva, A. (1967). Auditory adaptation at threshold intensities. *Acta Oto-Laryngol.* **S224**, 195–200.

Parker, W. P., Decker, R. L., and Richards, N. G. (1968). Auditory function and lesions of the pons. *Arch. Otolaryngology* **87**, 228–240.

Petty, J. W., Fraser, W. D., and Elliott, D. N. (1970). Adaptation and loudness decrement: a reconsideration. *J. Acoust. Soc. Am.* **47**, 1074–1082.

Pollack, I. (1948). The atonal interval. *J. Acoust. Soc. Am.* **20**, 146–149.

Raab, D. H., and Osman, E. (1962). Effect of masking noise on lateralization and loudness of clicks. *J. Acoust. Soc. Am.* **34**, 1620–1624.

Rayleigh, C. (1882). Acoustical observations. IV. *Philos. Mag.* **13**, 340–347.

Riggs, L. A., Ratliff, F., Cornsweet, J. C., and Cornsweet, T. N. (1953). The disappearance of steadily fixated visual test objects. *J. Opt. Soc. Am.* **43**, 495–501.

Scharf, B. (1970). Critical bands. *In* "Foundation of Modern Auditory Theory" (J. V. Tobias, ed.), pp. 157–202. Academic Press, New York.

Scharf, B. (1974). Loudness and noisiness—same or different? *Internoise 74: Proc. Inst. Noise Control Eng.*, pp. 559–564.

Scharf, B. (1978). Loudness. *In* "Handbook of Perception" (E. C. Carterette and M. P. Friedman, eds.), pp. 187–242. Academic Press, New York.

Scharf, B., and Horton, T. J. (1978). Scaling loudness and annoyance as a function of duration. *J. Acoust. Soc. Am.* **63**, S1 (S16).

Scharf, B., and Stevens, J. C. (1961). The form of the loudness function near threshold. *Proc. Int. Congr. Acoust., 3rd* **1**.

Schubert, K. (1944). Zeitschrift für Hals-Nasen-und Ohrenheilkunde. *Hörermüdung Hördauer* **51**, 19–74.

Sergeant, R. L., and Harris, J. D. (1963). The relation of perstimulatory adaptation to other short-term threshold-shifting mechanisms. *J. Speech Hear. Res.* **6**, 27–39.

Sewall, E. (1907). Beitrag zur Lehre von der Ermüdung des Gehörorgans. *Z. Sinnesphysiol.* **42,** 115–123.

Small, A. M., and Minifie, F. D. (1961). Effects of matching time on perstimulatory adaptation. *J. Acoust. Soc. Am.* **33,** 1028–1033.

Snyder, J. M. (1973). Threshold adaptation in normal listeners. *J. Acoust. Soc. Am.* **53,** 435–439.

Sorensen, H. (1960). A threshold tone decay test. *Acata Oto-Laryngol.* **S158,** 356–360.

Sorensen, H. (1962). Initial auditory adaptation I. In normal individuals. *Acta Oto-Laryngol.* **55,** 299–308.

Stephens, S. D. G., and Hinchcliffe, R. (1968). Studies on temporary threshold shift. *Int. Audiol.* **7,** 267–279.

Stokinger, T. E., and Studebaker, G. A. (1968). Measurement of perstimlatory loudness adaptation. *J. Acoust. Soc. Am.* **44,** 250–256.

Stokinger, T. E., Cooper, W. A., and Meissner, W. A. (1972a). Influence of binaural interaction on the measurement of perstimulatory loudness adaptation. *J. Acoust. Soc. Am.* **51,** 602–607 (a).

Stokinger, T. E., Cooper, W. A., Jr., Meissner, W. A., and Jones, K. O. (1972b). Intensity, frequency, and duration effects in the measurement of monaural perstimulatory loudness adaptation. *J. Acoust. Soc. Am.* **51,** 608–616 (b).

Teghtsoonian, R. (1971). On the exponents in Steven's law and the constant in Ekman's law. *Psychol. Rev.* **78,** 71–80.

ten Kate, J. H., Raatgever, J., and Bilsen, F. A. (1977). Neural responses to cosine noise in a wide range of intensity levels. *Int. Congr. Acoust., 9th, Madrid,* **4/9-VII,** J4, P512.

Thwing, E. S. (1955). Spread of perstimulatory fatigue of a pure tone to neighboring frequencies. *J. Acoust. Soc. Am.* **27,** 741–748.

Tsuiki, T. (1965). Studies on the perstimulatory loudness adaptation. *Int. Audiol.* **4,** 138–140.

Urbantschitsch, V. (1881). Zur Lehre von der Schallempfindung. *Arch. Gesamte Physiol. Menschen Tiere* **24,** 574–595.

Ward, W. D. (1973). Adaptation and fatigue. *In* "Modern Developments in Audiology" (J. Jerger, ed.), 2nd Ed. Academic Press, New York.

Weiler, E. M. (1972). Further consideration of adaptation and loudness decrement. *J. Audit. Res.* **12,** 212–215.

Weiler, E. M., and Gross, L. F. (1976). A positive measure of monaural heterophonic auditory adaptation. *J. Audit. Res.* **16,** 20–23.

Wiley, T. (1972). "Monaural Loudness Adaptation." Thesis, University of Iowa.

Wiley, T. L., Lilly, D. J., and Small, A. M. (1976). Loudness adaptation in listeners with noise-induced hearing loss. *J. Acoust. Soc. Am.* **59,** 225–227.

Wittich, B. A. (1966). Experimental studies in auditory adaptation. *Int. Audiol.* **5,** 7–47.

Wood, A. G. (1930). "A Quantitative Account of the Course of Auditory Fatigue." M.S. Thesis, the University of Virginia.

Wright, H. N. (1959). Auditory adaptation in noise. *J. Acoust. Soc. Am.* **31,** 1004–1012.

Wright, H. N. (1960). Measurement of perstimulatory auditory adaptation. *J. Acoust. Soc. Am.* **32,** 1558–1567.

Young, E., and Scahs, M. B. (1973). Recovery from sound exposure in auditory-nerve fibers. *J. Acoust. Soc. Am.* **54,** 1535–1543.

Zwislocki, J. J., and Goodman, D. A. (1980). Absolute scaling of sensory magnitudes: A validation. *Percept. Psychophys.* **28,** 28–38.

Speech-Cue Measures of Impaired Hearing

J. M. Pickett, Sally G. Revoile, and Ellen M. Danaher

Sensory Communication Research Laboratory
Gallaudet College
Washington, D.C.

This article describes studies of the discrimination of speech acoustic-cues by hearing-impaired persons and discusses the future potential of applying speech technology in auditory rehabilitation. We first give a brief sketch of the back-

57

HEARING RESEARCH AND THEORY, VOLUME 2

ground and theory of measuring speech perception by the hearing impaired. Then we describe some cue-discrimination tests that we and others have used, and some results obtained with hearing-impaired listeners. We also discuss the potential use of synthetic speech sounds for clinical tests of hearing. An appendix (Section X) describes methods of speech synthesis.

I. BACKGROUND

The early theoretical approach to the perception of speech acoustic properties was developed at Bell Laboratories, by Harvey Fletcher and his colleagues, from telecommunication theory and practice (Fletcher, 1929, 1953). This work designed an ''articulation index'' (AI) that would predict the level of speech communication that could be obtained through a given transmission channel. The AI takes into account the average frequency spectrum of speech and of any noise present, together with the frequency–amplitude characteristics of the channel. The index was constructed to predict the percentage correct word score that would be achievable over the measured channel.

Fletcher also adapted the AI theory for conditions of individual hearing impairment. For this purpose the threshold contour of an individual's hearing loss was transformed into channel limitations of noise and frequency range. The method successfully predicted sets of word-reception scores obtained from two persons with sensorineural impairments (Fletcher, 1953, pp. 435–436).

Articulation index has become a standard for predicting word scores for normal speech communication (ANSI S3.5-1969; S3.14-1977). However, AI has only recently been tested more intensively for predicting the effects of hearing impairment. For improved individual prediction, corrections to AI need to be developed for abnormal spread of masking and other auditory distortions of impairments (L. Braida, personal communication, 1978). The Fletcher approach has been modified successfully for use in determining the optimum frequency–amplitude corrections for individual hearing-aid amplification (Pascoe, 1978; Miller, 1982). However, even with optimum tailoring of the frequency– amplitude ranges of speech to the individual field of hearing, there is typically a reduced level of perception that cannot be explained solely on the basis of frequency–amplitude limitations (see Walden *et al.*, 1981, for a study related to this problem).

The classic measure of speech reception by the hearing impaired is the percentage of words understood, as spoken from a suitable list of words and heard at a suitable level of amplification. Using this measure the investigator and clinician can obtain some general indications of the difficulty encountered in understanding speech. Such a measure has a modicum of face validity. However, it provides little insight into the detailed auditory nature of the difficulty. The detailed auditory aspects would be expected to relate to the basic acoustic properties of speech, i.e., the particular acoustic features which distinguish the smallest units of words.

Theoretically the phoneme is a more basic unit in speech communication than the word: it is phoneme differences that distinguish words. About 1950, linguists and acousticians jointly began to consider relations between the phonemes and the acoustic patterns resulting from the production of the different consonant and vowel phonemes. A theory of phonemic acoustic features called distinctive feature theory was outlined by Jacobson *et al.* (1951). In this theory phonemes are distinguished by a few features of their articulation, such as the voicing, stop, and place features which are three major consonant features. The theory is to correlate feature production, the resulting acoustic patterns, and phoneme perception by listeners, to provide a complete, basic, and unified description of speech communication.

Subsequent research, stimulated in part by distinctive feature theory, has defined specific acoustic patterns that serve as auditory cues for phoneme identification; these cues can be described using only a few pattern categories (some particular acoustic cues are described below; for a more comprehensive review see Pickett, 1980; Borden and Harris, 1980). The phoneme cues are the ultimate basis of word discrimination and so they must be perceived correctly for completely normal development of language to occur (Liberman and Studdert-Kennedy, 1978; Studdert-Kennedy, 1980).

The work to be described here, although it is based on distinctive feature theory, and may provide new data bearing on the theory, is not aimed at theoretical development. Our approach is essentially opportunistic: current phonological theory in linguistics, and speech production theory in acoustics, provide new opportunities to develop a deeper understanding of the auditory factors in speech-perception problems of the hearing impaired.

Several investigators have recently analyzed impaired auditory aspects of speech reception along dimensions of distinctive features (Walden and Montgomery, 1975; Bilger and Wang, 1976; Wang *et al.*, 1978; Walden *et al.*, 1980; for a review of earlier studies see Pickett, 1979). However, these studies were aimed at general descriptions of phonemic-feature processing by the hearing impaired, so they did not attempt to measure auditory discrimination for variations in specific acoustic cues.

As modern speech acoustic theory developed further (beginning about 1935 at Bell Labs) a technology of speech processing also emerged. One technical development has provided very flexible techniques for synthesizing speech sounds and varying their perceptual cues in controlled ways (Klatt, 1980). These methods have been used extensively in the research on the normal acoustic cues in speech perception (Flanagan and Rabiner, 1973). Since about 1969 speech synthesis has also been used in studies of speech-cue discrimination by hearing-impaired listeners, at first especially in our laboratory.

We believe that eventually a detailed knowledge of impaired discrimination of speech acoustic cues can be developed that will contribute both to auditory theory and rehabilitation practice. On the theoretical side, we already have some rudimentary psychophysiological theories of impaired hearing (Evans and Wilson, 1977). We expect eventually to have physiological explanations of impairment effects on speech-cue discrimination.

On the practical side, a knowledge of impaired cue discrimination could serve to improve the habilitation of hearing impairment through aids to hearing, by contributing to advances in diagnosis, auditory training, and new designs for hearing aids. For example, if we had detailed descriptions of impairment in terms of speech cues we might be able to build special signal-processing aids that transform the received speech signal to enhance the cues for the hearing impaired. The technology exists but sufficient knowledge about impaired speech-cue discrimination does not.

We have begun to develop the required knowledge. We have concentrated on the phonemic cues, i.e., the cues that distinguish the different vowels and consonants. As will be seen, these cues are intricately patterned, and thus they are more likely to be critical for the hearing impaired than are the more grossly patterned cues of speech rhythms and voice intonations.

II. HEARING ACUITY FOR FORMANT FREQUENCY

The different vowels of speech are produced by voice transmission through different shape configurations of the vocal tract. Each vowel shape causes a unique frequency position of the vocal-tract resonances (formants). In particular the first and second resonances, formant one (F1) and formant two (F2), are known to provide major auditory cues that listeners use for vowel identification.

Thus for a start in relating acoustic cues to impaired hearing we measured the basic discrimination acuity for the frequency position of a formant-like resonant peak in the sound spectrum (Pickett and Mártony, 1970). We synthesized a test waveform with a single formant, the frequency of which could be shifted to different positions for discrimination tests. The spectrum shape of the test stimulus was like a single speech formant formed by a low-pass resonator that was excited by synthetic voice pulses having a speech-like wave-shape and frequency of repetition (125 Hz). Some spectrum plots of test stimuli are shown in Fig. 1.

The psychophysical procedure determined the formant-frequency discrimination threshold, that is, the smallest difference in frequency the listener could detect. On each test trial the listener was presented three successive stimuli, one

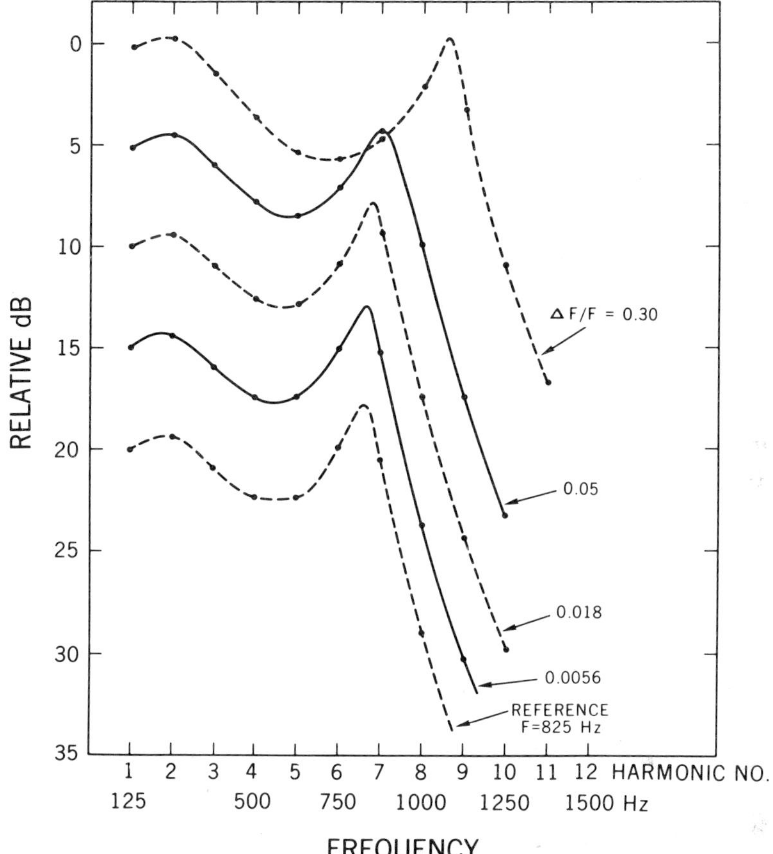

Figure 1   Spectra of a set of the synthetic, single-formant vowel sounds used in discrimination tests of formant frequency. Vowel spectra are shown for $F = 825$ Hz and for four different values of F labeled in terms of the proportion of frequency relative to $F(\Delta F/F)$. The plotted points give the measured relative amplitudes of the harmonics of each vowel at the input to the listener's earphone. The curves drawn through the points are the overall frequency responses of the synthesizer circuits fitted to the points. For better visual comparison, each curve is displaced upward 5 dB from the curve below. (From Pickett and Mártony, 1970.)

of which was different in formant frequency from the other two reference stimuli which were the same in formant frequency. The listener was required to identify which of the three stimuli was the different one and he was then informed of the correct answer. The amount of difference was adjusted between trials by an adaptive procedure which estimated the threshold as the amount of frequency difference necessary for 50% correct in the three-alternative response task. As an index of discrimination the threshold frequency difference was expressed as a

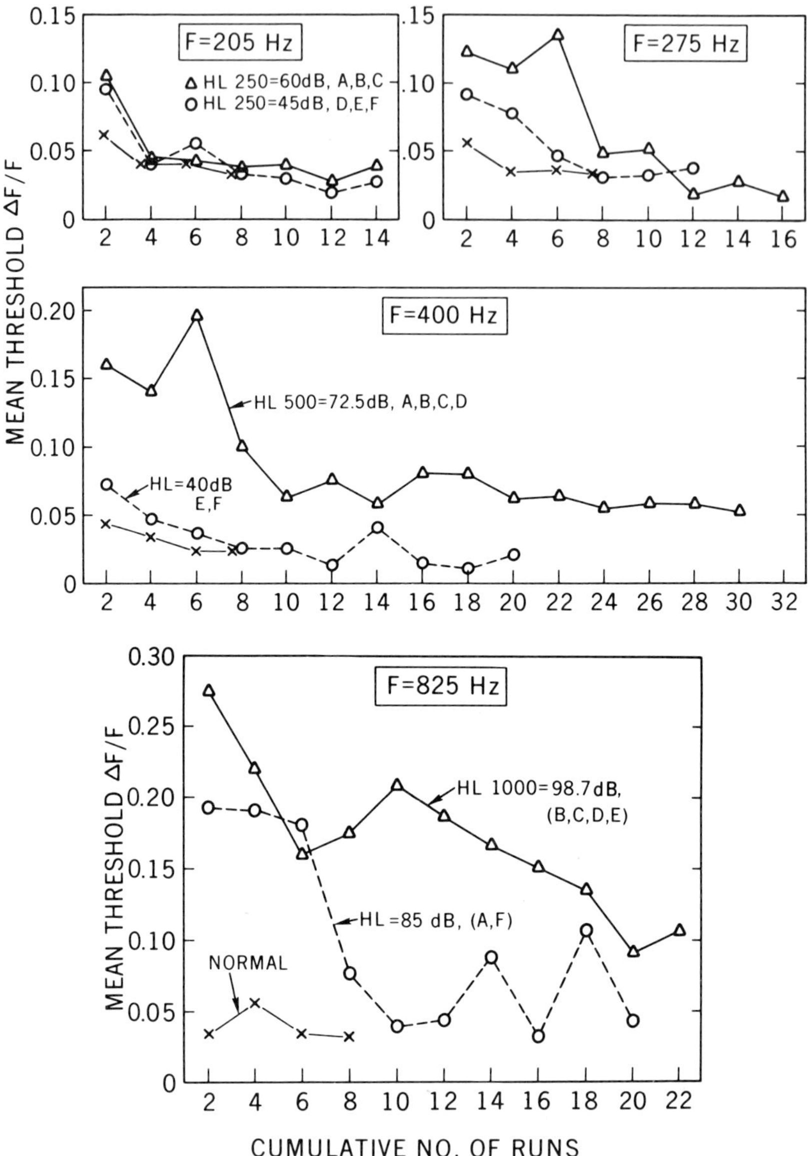

Figure 2 Vowel formant discrimination at four reference locations (F = formant resonance frequency) as dependent on experience in the experiment (cumulative number of runs) and on hearing loss (HL). Discrimination is plotted as the group mean threshold ΔF divided by F. The impaired subjects are divided into two groups according to amount of hearing loss at the audiometric frequency (250, 500, or 1000 Hz) nearest to the reference F frequency. The individuals of each group are identified by letter and the group mean hearing loss is given. The groups with severe hearing loss are plotted with triangles connected by solid lines; the groups with moderate loss are plotted with circles connected by dashed lines. A group of four naive normal listeners is plotted with ×s. (From Pickett and Mártony, 1970.)

difference limen, that is, the proportion of the difference relative to the reference frequency (F) of the two identical stimuli. F was set at a constant parametric value which was 205, 275, 400, or 825 Hz, for a given threshold determination.

The results showed that acuity, the $\Delta F/F$ at threshold, depended on the degree of hearing loss and on the formant frequency of the reference. The mean $\Delta F/F$ for listeners grouped as to degree of hearing loss is plotted in Fig. 2 as a function of experience in the experiment (cumulative number of runs). It will be seen in general that the two hearing-impaired groups, severe (triangles) and moderate (circles), both show very large learning effects, compared with the normals. Final practiced acuity was near normal (about 4%) if the hearing loss was only moderate and if tested in a low-frequency region (F = 205 or 275 Hz); acuity was poorer (5–10%) at the highest tested frequency (F = 825 Hz). For the severe group, the threshold acuity was very poor, about 10 to 15% at F = 825 Hz. These latter subjects obtained the same level of acuity through tactile vibration, felt as differences in intensity of vibration, when the earphone emitting the test sounds was impressed on their hands. Thus it appeared that the ear of the severely impaired listener may discriminate formant frequency only on the basis of tactile vibration.

Mártony and Agelfors (1974) carried out some tests of discrimination for two-formant synthetic vowels with deaf children ages 10–15. They found that those children with hearing loss less than about 100 dB had some residual auditory discrimination of low-frequency formant differences (testing range was F = 224 to 897 Hz; difference limens ranged from 5 to 21%). For children with losses greater than 100 dB the discrimination was very poor (greater than 30% difference limen) and discrimination appeared to be tactile.

III. DISCRIMINATION OF FORMANT TRANSITIONS

The formants also provide cues to perception of the consonants. For example in speaking the word *Bach,* the opening movement of the lips, going from the *b* to the *a,* causes the formants to go up in frequency; the formants make a rapid upward transition. In contrast when the tongue releases the *d* of *dock,* F2 goes down in frequency. The difference between *b* and *d* can be heard as a difference in the transition of the frequency of F2 at the beginning of the vowel: this frequency usually rises upon the opening into a vowel from lip constrictions, such as from *b, p,* or *w,* and either falls or is steady upon opening from tongue-tip constrictions such as *d, t,* or *y.* In general the different places of the main constrictions of the different consonants and vowels produce different formant-frequency patterns; these patterns may be transitional or steady. They are known to be one of the acoustic cues used by listeners for distinguishing the different places of articulation among consonants. [The other main cues to place of articulation are the frequency patterns of the brief release bursts (from stops), and of the friction noises of fricatives.] The formant transitions may also be responsible for the perception of speech as an integrated flow of sound (Cole and Scott, 1974) rather than the succession of silent gaps, transients, resonated buzzes, and hisses that it is acoustically. Because of the indicated importance of transitions in speech perception we next studied the acuity of discrimination for transitions in formant frequency with impaired listeners in two pilot experiments (Martin *et al.*, 1972).

A. Formant Transition Detection

We first measured acuity for detecting the occurrence of a formant transition. The transition to be detected was in the initial portion of a single-formant stimulus that was 500 msec in duration. This was compared with the same stimulus without any transition. The threshold amount of transition was measured using the same three-alternative procedure as for the steady-formant study; the two reference stimuli of a trial had no formant transition while the test stimulus had a constant-duration transition to an end frequency or steady state at the same formant frequency as the reference stimuli. The transition was rising; it was varied in frequency extent during a run of trials to determine the least amount of transition, ΔF, that could be detected.

The transition duration and steady-state frequency were varied parametrically over values found in speech. The transition duration was 50, 100, 300, or 500 msec. These values would be typical, respectively, of stops, glides, diphthongs, and very slow vowel glides. The steady-state frequency was 1.2, 2.0, or 3.0 kHz. As an example, in threshold runs with the 100-msec transition duration and 1.2-kHz end frequency, the stimulus having the transition began with an upward 100-msec F transition to 1.2 kHz and then continued for the remainder of the stimulus (400 msec) at $F = 1.2$ kHz. Examples of different 100-msec transitions may be seen in Fig. 4 where formant time-frequency tracks are shown to an end frequency of 1.5 kHz.

The extent of F transition was varied by changing the F frequency of the start of the transition. Each run began with a very large amount of transition on the first trial and the amount was then reduced following correct-response trials and increased after incorrect trials. The threshold index was the smallest transition extent that could be detected correctly on 50% of the trials; this was called the transition threshold, ΔF_{tr}.

Both normal-hearing listeners and moderate-to-severely impaired listeners were measured using stimulus levels that were adjusted to each listener's most comfortable level (MCL).

The results are shown in Fig. 3 in terms of the mean transition thresholds. It will be seen here that acuity for detecting the transition, in terms of the smallest

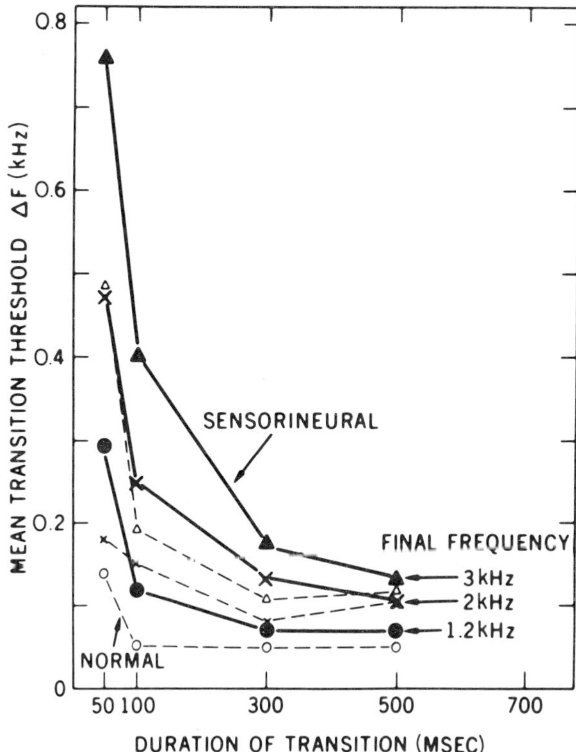

Figure 3 Effects of frequency location and duration of transition on formant transition detection threshold. Mean formant transition threshold, in terms of the frequency extent of transition that is just detectable from no transition, is plotted in kilohertz for three normal listeners and for three sensorineural hearing-impaired listeners with relatively flat contours of loss averaging 80 dB in the range 0.25–8 kHz. The frequency region in which the transition and subsequent steady state are located was varied as a parameter (indicated at the right by the "final frequency" values). Thresholds are generally higher (i.e., a larger transition is required for detection) for the hearing-impaired than for the normal group, and especially so with the briefer duration transitions in the higher frequency regions. (From Martin *et al.*, 1972.)

frequency extent or size of transition that could be detected, was better for long-duration transitions than for short ones, and better for transitions to a low steady-state frequency than to a high steady-state frequency. For example, with 100-msec duration the normal transition threshold, ΔF_{tr} of 50 Hz, was on the order of 5% of the 1.2-kHz steady-state frequency (called final frequency in Fig. 3). The impaired listeners' ΔF_{tr} was larger: on the order of 12%. Both normal and impaired listeners had less acuity, larger ΔF_{tr}, for transitions to higher final frequencies. With the very long transition of 500 msec, impaired and normal acuities were not significantly different at any frequency. For the 50- and 100-msec durations, which are very important in speech, the impaired listeners were considerably less acute than the normals.

We then made the test stimulus more speech-like by adding a lower steady formant (F1) to the stimulus, to study its effect on transition detection discrimination. F1 was steady in frequency at 489 Hz and simultaneous with the higher formant. The F2 steady-state reference frequency was 1.5 kHz. These two frequencies are approximately at the average of F1 and F2 in adult male voices. Both upward and downward transitions of 100 and 300 msec were tested.

Results are shown in Fig. 4 for 100-ms transitions. The plots show frequency tracks of the test stimulus having a transition extent of the threshold amount. It is

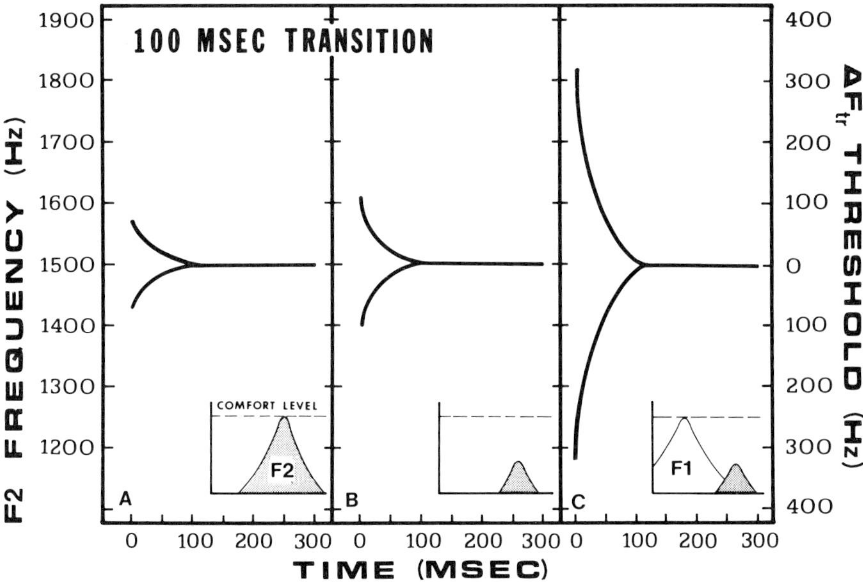

Figure 4 Frequency-time tracks of the second formant (F2) in stimuli where the F2 transition was just detectable (on the average) by six hearing-impaired listeners who had flat contours of hearing loss vs frequency of approximately 80 dB. Both upward and downward transitions were tested. The steady frequency of F2 was 1500 Hz following the completion of the 100-msec transition. Comparison stimuli for determining transition threshold had no transition, F2 being constant at 1500 Hz. F1, when present, was constant at 489 Hz. The inset graphs are diagrams of the spectrum relations for the three test conditions of amplitude/formant combination, one for each panel of the figure. (A) and (B) give the results for two baseline amplitude conditions in which F2 was presented alone. (B) is for the condition where F2 alone was presented at the same amplitude as it would occur in a representative speech stimulus (combined with F1) at the individual listener's comfortable amplified listening level, as was also done for the results with combined F1 and F2 shown in (C). The very large threshold transitions in (C) indicate the masking effect of the presence of F1, compared with the smaller threshold transitions in (B). (From Martin *et al.*, 1972.)

apparent that the presence of F1 caused a substantial reduction in F2 transition-detection acuity: compare the large extents of upward or downward threshold transitions in Fig. 4C with the small ones in Fig. 4B. The masking effect was greater for the hearing-impaired listeners than for normals: e.g., 350-Hz threshold transition vs the normals' 100 Hz when F1 was added.

Comparing upward and downward transitions, the transition thresholds and the masking effect were about the same even though the downward transitions began at higher frequencies. In this connection it should be noted that the impaired listeners were chosen to have relatively flat contours of loss vs frequency.

The F1 masking effect was studied in more detail in three further experiments (Danaher *et al.*, 1973). In the first experiment two frequency and amplitude relations between F1 and the higher formant, F2, were tested. A larger group of hearing-impaired subjects was divided into subgroups according to audiometric

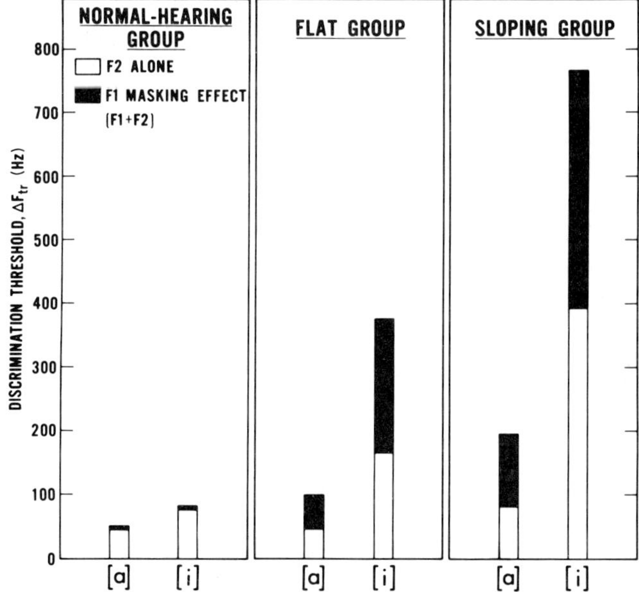

Figure 5 F2 transition detection threshold (discrimination threshold) in synthetic vowels [a] and [i]. The threshold is the amount of frequency transition in F2 that is just discriminable from no transition. The group mean thresholds, ΔF_{tr}, are plotted as histograms, overlapped between the two conditions, F2 alone (unfilled bars), and F1 plus F2 (filled bar behind the unfilled bar). Thus the filled distance showing is the amount of discrimination masking as measured by the difference in hertz between F2 alone threshold and F1 + F2 threshold. There is more masking by F1 for the impaired listeners (flat or sloping) than for the normal group (who were listening at their most comfortable level). The sloping group had poorer hearing than the flat group in the region of F2 and shows correspondingly more masking. However, see text for discussion of individual differences. (From Danaher *et al.*, 1973.)

contour of hearing: relatively *flat* ($N=11$), or *sloping* downward with progressively poorer hearing at middle and high frequencies ($N=13$). The steady-state portions of the stimuli simulated either the vowel /ɑ/ or the vowel /i/, with F1/F2 = 625/1100 Hz for [ɑ] and 375/2200 Hz for [i]. When a transition occurred in F2, F2 began at a lower frequency and reached the steady-state frequency in 100 msec.

There were four normal listeners; all listeners were tested at their individual MCL.

The results are shown in Fig. 5. They confirmed the existence of the F1 masking effect on transition detection in F2. F1 masking was found to be greater for listeners with sloping hearing losses; possibly this was because the sloping group had greater hearing loss at the F2 frequencies than the flat group. Acuity with [i] where F2 is high was less than with [ɑ], where F2 was lower. We had seen this frequency effect before with single-formant transitions.

There were very large differences in individual susceptibility to the masking, especially in the flat group where, with [i], a few of the listeners showed no more masking than normals. For [ɑ] most of the flat group were within the normal range of the masking effect for comparable levels. The individual differences within the two hearing-impaired groups showed little correlation with individual audiometric characteristics, such as level of MCL or hearing level in the F2 range.

B. Effect of Sound Level on Normal Performance

One might conclude from the group data at MCL that F1 masking effects occur only under hearing loss. However, the sound levels varied considerably among the three groups and the MCLs for the hearing-impaired subjects were at much higher intensity levels than those for the normal-hearing subjects. In fact, the hearing-impaired subjects preferred to listen at levels which were within the range where spread of masking normally occurs. The normals' MCLs were below those at which masking spread typically is found (Bilger and Hirsh, 1956; Martin and Pickett, 1970). If spread of masking is a factor in discrimination of formant transitions, then normal-hearing subjects likewise should demonstrate reduced discrimination at high sound levels.

To study this possibility, mean transition thresholds for the normal-hearing groups were obtained at overall levels of 75, 85, 95, and 105 dB SPL, as shown in Fig. 6; ranges are indicated by the vertical dashed lines. Mean F1 + F2 thresholds for the flat and sloping groups are plotted at their mean MCLs.

There is no evidence of spread of masking for normals at 75 and 85 dB. Their thresholds are essentially the same as those obtained at their MCLs. However, at 95 and 105 dB, substantial amounts of masking occur in some subjects. At these levels, the mean [ɑ] thresholds for the normal-hearing group are larger than those

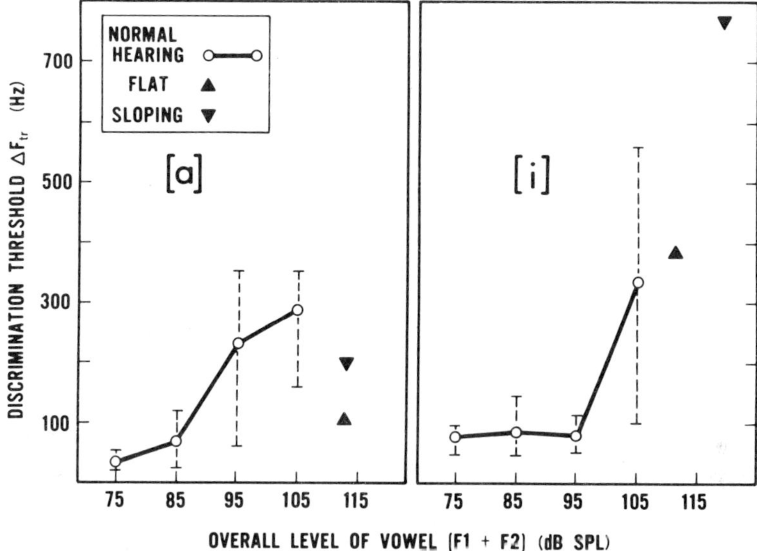

Figure 6 Comparative effect of vowel level on detection (discrimination) of F2 transitions by the subjects of Fig. 5; the normals' ranges of threshold span the dashed vertical lines through the plotted mean values. The mean thresholds for the sloping and flat impaired groups are the same as those in Fig. 5, plotted at the mean most comfortable listening levels (in the range 110–120 dB) for comparison with the normals' results. It will be seen that, when listening at high levels, the normals have large thresholds, comparable to the impaired listeners except for the sloping impaired with the vowel [i].

of the sensorineural groups. F1 masking effects in [i] occur only at 105 dB and are less than those in the sensorineural groups. Note that masking occurs at a lower sound level in [a], where the formants are in close proximity to each other. At 95 and 105 dB the range of the thresholds is wide and the variability within the normal-hearing group is as great as that which occurs within the sensorineural group.

These data indicate that reduced discrimination ability characterizes most persons who listen at high sound levels. The presence or absence of sensorineural loss does not seem to be a critical factor at these levels. The discrimination loss in the normal-hearing subjects probably is a result of the upward spread of masking produced by F1. Similarly, spread of masking might be the major factor for the impaired listeners. Therefore, the reduced discrimination ability that characterizes most persons with sensorineural loss might be attributed to a ''normal'' phenomenon that occurs at high sound levels, rather than to the sensorineural damage itself.

In studies of speech perception performance under conditions of high-level noise it has been found that normal performance deteriorates at levels above 85 dB SPL (Pollack and Pickett, 1958; Pickett, 1959). This reduction in speech perception may have been due to increased spread of masking from the F1 frequencies of the speech signal to the partially noise-masked F2 information in the mid-frequencies.

C. Effect of F1 Transition

Up to this point in our studies the F1 portion of the test stimuli had no frequency-transitions. In actual speech an F2 transition is usually accompanied by a simultaneous transition in F1 frequency. The F1 transitions are produced in articulating consonants, which are constrictive gestures as opposed to the more open vowel-like positions. Thus, in our previous tests the transition-containing stimuli, since they had no F1 transitions, did not give a consonant-like impression. In fact, we initially wanted to avoid having the stimuli sound like consonants because we hoped to measure the acuity of the ear, independent of the process of phoneme perception.

In the next study, different amounts of F1 transition were introduced as constant conditions on every stimulus of each trial, and the F2 transition acuity was

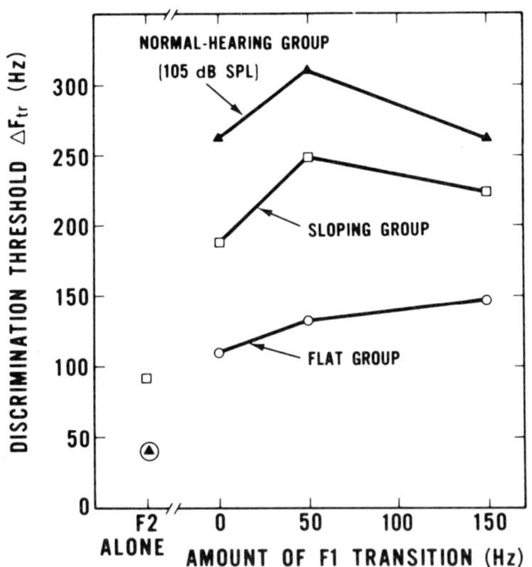

Figure 7   Effect of F1 transitions on detection of F2 transitions in [a]. Mean discrimination thresholds, ΔF_{tr}, for F2 alone was shown in the left of the figure to provide a basis for evaluating the amount of masking occurring in each of the test conditions. Eight subjects with flat sensorineural losses, seven subjects with sloping sensorineural losses, and four normal-hearing subjects were tested. The normal-hearing group was tested at 105 dB SPL. The amounts of masking with 0 Hz F1 transition are comparable to those in Fig. 6. Masking increased significantly (larger thresholds) with increased amount of F1 transition. (From Danaher *et al.*, 1973.)

measured as before. The results are shown in Fig. 7. It will be seen that the F1 transitions caused a small increase in the apparent masking effect of F1 on detection of a transition in F2. The increase between 0- and 50-Hz transitions was statistically significant.

In the third experiment of this series we studied the possibility of reducing the F1 masking effect by reducing the amplitude of F1. Only hearing-impaired subjects were measured, using the same procedure as before. The results appear in Fig. 8. The attenuation of F1 by 10 or 15 dB caused substantial reductions in masking, especially for the listeners who had flat contours of hearing loss. For these "flat" subjects masking was insignificantly small at 15-dB F1 attenuation when there was no F1 transition. The presence of an F1 transition again had the effect of increasing the masking.

A possibility for reducing F1 masking while retaining the loudness of F1 was to present the F1 portion of the signal to one ear and the F2 portion to the other ear. Tests were carried out with the usual monotic condition (F1 and F2 together in the listener's preferred ear), a dichotic condition (F2 to the preferred ear, F1 to the other ear), and with F2 presented alone to the preferred ear (Danaher and Pickett, 1975). Results are given in Fig. 9. Here there was often a substantial

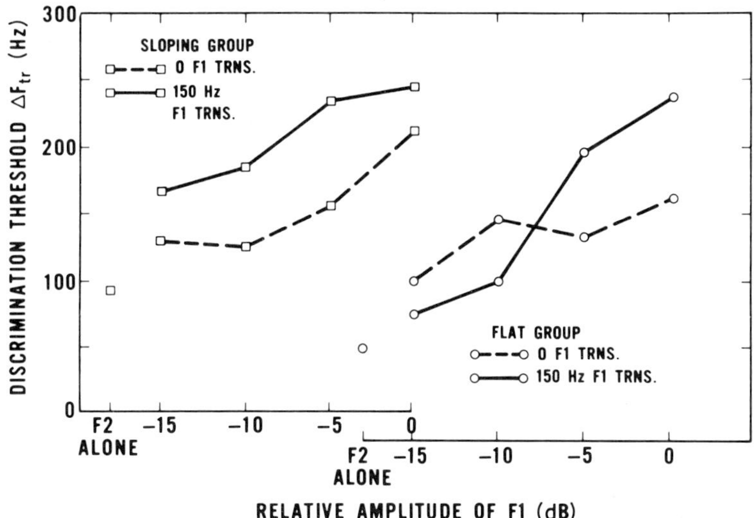

Figure 8 Effects of relative amplitude of F1 and frequency transitions in F1 on detection of F2 transitions in [a]. The zero reference for amplitude of F1 is that of natural speech. Seven subjects with sloping sensorineural losses and four subjects with flat sensorineural losses were tested. Mean ΔF_{tr} values for F2 alone are shown as a reference for evaluating the amount of masking produced by F1 in each of the test conditions. Attenuation of F1 by 10–15 dB significantly improves the F2 transition threshold to a smaller value. (From Danaher *et al.*, 1973.)

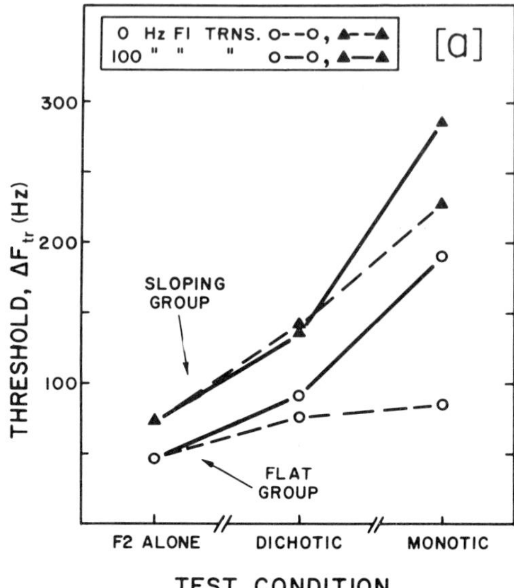

Figure 9 Effects of dichotic separation of F1 and F2 on the threshold amount of transition, ΔF_{tr}, for detecting a 100-msec upward transition in frequency of F2. The vowel was [a] (steady-state F1 = 650, F2 = 1200). There were eight listeners in the sloping group and seven in the flat group; the two groups' mean hearing loss was approximately 80 dB at 750 Hz. The differences between thresholds in the F2 alone condition vs the monotic condition indicate the amount of masking on the transition threshold; the differences are reduced by dichotic separation, especially when an F1 transition (of 100 Hz) was simultaneously present (data connected by the solid lines) and for the sloping listeners. (From Danaher and Pickett, 1975.)

dichotic release from the monotic masking. Apparently some of the masking effect is like the classical upward spread of masking (but for discrimination) and some of the effect is a general, more central type of masking that remains in effect under dichotic listening.

The presence of a transition in F1 did not increase masking of the F2 transition under the dichotic condition, suggesting that there might be some listeners who did not hear a consonantal effect in the dichotic stimulus.

Again, in general there were very large differences among subjects, differences that were unaccountable on the basis of the audiogram.

IV. BACKWARD MASKING OF TRANSITION DISCRIMINATION

In actual speech the F2 transitions caused by articulator movement sometimes precede the onset of F1 by an interval of about 50 msec. How much release from

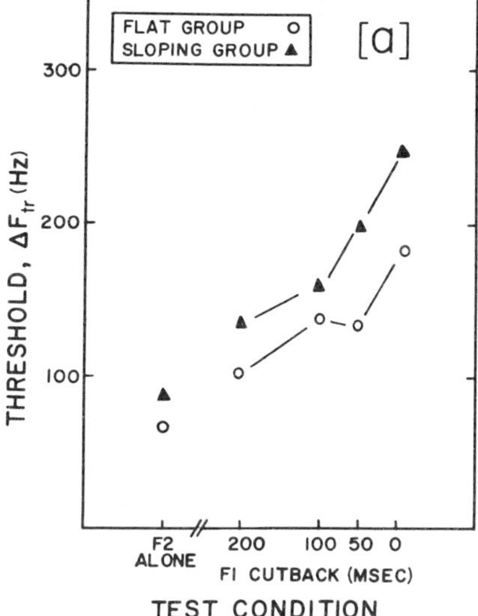

Figure 10   The effect of F1-onset delay on the discrimination of initial transitions in F2. Discrimination of F2 transitions was measured when the onsets of F1 and F2 were the same ("0 cutback") and when the onset of F1 was delayed (50, 100, and 200 msec) relative to that of F2. The F2 transition was 100 msec in duration. Steady-state F1 and F2 were at 650 and 1100 Hz, respectively. Twenty-three subjects with sensorineural losses, like those in Fig. 9, were tested. Backward masking from F1 is seen by comparing the F2 alone thresholds with F1 + F2 thresholds, where F1 is cut back (delayed) in onset relative to F2. With 100 msec cutback the entire F2 transition occurs before the onset of F1, yet F1 has caused a fairly large increase in the transition detection threshold. (From Danaher and Pickett, 1975.)

F1 masking would this provide? We studied this question by measuring transition detection in F2 under different amounts of delay of the onset of a steady F1 relative to the onset of the F2 transition. The results appear in Fig. 10. As before F1 had a backward masking effect on detecting the occurrence of the F2 transitions. A larger F2 transition was necessary for detection in the presence of a delayed F1 onset than with no F1 present. Even when F1 was delayed as much as 100, or even 200 msec, there was a transition-detection masking effect for some impaired listeners (Danaher and Pickett, 1975).

Temporal masking effects on audibility, both backward and forward in time, are well established in the psychoacoustic literature (see Elliott, 1967, for example). We asked ourselves whether the backward masking we had found on discriminating the occurrence of an F2 transition would be explainable as an effect of reduced audibility. Therefore, we compared the F1 backward and foward masking on F2 with the masking produced by an F1-shaped noise on pure tone thresholds at frequencies above the F1 resonant frequency (Danaher *et al.*, 1978). It was found that significant amounts of masking on tone sensitivity extended only as far as about 50 msec backward and forward in time relative to the onset or offset of the F1 noise masker. In contrast, masking for the detection or occurrence of an F2 transition had extended in our previous experiment, for intervals up to 100 and 200 msec before and after the onset or offset of F1. Therefore it appeared that masking of F2 transition discrimination could not be entirely explained in terms of a shift in audibility.

V. DISCRIMINATION FOR RATE OF FORMANT TRANSITION

The rate of formant transition serves as a cue for differentiating the glide consonants, which are articulated with a moderate rate of movement, from the stop and nasal consonants, which are articulated by a faster movement. Also these rates vary somewhat with the overall rate of speaking, and thus sensitivity

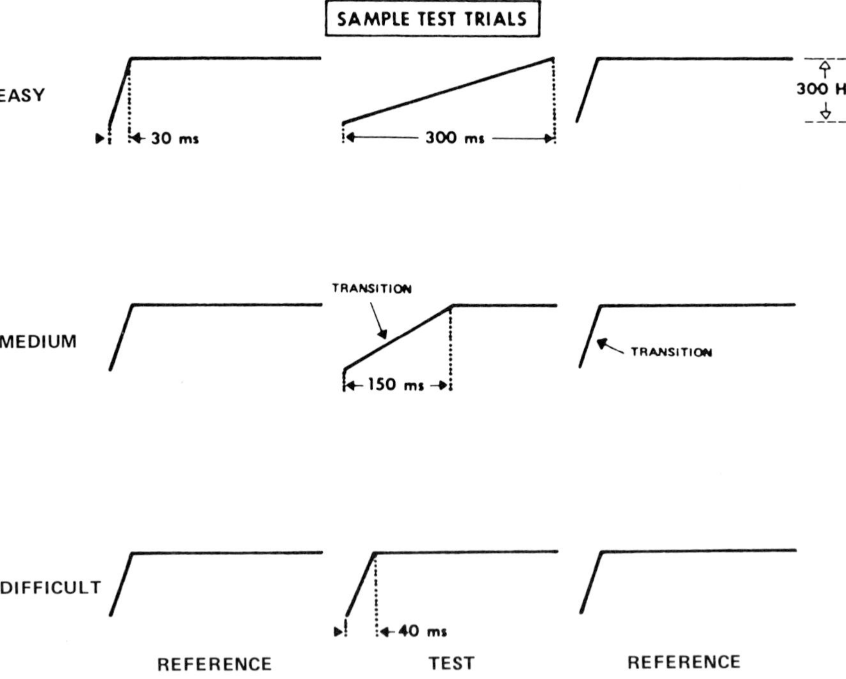

Figure 11 Frequency-time formant tracks of some stimulus triplets for testing discrimination for rate of formant transition. Three triplets are shown in which the second "test" stimulus is different from the other two "references" stimuli which are identical. "Easy," "medium," and "difficult" triplets are shown corresponding, respectively, to a test-transition duration of 300, 150, or 40 msec.

to the transition rate may serve as a normalizer for speaking rate in the speech-understanding process.

We recently carried out some tests with hearing-impaired listeners for discriminating differences in the rate of frequency change in the transition of a single formant. A reference stimulus with a fast transition, and different comparison test stimuli with slower transitions were used in an adaptive procedure similar to that used previously for transition detection. The transitions either preceded or followed the formant steady state.

Examples of formant tracks for upward transitions are shown in Fig. 11. In each trial of a run to threshold all three stimuli were constant in total duration and had transitions of the same frequency extent (300 Hz in Fig. 11). The steady-state frequency was 1000 Hz. The two reference stimuli in each trial contained transitions that were the same duration throughout a run. The different or test stimulus in each trial contained a transition that was longer in duration than the reference-stimuli transitions. The test-stimuli transitions varied in duration, during the run to thresholds, based on an adaptive procedure. The task of the listener on each trial was to identify correctly which of the three stimuli had the longer transition. Feedback of the correct answer was provided.

Since the transition frequency-extent was kept constant, transition rate discrimination can be described in terms of the threshold transition duration. Some preliminary results for two groups of hearing-impaired listeners are shown in Fig. 12. Both upward and downward transitions were tested that occurred either at the beginning or at the end of the formant steady state; the corresponding four reference transition patterns, with 30-ms transitions of 100 Hz, are shown at the left. Opposite each pattern the horizontal bars show the mean longer transition duration that was necessary for threshold performance.

Generally, both impaired groups of listeners performed similarly but more poorly than a control group of normal listeners not described here. The best impaired thresholds of 70–100 ms would be only just adequate for discriminating the longer transitions of glide consonants from the brief ones of stops, where the adjacent vowel-formant transitions are on the order of 30–50 ms. The long thresholds of about 200 ms would not support discrimination of glides from diphthongs.

Comparing initial vs final transitions, the impaired groups tended to show better discrimination for final transitions falling in frequency from the formant steady state, than for transitions rising from the steady state. For transitions rising in frequency, there was a marked superiority in duration discrimination of initial over final transitions. However, these effects are probably peculiar to these particular listeners. In a larger body of hearing-impaired data that is currently undergoing analysis, and in data for normal-hearing listeners, there is no general superiority in transition cue duration discrimination between initial vs final transitions in the same frequency range.

                        J. M. Pickett, Sally G. Revoile, and Ellen M. Danaher

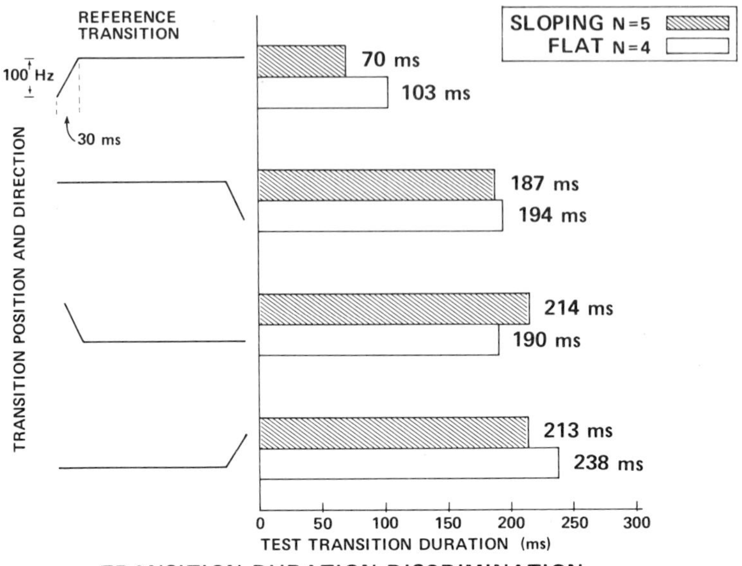

Figure 12 Stimulus reference patterns (on the left) and corresponding mean transition-duration values at threshold for two groups of hearing-impaired listeners. The reference transition duration was 30 msec. The first two reference stimuli in the column of patterns have 30-msec transitions between 900 and 1000 Hz: initial upward for the first pattern and final downward for the second pattern. The 70- and 103-msec test transitions were the mean durations discriminable from the initial upward reference transitions for sloping and flat listeners, respectively. In other words the sloping listeners could discriminate a transition closer in rate to the 30-msec transition than the flat listeners. Other comparisons are described in the text.

Individually the present results showed that one-fourth of the subjects had minimal discrimination differences ($\pm 10\%$) between initial and final transition rate. Nearly one-half of the subjects showed faster rate discrimination for initial than for final, while about one-fourth showed slower discrimination for initial than for final transitions.

These results suggest that different hearing-impaired persons may not discriminate the durations of initial and final transitions equally well. For some hearing-impaired listeners the duration cues provided by initial transitions may be easier to hear than final transitions. Other listeners may hear final transition cues more easily than initial cues.

VI. CUES TO CONSONANT VOICING

The voicing of consonants, i.e., the contrast between the unvoiced consonants /p,t,k,s,ʃ,f,θ,h/ and the voiced consonants /b,d,g,z,ʒ,v,ð/, is an important distinction in speech communication (Denes, 1963; Carterette and Jones, 1974, Table 7.4). How well is the voicing distinction perceived by persons with hearing impairment? Previous studies indicate that perception of consonant voicing is better than perception of place of consonant articulation in hearing-impaired listeners (Rosen, 1962; Schultz, 1964; Owens and Schubert, 1968; Cox, 1969; Pickett, 1979). We would like to be able to explain this effect in terms of discrimination of specific types of acoustic cues. The most important acoustic cues to consonant place are spectral cues in the middle and high frequencies, such as the F2 transitions of adjacent vowels and the spectral composition of stop release bursts and fricative noises, as we noted earlier. The acoustic cues that convey voicing are both spectral and temporal; however, the spectral cues tend to be low in frequency, primarily in the first formant region and below.

The consonant voicing cues depend mostly on the speaker's temporal control of the source of sound production in the vocal tract, relatively independent of the shape or place of articulation. For voiced/unvoiced consonants, respectively, the presence/absence of vocal-fold vibration causes temporal differences in the formant patterns of the adjacent vowel and duration differences in the consonant constriction and consonant release burst of noise. The pattern of spectral cues to voicing is relatively independent of the place of articulation. Such cues are in the low frequencies of the voice pitch, in the type of sound source, and in the transition of the first formant of the adjacent vowel (for further explanation see Pickett, 1980, pp. 133–145, 188).

These spectral cues to voicing might be more affected by hearing impairment than the temporal cues. For example, discrimination of the formant-transition differences in F1 might be degraded more than discrimination of the gross temporal cues such as the vowel lengthening that occurs before final voiced consonants but not before unvoiced.

We studied the importance of temporal and spectral cues to consonant voicing for hearing-impaired listeners. In naturally spoken syllables, voicing cues for final stop consonants were sytematically altered. Although natural variations occurred in the syllables, certain cues were "neutralized" to examine their effect on voicing perception.

We believe it is important to use corpuses of natural syllables in studies of speech-cue perception by the hearing impaired. As cues are deleted, or if cues are unavailable due to the impairment, impaired listeners may be confused by the natural variations in the remaining cues because the total information they receive is less redundant than for normals.

We expected that the discriminative power to the hearing impaired of the three types of major voicing cues would be, from strongest to weakest: (1) vowel duration, (2) the voiced murmur during the constriction of the voiced stops, and (3) differences in the spectrum during the off-going vowel transition into the consonant. Therefore, if the murmur and burst were removed, voicing should still be perceived fairly well on the basis of vowel duration and information in the vowel off-going transition. However, if vowel duration cue differences were reduced, presumably voicing perception would depend only on the differences in transient spectral structure in the vowel transitions preceding voiced vs voiceless consonants. Below we describe the method and preliminary results only for the modifications to vowel duration, and to occlusion duration and voicing murmur during the consonant constriction. Further details and results will be found in Revoile *et al.* (1982).

The set of syllables used for recording speech material was *pad, cad, tad, bad, gad, dad, dap, dak, dat, dab,* and *dag,* with the vowel pronounced as /æ/. Ten successive randomizations of these syllables were recorded by a speaker, thus providing a stimulus set with 10 different spoken tokens of each syllable. Only the subsets of stimuli with contrasting final consonants, *dap, dak, dat, dab, dag, dad,* were used in this experiment.

It was desired to retain some natural variation in the syllables. Thus the adjustments to acoustic cues were made for each pair of contrasting syllables, the pairs being chosen according to the order in which they were spoken in the original randomized list. For example the first *dat* spoken was paired with the first *dad.*

The acoustic-cue modifications were made by waveform deletion and splicing of segments of the syllables after they had been digitized and deposited on a computer-disk system. The deletion and splicing points were at near-zero amplitude points. These occur for vowels just before the start and end of each pitch period, the time period of one vocal tract excitation by a glottal pulse. For the condition neutralized vowel duration, the two vowels in each pair were adjusted to be as equal as possible by deleting or iterating pitch periods within each syllable. For example, in one pair the vowel in *dat* had a duration of 251 msec compared with the 352-msec vowel in *dad;* then, since the talker's pitch (fundamental frequency) was about 100 Hz, five pitch periods deleted from *dad* and five pitch periods iterated in *dat* adjusted both vowels to approximately 300 msec in duration (see Fig. 13). In another condition closure was equalized in each vowel-adjusted pair and the closure murmur deleted from the voiced member of the pair, as seen in Fig. 13.

The results of the hearing-impaired listeners were analyzed separately into a high-performance group and a low-performance group with similar losses (Fig. 14). Percentage correct voicing perception was scored separately for voiced (V) and unvoiced (UV) stimulus consonants; the results appear in Fig. 15. When only vowel duration was neutralized, voicing perception was much poorer for the low-performance group than for the high-performance group of hearing-impaired listeners. For the low-performance group, voiced stops were perceived somewhat better than unvoiced. This suggests that increasing the shorter vowel duration of the unvoiced stimuli degraded perception somewhat and caused some unvoiced stimuli to be heard as voiced. When vowel and closure duration were

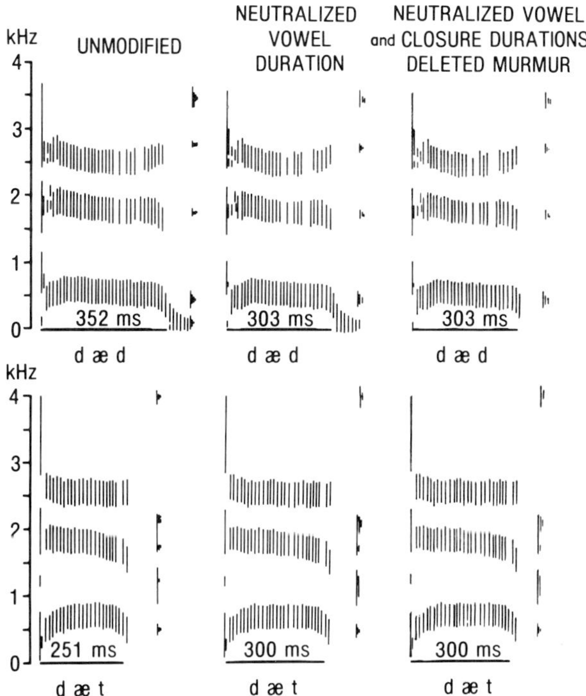

Figure 13 Examples of how a pair of test syllables was modified for conditions to test the effects of neutralizing or deleting cues to the voicing perception of final stop consonants. Schematic spectrograms are shown of one pair of test syllables, *dad* (top row) and *dat* (bottom row). The unmodified final consonant closure intervals appear, for *dad*, as a low-frequency murmur ending at a burst when the ''d''-closure is released and, for *dat*, as a silence during a somewhat longer closure interval ending in a somewhat stronger release burst. The vowel in *dad* was 352 msec in duration compared with the *dat* vowel of 251 msec duration. For the condition of neutralized vowel duration the vowels of this syllable pair were altered to the values shown in the middle. To this alteration was then added the condition of equated closure duration and murmur deletion seen on the right for a third test condition.

neutralized and the voiced murmur omitted, the high-performance group showed reduced perception, especially for the voiced stops. Apparently, the high-performance group used the murmur accompanying the final voiced stops to identify them as voiced.

It will be noted in Fig. 15 that the normals' voicing perception is still better than 90% correct with only the vowel spectral cues remaining. The high-performance hearing-impaired group also perceived unvoicing very well on the spectral cues but scored only 78% correct on the voiced consonants; apparently they could not always respond to the correct spectral cues for the voiced consonants in the face of the shortened vowels that were cueing unvoiced responses. The

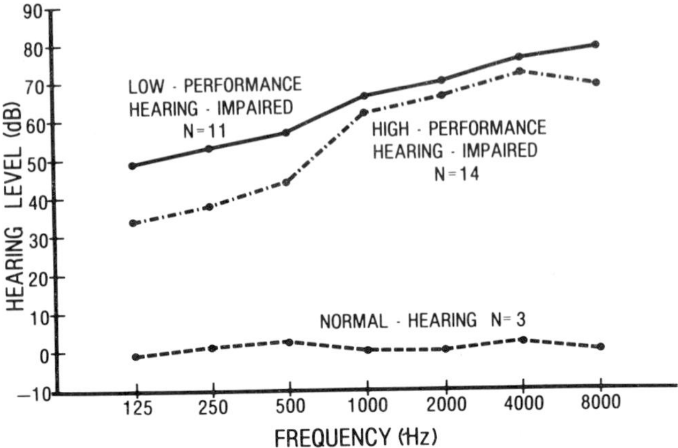

Figure 14 Group mean audibility thresholds at audiometric test frequencies. The two impaired groups were formed on the basis of relatively high vs low performance in the identification of the voicing of final stop consonants, as will be seen in Fig. 15. The hearing of these two groups is similar at 1000 Hz and above, but the high-performance group has better hearing below 1000 Hz.

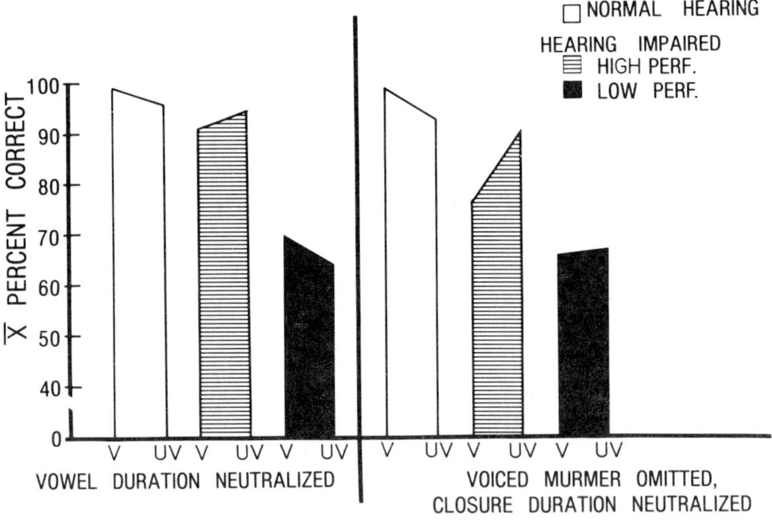

Figure 15 Group performance in identification of stop voicing under the three conditions of cue-modification illustrated in Fig. 13. Performance scores may first be combined for voiced and voiceless consonants. Normals were not greatly affected by neutralization of the vowel duration cue, nor by the *additional* omission of the voiced-consonant murmurs and neutralized duration of the consonant closure intervals. The low-performance impaired group was significantly dependent on the vowel duration cue. The high-performance group was less sensitive to vowel duration neutralizations but more sensitive to the cues of consonant murmur and duration. Looking at performance in identification of stop voicing, separately for voiced (V) and unvoiced (UV) stops, the voiced murmur omission greatly reduced identification of the voiced stops by the high-performance impaired group but had little effect on the normals or on the low-performance impaired group.

low-performance hearing-impaired group scored only a little above chance; apparently they could make relatively little use of the remaining spectral cues.

VII. VOICING-CUE DECODING TO PHONEME PERCEPTION

The speech-cue decoding process exhibits discontinuities with reference to the physical continua along which certain phoneme differences are constructed. Let us examine this rather unusual characteristic of speech perception because it may be used as an index of normality of auditory processing of speech. For example, the identification of the voicing of stop consonants in consonant–vowel syllables is a discontinuous function of the amount of delay between the release of the stop closure and the beginning of the vowel. This delay is called voice onset time (VOT). The VOT interval is occupied by a very brief but strong transient lasting about 10 msec, followed by either a long or short interval of weaker aperiodic excitation of the vocal tract, before the strong periodic voicing excitation of the vowel begins. In English, VOT is brief for voiced stops [b,d,g] and long for unvoiced stops [p,t,k].

In studies of the perception of stop voicing, the VOT cue has been varied to determine the relation between the perception and the acoustic pattern changes resulting from changes in VOT. It is found that the perception is unchanging above or below a narrow "boundary" region of VOT between about 20 and 40 msec. Any value below the region is heard as voiced and any value above as unvoiced. Furthermore, any 20-msec difference in VOT outside the boundary region is poorly discriminated by listeners, whereas a 20-msec difference across the boundary is highly discriminable (Abramson, 1977; Lisker, 1975; Summerfield and Haggard, 1977).

These perceptual effects in normal phoneme decoding were first tested with severely hearing-impaired children by Bennett and Ling (1973). A speaker created different amounts of VOT in test syllables. The syllables' initial stop consonants had to be identified by normal and hearing-impaired listeners. When percentage correct voicing was plotted vs VOT, the normal group showed a normal boundary between 20 and 40 msec VOT. However, the impaired group showed little change from chance performance in perceiving voicing. Although this study has the advantage that natural syllables were used, the speaker's task was unnatural in that he had to produce extreme and intermediate values of VOT which only rarely occur in speech.

Parady *et al.* (1981) carried out an experiment using a continuum of 10 synthetic syllables having VOTs of −10, 0, 10, 20, 25, 30, 35, 40, 50, and 60 msec. Both identification and discrimination tasks were used, for groups of normal, moderate, severe, and profoundly impaired listeners.

They found that the identification and discrimination of stop voicing vs VOT was normal, with a boundary region between 20 and 40 msec, for listeners with only moderate impairment and for 5 of the 10 listeners with severe impairment. The other five showed either a diffuse, lengthened boundary or no boundary effect at all.

One profoundly deaf subject had normal characteristics of response to the VOT cue for voicing while another could discriminate well between two stimuli across the boundary but did not correctly assign the longer VOTs to an unvoiced category. Also one profound listener showed good discrimination of VOT which he apparently had never learned to use as an identification cue.

Why, in a group of equally severely impaired listeners, should some listeners show abnormal decoding of VOT while others show the normal boundary effect? On the current evidence we can only speculate. Certainly both auditory and learning/experiential factors could be involved. On the auditory side possibly some listeners are subject to a backward masking effect of the vowel on the brief transient which marks the beginning of the VOT interval. On the learning side, some listeners may never have experienced faithful amplification of the transient because of the distortions inherent in hearing aids.

VIII. SPEECH TECHNOLOGY AND HEARING HABILITATION

A. Resynthesis of Natural Speech

The artificial constancy of synthetic speech stimuli may be an undesirable circumstance for the study of impaired speech perception. The constant stimuli could cause overestimates of the availability of a cue for the impaired listener as compared with his functional use of the cue in real-life situations where the cues vary with rate and style of utterance. Recent developments in speech technology make it quite feasible to use natural utterances in studies of the speech cues. In addition to the waveform-splicing approach, as used in our study of consonant voicing above, we have also used resynthesis of natural speech tokens. The data for resynthesis are derived by analyzing the natural tokens using the procedure of linear prediction coding (LPC). This provides a succession of resonance patterns representing the speech spectrum at successive time points. For resynthesis, the sequence of resonance patterns is successively excited by the voice pitch as analyzed at each time point or by an aperiodic source for the aperiodic portions of the original. All of this is carried out automatically by a computer (see X.D).

In a pilot study of voicing cues in initial stop consonants we tested the voice-pitch initial contour as a cue by setting the pitch for resynthesis constant at the mean pitch for each test syllable, thus retaining some of the pitch variation from token to token, and all variations of the other cues, but obliterating the pitch contour of the vowel which normally starts at a higher frequency after unvoiced stops than after voiced stops. We also attempted to switch the type of excitation of the resonance patterns between the initial portions of voiced–unvoiced pairs. For this the pitch excitation from the voiced onset was applied to the resonance patterns of the unvoiced onset, and the noise excitation of the unvoiced onset was applied to the patterns of the voiced onset. This was carried out for each pair of tokens.

Our results thus far are incomplete. However, it appears that very few hearing-impaired subjects are sensitive to the neutralization of the pitch cue alone. This would suggest that they can utilize either the cue of voice onset time from release to vowel or the cue of lower starting frequency of F1 upon release of the voiced consonants. We can manipulate the F1 cue through synthesis of natural-based syllables using formant-coded instructions, e.g., with the Klatt (1980) synthesizer. The instructions can be derived automatically from the LPC analysis data, followed by hand correction of any errors made in automatic picking of formants. Using this approach we can also obtain better control of the synthesis with switched excitation than we have experienced with LPC resynthesis (see X.D).

B. Synthetic Speech Stimuli for Diagnostics

The technology of speech processing currently provides an array of methods for synthesizing speech. Some of these are available as highly efficient, easy-to-use software for minicomputer systems (see Section XIII). Others are portable special-purpose synthesizers for voice response under control of keyboard inputs, such as Texas Instruments' *Speak & Spell* and Phonic Ear's *Handi-Voice*, a synthesizer for use by nonoral persons.

This technology can also be applied to the treatment of hearing loss and remediation of impaired speech discrimination. We believe that the most basic problem in remediation is to optimize the patient's understanding of speech signals. Ideally, diagnostic methods should be as closely related as possible to the acoustic-cue information of speech. Similarly, the habilitation treatment, consisting of hearing-aid fitting and listening training, should try to optimize the patient's use of the cue information.

Presently there is not much basis for using speech technology in diagnosis and habilitation. Test and training methods using cue-controlled speech material need to be developed especially for use in the clinic and school. For example, the individual patient's susceptibility to within-speech discrimination masking and its release by suppressing F1 might be measured in the clinic as an indicator of the potential advantage of prescribing a hearing aid that suppresses the low frequencies.

With this last possibility in mind, we undertook to develop and validate a rapid test for measuring the F1 masking effect on detection of F2 transitions. A synthesizer was provided that produced, on each trial, a pair of two-formant stimuli. The first stimulus had no transition in F2 and the second stimulus had a transition in F2 during the initial 100 msec. To determine an initial threshold, the frequency extent of this transition was reduced in successive trials until the listener indicated that the two stimuli sounded the same (thus at this point the transition was not detectable). A few such runs could establish the threshold amount of F2 transition for detection. Then F1 would be attenuated and the threshold redetermined. If a substantially smaller threshold was found, then it would indicate that the patient was susceptible to spread of masking from F1. Then the plan was to validate this procedure by determining whether the patient would also benefit from applification of speech by an amplifier that suppressed the F1 range of frequencies, as compared with a flat-response amplifier.

A thorough piloting of the threshold method with naive normal-hearing subjects revealed that it was highly unreliable in comparison to our earlier "laboratory" method, which had used feedback and was repeated many times for each listener. The subjects reported that the pair of stimuli never sounded exactly the same, even when they were physically identical (i.e., when the F2 transition was set to zero). This caused the judgment of "same" to be very difficult. Thus it would appear that tests of fine auditory discrimination between successive stimuli are not suitable for use with the naive clinical listener. It will probably be necessary to devise tests of masking that require only the detection of the presence or absence of a very salient sound component. This may be difficult to arrange for acuity tests of changing sounds as they occur in speech.

C. Potential of Synthetic Speech for Listening Training

We believe that the current development of speech technology creates a potential field of application for auditory training, i.e., the training of a hearing-impaired person to maximize the use of the speech-cue patterns his ear provides under amplification. Currently auditory training employs natural speech stimuli that are not well controlled as to embodiment of essential cues. However, the listener differences in cue discrimination, as seen in our research, would indicate that the use of carefully controlled, individually tailored training materials and procedures could improve the efficiency and outcomes. Although the types of listener differences in cue discrimination need much further exploration and study, it is apparent at this stage that some patients show within-speech masking of cues, both simultaneous and serial.

In our formant transition studies we often found that a listener improved in discrimination performance, presumably because of the clearly isolated cue and the procedure of answer feedback. How might this improvement in synthetic cue discrimination be made to carry over to speech perception? In the case of F2 transitions, cue discrimination might be trained with F1 suppressed at first and then increased progressively. Another gradable cue parameter is the rate of formant transition. Slow transition rates might first be presented in isolation. When faster, speech-like rates could be perceived, gradually the transition would be imbedded in contexts. Real-speech context, because of the overlapping of speech movements, changes the extents of transition and sometimes the directions and rates. These changes may make some cues ambiguous, but these interactions also provide serial pattern information about the adjacent phoneme articulations. All of these complex interactions must be accommodated and used in decoding the message (Liberman and Studdert-Kennedy, 1978).

Speech synthesis with natural variations can provide training material that is systematically programmed and adapted for individualized auditory training. Hand-held and desk-size synthesizers could be developed for practice at home and for training in the clinic.

D. Prosodic Cues from Electrical Stimulation

Most of our discussion above applies mainly to the phonemic (consonant and vowel) cues. The overall rhythms of speech and the tonal variations among the syllables provide cues that are necessary for the perceptual marking of the syllable boundaries in the stream of phonemic patterns. These are called prosodic cues. Among the hearing impaired probably only the severe-to-profoundly impaired suffer deficiencies in the receptive discrimination of prosodic cues (Risberg, 1979; Erber, 1983).

In a recent study with profoundly deaf subjects who had had normal hearing until shortly before the experiment, the voice-tone or pitch of the speaker, i.e., the fundamental frequency alone, was impressed on the auditory nerve through an electrode placed on the round-window area just outside the cochlea. The subjects reported that they could perceive "the voice" of the speaker. They were tested for their ability to label upward pitch tracks as "questions" and downward pitch tracks as "statements." They were reasonably accurate in this task. This indicated that some prosodic cues might be provided electrically for the totally deaf (Fourcin *et al.*, 1979). A simulation experiment with normal-hearing listeners indicated that receiving the voice pitch alone, when added to lipreading of a speaker reading continuous text, increased the correct word-reception rate by nearly a factor of two. Thus it appears that provision of only limited prosodic information for the newly but profoundly deafened person, through external electrical stimulation, would improve lipreading success considerably (Rosen *et al.*, 1981).

IX. CONCLUSION

To summarize, what is the state of knowledge and art in the study of speech-cue discrimination by the hearing impaired? From speech-cue research we now know that there may be numerous types of individual hearing problems as related to speech communication. Listeners with the same apparent hearing loss, for example, can show very different degrees of within-speech masking of cues, either simultaneous or backward or forward (Danaher *et al.*, 1978). Some of the cue-masking problems may be due to the damaged ear, but some may be due to lack of sufficient experience with high-quality amplification; very little is known about the role of experiential factors.

However, very powerful computer methods may be used in delineating specific factors better than we can at this time. Speech technology has provided us with methods for designing new diagnostic tests and new types of hearing aids for correcting hearing.

Methods for clinical tests with naive listeners must be developed which, unlike our laboratory discrimination tests, require no training of the listener. Probably a judgment task of whether or not a sound is fluctuating in some aspect will be the most complex discrimination that can be used in the clinic. Such tests would then have to be correlated with cue discrimination.

X. APPENDIX: METHODS OF SPEECH-CUE CONTROL

This appendix describes methods currently available for using computers to manipulate and generate various perceptual cues in speech. Of particular interest are methods using natural speech. Three methods of synthesis are described for natural-based synthetic stimuli. The scope of each method is discussed as well as its advantages and disadvantages.

A. Manipulation of Natural Speech Waveforms

The method of deleting or iterating natural speech waves provides stimuli having high face validity except, of course, for the fact that original stimulus continuity of changing spectral patterns may be interrupted. Deleting distributed pitch pulses helps to maintain continuity. The perceptual system for speech does not seem very sensitive, in causal listening, to moderate discontinuities with central portions of vowels and fricative noises. The rationale for using this method with the hearing impaired is described in Section V.

Cue deletion or alteration by iteration in particular segments of the original speech waveform is particularly easy to accomplish through editing and reassembly of digitized waveforms using an appropriate minicomputer system with a scope display of the waveform. Manipulated segments may be stored separately before reassembly and thus they may be filtered or altered in ways other than by simple deletion, if so desired. There are software systems available for speech-wave editing and reassembly as well as for the speech analysis and synthesis procedures described below [for example see the Interactive Laboratory System developed by Markel and co-workers (ILS, no date)].

B. Theory of Speech Synthesis

Speech synthesis methods are based on an acoustic theory of speech production called the source-filter theory. This theory accounts for the various sound-spectrum patterns seen in speech as resulting from the combinations of the spectrum of a source sound and the spectrum-modifying action, the filtering or transfer response, of all the vocal-tract spaces affecting the propagation of that sound to the outside air. In research on the adequacy of the theory (Fant, 1960, and references there) it was found that the sound source of the voicing phonation, produced in the larynx, consisted of a wave of periodic pulses. The pulses were roughly triangular in shape and could be idealized for a "standard" voice source to have a simple downward-sloping spectrum. Then if this wave of pulses is applied to the bottom of a tube shaped as is the vocal tract of a speaker producing a given vowel, the output sound from the shaped tube has a spectrum very similar to the natural vowel. It was also found that the acoustic transfer response of the vocal tract could be very concisely approximated as the filtering effects produced by a series of elementary resonances connected in series. Various vowel and consonant articulations were modeled in this way to confirm the appropriateness of this source-filter theory. Some of the modeling was used to produce audible synthetic vowels and consonants, and thus synthetic speech had its beginning (the classic technical book on source-filter theory is Fant, 1960; a reader who is unfamiliar with acoustic theory should see Pickett, 1980).

Generally speaking, three types of speech synthesis have been used to generate stimuli for controlled acoustic studies of speech cues: (1) formant synthesis, (2) synthesis from linear prediction coding (LPC) of natural speech, and (3) articulatory synthesis.

Using formant synthesis, artificial acoustic cues can be manipulated throughout the range of values found in speech (and even beyond the normal ranges). LPC synthesis uses natural speech as a basis and can be used to easily incorporate, in studies of perception, some of the natural variations in speaking and among speakers. Special LPC cues that are easy to manipulate are those related to voice pitch and the nature of vocal-tract excitation, i.e., whether excitation is periodic from voicing phonation, or aperiodic due to friction and air-stream turbulence. It is difficult to manipulate the formant frequencies in LPC re-synthesis. This is better done through formant synthesis based on an LPC-coded analysis of speech, as explained further below.

C. Formant Synthesis

The simplest formant synthesizer, one that is easy to control for variations of major cue parameters, approximates the transfer response of the vocal tract by using three resonant circuits in series, representing the lowest three resonances of the vocal tract. The frequency of each resonance is variable and is controlled in time by a function (i.e., a time track) selected by the experimenter. The control functions used are often more-or-less standard ones from the literature, which in turn were simplified tracks originally derived from spectrographic studies of speech.

The representativeness of three-formant serial synthesis is good considering the very small number of parameters (six) that need to be specified: voicing pitch and voicing amplitude, frication amplitude, and three formant frequencies. The theoretical basis for this reduced representation of vocal-tract acoustics was developed by Fant (1960).

Obviously the three-formant series-connected synthesizer is well suited to the study of formant cues and it has been widely used for this purpose. A recent system for formant synthesis that is slightly more complex, but more flexible, and easy to use on minicomputers, was designed and published by Klatt (1980).

D. Synthesis from LPC Data

The linear prediction method represents speech by calculating, for successive samples of the original wave, sets of many resonances (seven in the typical case). Each sample's set of resonances is adjusted to represent the original spectrum in its amplitude-frequency pattern assuming that a standard source wave of fixed spectrum was exciting the vocal-tract resonances. The LPC-calculated reso-nances often are close to the real formants of the utterance, but they are not necessarily the same because they are adjusted to match the details of the original's spectrum and spectral balance; these details are a function of the individual speaker's source spectra as well as his formant frequencies and amplitudes. Nevertheless, since the main peaks and valleys in the spectrum, and its general shape, are usually well represented, a very realistic synthesis of the utterance can be obtained by calculating the waveform that would result from appropriately exciting the successive sets of LPC resonances with the standard voicing phona-tion or friction noise. A natural-sounding synthesis is achieved because the individual speaker's vowel formants, especially the upper ones F4 through F7, and particularly their general amplitudes relative to the lower formants, are rather accurately reproduced due to the optimum-match procedure of the linear prediction. With a three-formant synthesizer the upper spectrum of the vowels is synthesized with a standard F4–F7 spectrum that does not change except in amplitude under the automatic influence of the frequency positions of the lower formants; thus variations in speakers' upper spectrum are not represented.)

The linear-prediction-coded data are easy to derive for extended utterances or for large collections of short utterances. This makes it possible to synthesize test stimuli which contain natural variations in expression, rate, style, different speakers, and so on. However, the cue manipulations that can be easily made in LPC synthesis are limited to changes in the source-sound characteristics of voice pitch and friction noise. LPC "formant" structure could also be manipulated but not with the ease of formant-coded synthesis, because when any LPC "formant" frequency is changed, all the other resonances, their bandwidths, and amplitudes might have to be readjusted. In formant-coded synthesis the amplitude adjustment is made automatically and no other changes are necessary.

However, one can manipulate formants and still retain some natural variations by using the data from a linear prediction analysis and then arranging a formant-coded synthesis by using the LPC analysis data as a base from which to derive formant-frequency control signals for the formant synthesizer. This can be done by accepting the frequencies of the first three or four LPC resonances as F1, F2, F3, and F4. These data may then be examined for any unreasonable discontinuities or absurdities in formant tracks and the tracks can be smoothed by inserting new F values where necessary. Then one is ready to manipulate formant frequency cues, as desired, to test cue dependencies. The pitch and durational variations of the original natural utterances are normally retained in the synthesis, but they could also be manipulated as well.

E. Articulatory Modeling Synthesis

In a sense the early modeling of vowels described above under the source-filter theory was articulatory synthesis. The vocal-tract shape was modeled electrically and synthetic vowel sounds were produced for perceptual experiments. However, only static articulatory shapes were employed at first. K. N. Stevens and co-workers developed the first dynamically controlled electrical model of vocal tract shape (Rosen, 1958; Rosen and Stevens, 1959). This model was further developed by Hecker (1962) for studies of nasalized vowels and nasal consonants.

Articulatory synthesis is now accomplished by computer simulation of vocal-tract movements and coordinated changes in the source sounds for tract excitation; as a recent example see Rubin *et al.* (1981). With this method the spectral cues per se, for example, the formants, are not easily manipulated. If natural-based examples were needed, the control signals to the articulatory synthesizer would have to be derived by movement analyses and X-ray studies of each speaker's utterances. However, the articulatory method is of great importance in furthering our knowledge of speech and has been used in studies of those cues, such as cues to nasalization, which are not understood well enough in acoustic production to model adequately by formant-coded synthesis (Abramson *et al.*, 1981).

Acknowledgments

This article was prepared with support from the Gallaudet College Research Institute and grants to Gallaudet College from the U.S. Public Health Service and the National Institute of Handicapped Research (Grant G008103979 for the Rehabilitation Engineering Center for the Deaf and Hearing-Impaired). The research reported from our Laboratory was supported by the Research Institute and by Grants NS-05464 and NS-13190, and Fellowship 5F32 NS-06025, from the National Institute of Neurological and Communicative Disorders and Stroke.

References

Abramson, A. S. (1977). Laryngeal timing in consonant distinctions. *Phonetica* **34,** 295–303.

Abramson, A. S., Nye, P. W., Henderson, J., and Marshall, C. W. (1981). Vowel height and the perception of consonantal nasality. *J. Acoust. Soc. Am.* **70,** 329–339.

ANSI (American National Standards Institute). (1969). Standard for Methods for Calculation of the Articulation Index, S3.5.

ANSI (American National Standards Institute). (1977). Standard for Rating Noises with Respect to Speech Intelligibility, S3.14.

Bennett, C. W., and Ling, D. (1973). Discrimination of the voiced-voiceless distinction by severely hearing-impaired children. *J. Auditory Res.* **13,** 271–279.

Bilger, R., and Hirsh, I. (1956). Masking of tones by bands of noise. *J. Acoust. Soc. Am.* **28,** 623–630.

Bilger, R., and Wang, M. (1976). Consonant confusions in patients with sensorineural hearing loss. *J. Speech Hear. Res.* **19,** 718–748.

Borden, G., and Harris, K. (1980). "Speech Science Primer." Williams & Wilkins, Baltimore, Maryland.

Carterette, E. C., and Jones, M. H. (1974). "Informal Speech." Univ. of California Press, Berkeley, California.

Cole, R., and Scott, B. (1974). Toward a theory of speech perception. *Psychol. Rev.* **81,** 348–374.

Cox, B. P. (1969). "The identification of unfiltered and filtered consonant-vowel-consonant stimuli by sensorineural hearing-impaired persons." Unpublished Ph.D. dissertation, University of Pittsburgh.

Danaher, E. M., and Pickett, J. M. (1975). Some masking effects produced by low-frequency vowel formants in persons with sensorineural hearing loss. *J. Speech Hear. Res.* **18,** 261–271.

Danaher, E. M., Osberger, M. J., and Pickett, J. M. (1973). Discrimination of formant frequency transitions in synthetic vowels. *J. Speech Hear. Res.* **16,** 439–451.

Danaher, E. M., Wilson, M. P., and Pickett, J. M. (1978). Backward and forward masking in listeners with severe sensorineural hearing loss. *Audiology* **17,** 324–338.

Denes, P. (1963). On the statistics of spoken English. *J. Acoust. Soc. Am.* **35,** 892–904.

Elliott, L. L. (1967). Development of auditory narrow-band frequency contours. *J. Acoust. Soc. Am.* **42,** 143–153.

Erber, N. (1983). Speech perception and speech development in hearing-impaired children. *In*

"Speech of the Hearing-Impaired: Research, Training, and Personnel Preparation." (I. Hochberg, H. Levitt, and M. Osberger, eds.) Univ. Park Press, Baltimore, Maryland.

Evans, E. F., and Wilson, J. P., eds. (1977). "Psychophysics and Physiology of Hearing." Academic Press, New York.

Fant, G. (1960). "Acoustic Theory of Speech Production." Mouton, The Hague.

Flanagan, J. L., and Rabiner, L. R., eds. (1973). "Speech Synthesis." Dowden, Hutchinson, & Ross, Stroudsburg, Pennsylvania.

Fletcher, H. (1929). "Speech and Hearing." Van Nostrand/Reinhold, Princeton, New Jersey.

Fletcher, H. (1953). "Speech and Hearing in Communication." Van Nostrand–Reinhold, Princeton, New Jersey.

Fourcin, A. J., Rosen, S. M., Moore, B. C. J., Douek, E. E., Clarke, G. P., Dodson, H., and Bannister, L. H. (1979). External electrical stimulation of the cochlea: Clinical, psychophysical, speech-perceptual and histological findings. *Br. J. Audiol.* **13,** 85–107.

Hecker, M. (1962). Studies of nasal consonants with an articulatory synthesizer. *J. Acoust. Soc. Am.* **34,** 179–188.

ILS. "Application Note No. 1: Speech Analysis and Synthesis." Signal Technology, Inc., 15 West De La Guerra Street, Santa Barbara, California, 93101.

Jacobson, R., Fant, G., and Halle, M. (1969). "Preliminaries to Speech Analysis." MIT Press, Cambridge, Massachusetts (1st published 1951).

Klatt, D. H. (1980). Software for a cascade/parallel formant synthesizer. *J. Acoust. Soc. Am.* **67,** 971–995.

Liberman, A., and Studdert-Kennedy, M. (1978). Phonetic perception. *In* "Handbook of Sensory Physiology, Vol. 8: Perception." (R. Held, H. Leibowitz, and H. Teuber, eds.). Springer–Verlag, Berlin and New York.

Lisker, L. (1975). Is it VOT or a first-formant transition detector? *J. Acoust. Soc. Am.* **57,** 1547–1551.

Martin, E. S., and Pickett, J. M. (1970). Sensorineural hearing loss and upward spread of masking. *J. Speech Hear. Res.* **13,** 426–437.

Martin, E. S., Pickett, J. M., and Colten, S. (1972). Discrimination of vowel formant transitions by listeners with severe sensorineural hearing loss. *In* "Speech Communication Ability and Profound Deafness" (G. Fant, ed.), pp. 119–133. Bell Assoc. Washington, D.C.

Mártony, J., and Agelfors, E. (1974). Two psychoacoustic tests with severely hard-of-hearing children. Speech Transmission Laboratory, Quarterly Progress and Status Report 1/1974. Royal Institute of Technology, Stockholm.

Miller, J. D. (1982). Paper on frequency-amplitude adjustments in amplification for the hearing-impaired, presented at the Meeting of the Committee on Hearing Bioacoustics and Biomechanics, National Research Council, National Academy of Sciences, Washington, D.C.

Owens, E., and Schubert, E. D. (1968). The development of constant items for speech discrimination testing. *J. Speech Hear. Res.* **11,** 656–667.

Parady, S., Dorman, M. F., Whaley, P., and Raphael, L. J. (1981). Identification and discrimination of a synthesized voicing contrast by normal and sensorineural hearing-impaired children. *J. Acoust. Soc. Am.* **69,** 783–790.

Pascoe, D. P. (1978). An approach to hearing aid selection. *Hear. Instrum.* **29,** 12–16, 36–37.

Pickett, J. M. (1959). Low-frequency noise and methods for calculating speech intelligibility. *J. Acoust. Soc. Am.* **31,** 1259–1263.

Pickett, J. M. (1979). Perception of speech features by persons with hearing impairment. *In* "Current Issues in Linguistic Theory." (H. Hollien and P. Hollien, eds.), Vol. 9, pp. 721–736. Benjamins, Amsterdam.

Pickett, J. M. (1980). "The Sounds of Speech Communication." Univ. Park Press, Baltimore, Maryland.

Pickett, J. M., and Mártony, J. (1970). Low-frequency vowel formant discrimination in hearing-impaired listeners. *J. Speech Hear. Res.* **13**, 347–359.

Pollack, I., and Pickett, J. M. (1958). Masking of speech by noise at high sound levels. *J. Acoust. Soc. Am.* **30**, 127–130.

Revoile, S., Pickett, J. M., Holden, L. D., and Talkin, D. (1982). Acoustic cues to final stop voicing for impaired- and normal-hearing listeners. *J. Acoust. Soc. Am.* **72**, 1145–1154.

Risberg, A. (1979). "Bestämning av Hörkapacitet och Talperceptionsförmåga vid Svåra Hörse-lskador (Defining Hearing Capacity and Speech Perception Ability in Severe Hearing Impairment)." A collection of articles in English, presented for the doctorate to the Department of Speech Communication, Royal Institute of Technology, Stockholm.

Rosen, G. (1958). Dynamic analog speech synthesizer. *J. Acoust. Soc. Am.* **30**, 201.

Rosen, G., and Stevens, K. N. (1959). Apparatus for the generation of psychoacoustic stimuli varying in complexity from noise bursts to syllables. *J. Acoust. Soc. Am.* **31**, 114 [Abstr.].

Rosen, J. (1962). "Phoneme Identification in Sensorineural Deafness." Ph.D. thesis, Stanford University, Palo Alto, California.

Rosen, S. M., Fourcin, A. J., and Moore, B. C. J. (1981). Voice pitch as an aid to lipreading. *Nature (London)* **291**, 150–152.

Rubin, P., Baer, T., and Mermelstein, P. (1981). An articulatory synthesizer for perceptual research. *J. Acoust. Soc. Am.* **70**, 321–328.

Schultz, M. C. (1964). Suggested improvements in speech discrimination testing. *J. Aud. Res.* **4**, 1–14.

Studdert-Kennedy, M. (1980). Speech perception. *Language Speech* **23**, 45–66.

Summerfield, Q., and Haggard, M. (1977). On the dissociation of spectral and temporal cues to the voicing distinction in initial stop consonants. *J. Acoust. Soc. Am.* **62**, 435–448.

Walden, B., and Montgomery, A. (1975). Dimensions of consonant perception in normal and hearing-impaired listeners. *J. Speech Hear. Res.* **18**, 445–455.

Walden, B., Montgomery, A., Prosek, R., and Schwartz, D. (1980). Consonant similarity judgments by normal and hearing-impaired listeners. *J. Speech Hear. Res.* **23**, 162–184.

Walden, B., Schwartz, D., Daniel, M., Montgomery, A., and Prosek, R. A. (1981). Comparison of the effects of hearing impairment and acoustic filtering on consonant recognition. *J. Speech Hear. Res.* **24**, 32–43.

Wang, M., Reed, C., and Bilger, R. (1978). A comparison of the effects of filtering and sensorineural hearing loss on patterns of consonant confusion. *J. Speech Hear. Res.* **21**, 5–36.

Applied Research on Competing Messages

J. C. Webster

Communications Research Department
National Technical Institute for the Deaf
Rochester Institute of Technology
Rochester, New York

I. INTRODUCTION

Garner (1972) delivered a treatise on the acquisition and application of scientific knowledge exposing as a myth the fable that "scientists" acquire knowl-

93

HEARING RESEARCH AND THEORY, VOLUME 2

edge and put it into the public realm and "problem solvers," uttering words of gratitude, extract it. The myth is that the dichotomous breakdown between pure (basic) and applied research is not logically correlated with laboratory versus field studies, analytic versus wholistic approaches, general versus specific knowledge, and experiment versus observation. He then selected five psychological problems and/or concepts to show how applied research carried out by scientist problem solvers in laboratory experiments generated both specific and general knowledge. The first of his topics was "selective attention" which he said "was essentially banned in modern American psychology . . . [since] . . . it . . . went on inside the head [and] was not available for direct observation." Noting that today it is a very active research area and "many . . . feel it is the central problem in cognitive psychology, [he asks], What brought the concept . . . back into psychology?"

His answer is "a man with a real problem and not enough knowledge to solve it." He cites two references, Broadbent (1952a) and Webster and Thompson (1954), to substantiate his statement that, "in the middle 1950s the topic began to be researched actively." In his answer I would amend his "a man" with "two groups of men" and add a clause which in this case was not a myth and is often the case, "independently in two different countries."

In the remainder of this article I will review my own work on selective attention quite extensively. I will refer to others' work including the work of Broadbent and Poulton in England less extensively since along with my work it is well summarized and used as the basis for a filter theory by Broadbent (1958). Broadbent's filter theory in turn set up a theoretical challenge that generated extensive basic research particularly by Moray and Treisman in the 1960s. Since Broadbent (1971) covers these studies extensively in enlarging and/or clarifying his filter theory, I will refer to them only to the extent needed to set the stage for my latest applied selective attention research on bilingualism. I will conclude by describing how I used the selective attention paradigm to develop a test to evaluate the degree of bilingual interaction.

I was introduced to the competing message problem at the Navy Electronics Laboratory in 1951 with the assignment of a project concerning human factor considerations in air control towers. At that point in applied military research problems the principal researcher was allowed and encouraged to (1) go into the field and witness the extent and operational implications of the problem, (2) delineate and formulate the crucial parameters in forms amenable for laboratory experiments or simulations, (3) design an experiment usually around the statistical technique of an analysis of variance (ANOVA), (4) run, analyze, and interpret the results, and (5) follow through, at least initially, on the application of the results back in the field.

Some of the major problems originally assigned to be answered in the air control environment included (1) acceptable background noise levels, (2) minimum acceptable speech-to-noise ratios (S/N), (3) configuration and numbers of loud speakers, and (4) optimum watch lengths. Observations in Navy, Air Force, and Civil Aeronautics Administration (CAA) towers (Los Angeles, Chicago Midway, Washington National) indicated that the majority of objectional noise was coming from the loudspeakers themselves. Outside aircraft noise or voices of other tower operators was not of the same order of magnitude as the chatter and noise received over the radio. It was also apparent that whereas many towers monitored as many as 15 channels, the load was not evenly distributed. Indeed, in most towers 95% of the load was limited to six or fewer channels. However, it was also obvious that in many cases the messages overlapped each other, that there was in fact a competing message problem. With this knowledge of the observed conditions in air control towers in hand, the formulation of the crucial problems and the design of the applied experiment were in order. Although not systematized as well in 1951 the factors detailed in the next section were taken into account.

II. FACTORS IN AN APPLIED EXPERIMENT

Human Factors

Some of the independent, intermediate, and dependent variables that have to be considered and controlled in any psychoacoustic experiment are listed in Table I (adapted from Gulian, 1973, and Webster, 1975). At the bottom are the dependent variables, or outputs, or the effects that sounds may have on a human being and for which the experimenter has to find some measurable aspects. Often it is the accuracy of performance that is measured, for example, syllable, word, or sentence intelligibility, or paragraph comprehension. Sometimes it is both speed and accuracy that are measured, for example, when the problem is the effects or consequences of noise and/or competing speech messages on work performance. In the air control tower case it was assumed that the speed and accuracy of perceiving speech messages in noise would correspond with work performance.

The effects on sleep, relaxation, and annoyance, although hard to measure and interpret, are at least easy concepts to understand. In the air control tower case, annoyance and/or fatigue were the important variables and not many people deny that overlapping speech messages and noise can and do affect them. Action refers to what an individual or group might do in response to the speech and noise: kick the console, smoke too many cigarettes and/or drink too much coffee, write a memo to the supervisor, complain to the union, etc.

In the middle of the table are the intermediary or intervening, sometimes called moderator, variables which historically are often not considered or are relegated to insignificance. The physiologic variables are easy to understand; for example, the following statements are often seen, "normal young adults with no hearing loss," the converse "students at a residential school for the deaf," or in the air control tower case, "actual Navy and CAA air controllers."

Concerning individual differences, sex and age are usually considered and

TABLE I

INTERACTIONS OF SOUND AND HUMAN ACTIVITIES

Independent Variables (Input)		
Sound Stimulus	Task	Environment
Intensity	Information source	Sociocultural variables
Frequency	Duration	Time
Complexity	Temporal characteristics	Location
Duration	Paced/unpaced	Home/work
Location	Stimulus rate	Inside/outside
Type	Type (work and relaxation)	Ambient factors
Speech	Language-related	Noise
Music	Non-language-related	Vibration
Noise	Intellectual	Light
Temporal characteristics	Psychomotor	Temperature
Steady state	Psychophysical	Humidity
Time varying		

Intermediary Variables		
Physiological	Psychological	Individual Differences
Arousal level	Perceptual capabilities	Intraindividual
Health state	Meaningfulness of stimulus	Age
General	Motivation	Interindividual
Auditory	Attitude	Sex
Other sensory modalities	Arousal level	Neurohumoral reactivity
Accumulated efforts	Previous experience	Personality traits
Fatigue	With task	
Lack of sleep	With noise	

Dependent Variables (Output, Effects)			
Speech and Performance	Sleep and Relaxation	Annoyance	Action
Accuracy		Individual	Complaints
Speed		Group	Physical
Discrimination		Fatigue	Legal
Output			

personality traits are usually the least well accounted for. The perceptual capability, motivation, attitude, arousal level, and past experience of the individuals, or the meanings associated with the sounds, should be controlled and often are not.

Table I is meant to be general so that it can be used as a checklist for any experiment, survey, or field study on the effect of sound on humans. It could be used to help lay out a study of the effects of (1) complex overlapping speech messages and/or noise on controlling aircraft in the vicinity of and on the ground at busy airfields, (2) the community response to industrial, vehicular, or airport noise, (3) operating a weaving machine, (4) performing in a symphony orchestra, or (5) teaching (deaf) students in a classroom.

Concerning the independent variables, language or communication-related tasks, such as a teacher in a classroom, a pilot in an aricraft, or a controller in the air control tower are probably the most difficult to specify completely because the perception of spoken language depends on so many nonacoustic events. Problems of dialect, grammar, linguistics, phonetics, and semantics immediately come to mind. Specifying the pertinent physical characteristics of a speech signal is far from a closed book. An average speech spectra can be derived and suitable peak factors added. Vowel-to-consonant ratios can be established. A root-mean-square overall intensity can be, and usually is, the value most typically used to describe speech level. The bandwidth and/or weighting network used should correlate highly with the perception of speech and the noise level should be measured using the same bandwidth, as was used to measure the speech. Although instantaneous displays of the speech signal can be shown, the preceding and/or following phoneme can alter drastically the instantaneous acoustic portrayal of any given phoneme.

The voice or speech message input in the air control tower study begged many of the problems just discussed by relying on pseudo-realism and a face validity. The voice messages from mock pilots in aircraft were recorded by eight different ''typical general American dialect'' voices on four typical aircraft microphones in a background of cockpit noise at a level of 110 dB(C). The noise levels should have been specified in dB(A) not dB(C). However, in 1951 the results of a series of experiments by Klumpp and Webster (1963) and Webster and Klumpp (1963, 1965) and other evidences, Young (1964) and Botsford (1969), of the advantages of A-weighting as opposed to C-weighting were not known.

Just as specifying the physical characteristics of the speech signal is a can of worms, so is specifying the task. It is much easier to measure a speech task that is divorced from all higher order language-related factors (linguistics . . . dialects) but much harder to interpret the results in terms of the real world. On the contrary, it is much more difficult to make meaningful measures on everyday redundant, running speech but easier to generalize the results. The information input for language-related tasks can be either auditory (speech) or visual (reading, writing) and paced or unpaced. Listening to speech on radio or TV is paced. Since the listener in a face-to-face, two-way radio or telephone conversation may ask the talker to repeat or to slow down, the task may be considered unpaced.

In the air control tower study the messages were recorded and no provisions were made for asking for repeats. The task performance was definitely paced. In an actual operating pilot/control tower exchange repeats can and may be requested. However in general, the channel and ID of the communicators must be perceived before a repeat can be requested. This factor determined the paced task chosen for this experiment.

Specifying the speech-interference aspects of the ambient noise is complex although it is better understood than specifying the work-performance, interference, or annoyance aspects of sound. Like the musical signal, the speech signal is influenced (adversely) by reverberation and perhaps by vibration. These parameters were not controlled or varied in the control tower experiment but background levels probably minimized any undo influences of reverberation.

An intermediate variable of importance to tasks related to spoken language is auditory perceptual capability which is related to degree of hearing impairment and often to age because of progressive loss of hearing (presbycusis). The real-world language-related control tower task must be classified as a very complex intellectual task. Any intermediary variable that can be shown to affect an intellectual task will almost certainly affect a speech reception task. These might include physiologic or psychologic arousal level, fatigue or lack of sleep, motivation, attitude, and meaningfulness of (competing) stimuli. The degree of sensory interaction is very important, particularly to people conversing in their nonnative language. A person who knows no Russian can quite easily read or write English while two colleagues converse in Russian, in his presence. If they conversed in English or German, if German had been their original native language, their reading or writing task would very likely be interfered with. There is probably no area where selective attention (sensory interaction) is of more importance than in the study of language-related tasks.

Dependent variables most often measured are the accuracy of lists of words, sometimes sentences or nonsense syllables. Speed in the sense of correct words per minute is not usually important but the reaction time of a response may be a very sensitive measure. The controversies in speech intelligibility testing deal with how detailed an accuracy measure should be. Is a correct/incorrect score for a word (sentence) sufficient, or should a confusion matrix be run on individual phonemes (words). Annoyance is very seldom measured although in the reverse case where annoyance is the object, for example, in an airport noise survey, interference with the speech (TV, radio, telephone, conversation) is always high on the list. With the possible exception of interference of noise on sleep, interference with auditory language-related tasks is often the most annoying. In the air control tower study the question asked by the sponsor dealt with fatigue not annoyance per se. This was designed into the experiment by running 4-hour-long test sessions.

III. EXPERIMENTAL DESIGN

In the air control case defining a realistic and measurable task involved simulating the listening conditions of a tower and creating stimuli that required responses that could be scored. Two major limitations in scope resulted from the field observations: the use of only six channels for information transfer, and the use of these channels for the introduction of background noise. Two towers were mocked up; one had an individual loudspeaker for terminating each of the six incoming channels and the other had only a single loudspeaker for all six channels. Each had a provision for pulling down one channel into an earphone. Both had switching consoles for placing the answering microphone into the proper channel (and measuring the channel agreement between incoming and outgoing messages). In each tower the loudspeaker(s) could be mounted (1) directly ahead, (2) directly overhead, or (3) at the wall–ceiling junction. A picture of the single loudspeaker tower is shown in Fig. 1.

The task required of the mock tower operators was (1) to identify the calling aircraft by name and number (United 629), (2) to read time off a clock and footage off of a mock altimeter both of which allowed a gross measuring of response time (RT), (3) to repeat back key words of the incoming message, and (4) to do this on the same channel the aircraft called in on.

To minimize intervening variables as much as possible, actual Navy and CAA air control operators acted as listeners and worked a 4-hour shift (experimental session) for one or two 5-day weeks.

The speech and noise variables were designed into the stimulus material which were recorded on 16 reels of 35-mm magnetic tape. The speech and noise variables included the use of eight different talkers, who talked over four different microphones, at eight different vocal levels covering a 28-dB range, and a choice of actual control tower vocal babble or thermal noise for background noise. Information rate per channel was accounted for by using four channels for scoreable items and distributing the items equally among the channels for half of the tests (0.25, 0.25, 0.25, 0.25) and realistically unequal for the other half of the tests (0.70, 0.05, 0.20, 0.05). The details of the whole experiment including how these stimulus variables were counterbalanced can be found in Webster and Thompson (1953a,b).

In summary there were variables that were changed from day to day [loudspeaker placement, overall level (and type) of noise, relative S/N], those that changed within a day (proportion of messages per channel, use of the pull-down facility, or choice of pass-band), and those that changed within a reel

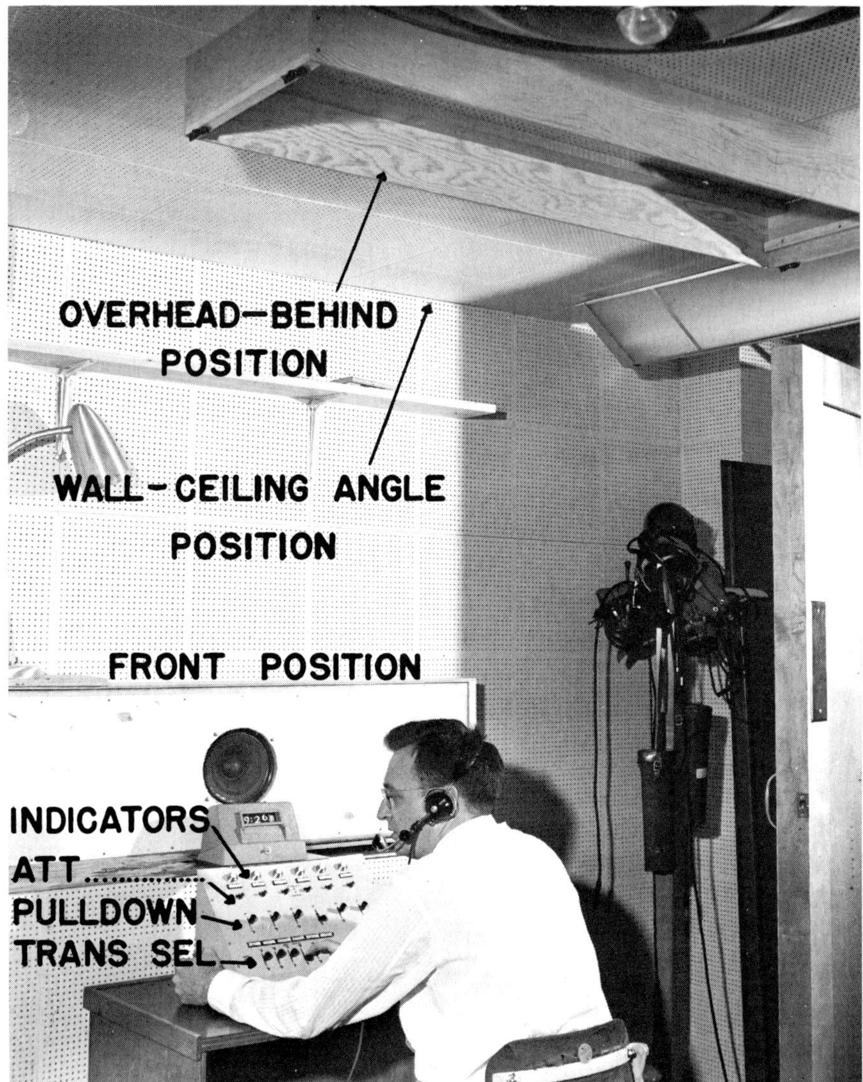

Figure 1 Picture of single loudspeaker mock control tower. All six audio channels are heard from a single loudspeaker, which on various days was located in front of the operator (as shown), on the wall–ceiling angle, or on the ceiling above the operator's head. On the console are channel identification (indicator) lights, attenuator pads, pulldown switches, and transmitter channel selector switches (From Webster and Thompson, *J. Aud. Eng.* **1,** 172, 1953b.)

(talker, microphone, relative speech level). Scores could be analyzed by type or mock tower (number of loudspeakers), operator, and all of the variables mentioned above.

There were four messages per aircraft that called in and these were of two types sequenced into five different orders. The first message of each set was of the type "Lindberg Tower, this is United 461, over." The correct response was "United 461, Lindberg Tower, Altimeter 566, Time 1426." The remaining three messages were of the second type. They used the same address and ID as the first but had a three-word message. The response to this was to identify the calling aircraft and to repeat the three-word message. The three words were in fact taken from Haagen's (1945) "Twenty-four word multiple choice tests" which were the original lists A and B to which Black (1957) added lists C and D and used extensively to select and/or train naval aviation cadets to talk and listen more effectively in cockpit noises.

Four of the five sequences of four messages per aircraft consisted of three aircraft calling in succession and each delivering one to four of his messages before the next aircraft called in. These are the nonoverlapping sequences. In the fifth sequence, a fourth aircraft called in and his messages overlapped those of

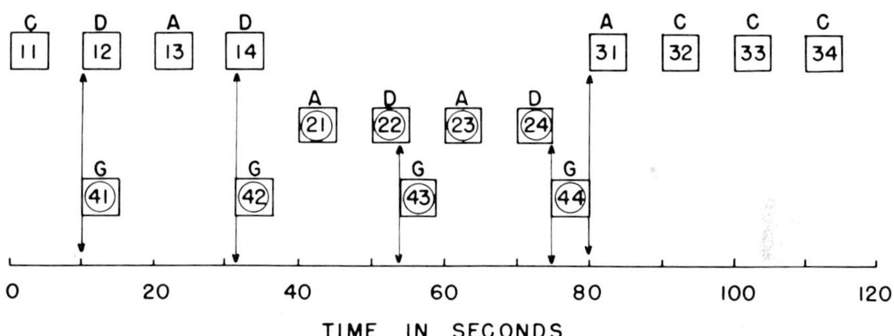

CONDITIONS

I   CONTROL (NO 41,····44 MESSAGES)

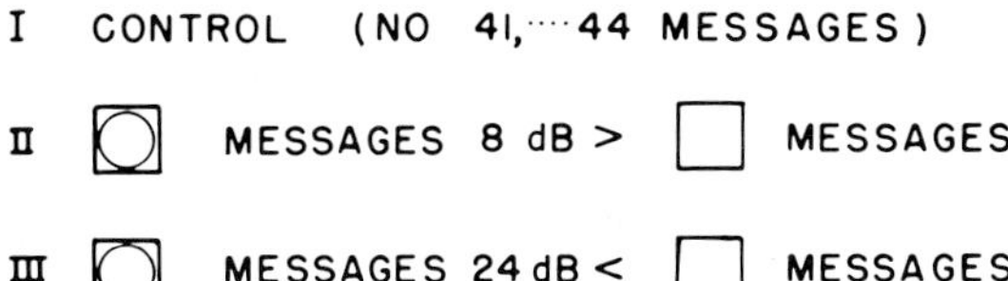

Figure 2 Schedule of competing messages, showing how the four messages of planes 1, 2, and 3 are overlapped by the four messages of plane 4. Those messages labeled "C" were heard in the clear; those labeled "A" were heard after a competing pair (presumably while the operator was speaking his response); those labeled "D" are overlapped by the overlapping messages, "G." (From Webster and Thompson, *J. Acoust. Soc. Am.* **26,** 398, 1954.)

the other three. This sequence, shown diagrammatically in Fig. 2, was very realistic in terms of actual operations in control towers. These competing messages started a series of studies on the processing of competing messages or selective attention that continued for over a decade.

A few of the results of this very complex experiment are shown in Figs. 3 and 4. The results, in terms of the percentage of words repeated back correctly, for three pairs of air controllers, over a 5-day period are shown in Fig. 3. The effect of thermal noise and/or control tower babble [at a level of 70 dB(C), which was probably 67 ± 2 dB(A)] on overall word intelligibility and learning is quite apparent. This leads to a major conclusion that noise levels in communicating spaces of this type should not exceed 70 dB. Other conclusions of the study evident in Fig. 3 are the advantage of being able to ''pulldown'' one channel into (earphone), or close to (loudspeaker), one ear (∇); use of individual loudspeakers on each channel ($\square$); and the irrelevancy of loudspeaker array placement (F,$\angle$, $\uparrow$). Preference questionnaires confirmed all three objective results.

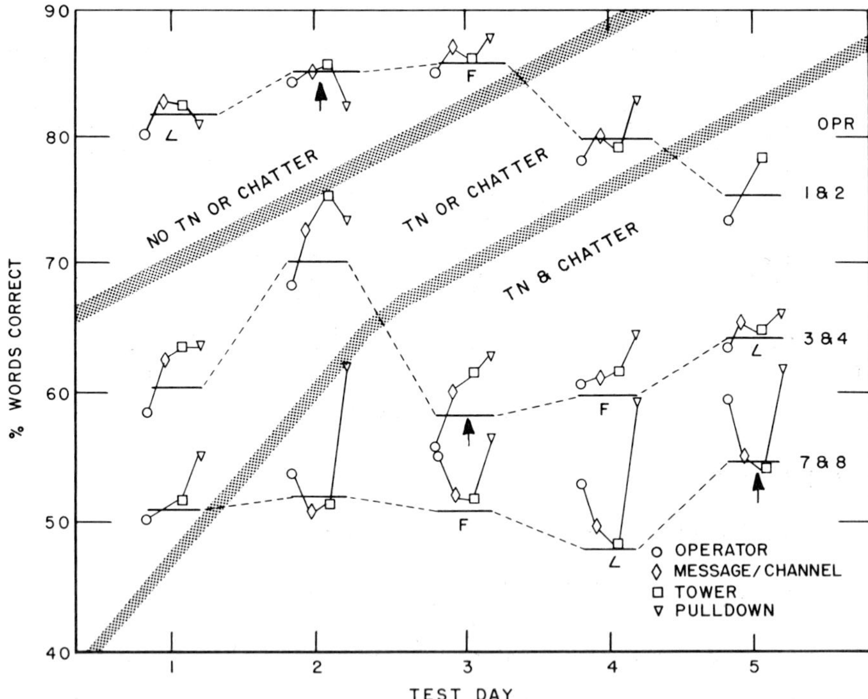

Figure 3 Percentage of words repeated back correctly for each of the five test days, for three pairs of operators. Within each day comparisons are made between operators, the distribution of messages per channel, the towers (six loudspeakers vs one), and the use of the ''pulldown'' facility. (From Webster and Thompson, *J. Aud. Eng.* **1**, 173, 1953b.)

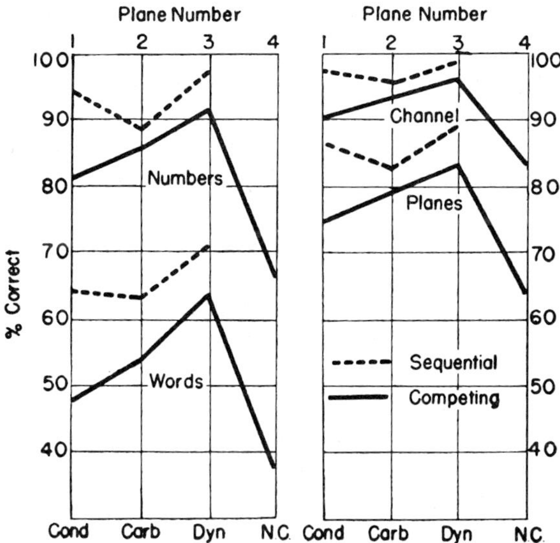

Figure 4   Percentage of correct responses for channel identification, plane name, plane numbers, and words averaged over the four messages of each plane. The recorded messages were originally spoken into a condenser (Cond) microphone for plane 1, a carbon (Carb) microphone for plane 2, dynamic (Dyn) for 3, and noise canceling (N.C.) for 4. Messages of plane 4 competed with those of planes 1 and 2 as shown in Fig. 2. (From Webster and Thompson, *J. Acoust. Soc. Am.* **26,** 399, 1954.)

Figure 4 shows the percentage of correct responses for only that sequence of messages that overlapped, as shown in Fig. 2. Each section of the message, including which (of the four) channels it came in on, and/or the microphones used for recording it, is shown separately. If the incoming message, on channel 1 was "North Island Tower, this is Navy 461, System, Foam, Banner" the correct (1) "Channel selection switch" was 1; (2) "plane response," was Navy (of four possible callers); (3) "number response" was 461; and (4) "word response" was System, Foam, Banner. The percentage of correct responses of this overlapping sequence is always less than for the nonoverlapping sequences. However the total amount of information transmitted per unit time was higher in the overlapping sequence since one-third more information (four messages instead of three) was transmitted and the increased error rate did not approach 1.33.

This whole aspect of the study, responding to both of two overlapping messages, is described in greater detail by Webster and Thompson (1954). They report that the greater the degree of overlap, or simultaneity, of the two messages the greater the interference. The overlapped message showed less interference than the overlapping because (1) in the case in which there was complete simultaneity the overlapped message was the second in a sequence of four [a message where that voice on that channel with that microphone and that (ID) had already been heard once] whereas the overlapping message was the first of the four message set, and (2) in the case where there was not complete simultaneity the overlapped message started before the overlapping message came in. Some interference was also caused by messages that did not overlap each other but the second one overlapped the response to the first. The amount of interference for each of these cases is shown in Fig. 4.

IV. CUES THAT AID IN LISTENING TO ONE OF TWO SIMUTANEOUS VOICE MESSAGES

At the same time the air control study was being performed at NEL work on competing messages was being carried on by Broadbent and Poulton at the Applied Psychology Research Unit in Cambridge, England. The earliest published papers, Broadbent (1952a,b) and Poulton (1953), agreed with our finding, namely, that a multiple loudspeaker array gave better results than a single loudspeaker, and that horizontal separation of the channel sources aided reception. They also found that a visual indication of the channel on which the message appeared aided reception. For practical reasons the application of this visual indication cue is limited mainly to wired systems such as interphones and intercoms and not radio systems. Questions arose as to how much spatial separation of channel sources is necessary and what other cues for competing message reception might exist.

To verify and/or refine the existence of visual and horizontal separation cues and to determine if and how much, selective bandwidth restriction might aid simultaneous voice message reception, Spieth *et al.* (1954) performed a more "basic" experiment. They used a performance task patterned after PAL Auditory Test 4 (see Karlin *et al.*, 1944), instead of a speech or word discrimination task. The task was to answer questions about a visual display consisting of 16 geometric entities in five positions of five different boxes. For example, two competing messages might ask "Where in box 5 is the triangle," and "What figure is in the upper left of box 1." These two messages could come in on two of three channels. Each message had an address and an ID. One message would have the address of the operator (subject) and required a response over the correct channel.

There were three loudspeaker separations: (1) none (a single loudspeaker), (2) 10–20° (10° between adjacent loudspeakers), or (3) 90–180° (90° between adjacent loudspeakers). Three bandwidth conditions were chosen and assigned to individual channels, namely (1) wideband (100–5000 Hz), (2) low pass (100–1600 Hz), and (3) high pass (1600–5000 Hz). In a control condition all channels were wideband. Twenty relatively untrained listeners answered one of two messages. Data from 16,880 message pairs verified that horizontal separation, even as little as 10°, the pulldown facility, and the selective use of bandwidth restriction aided message reception. Visual cues aided in correct channel selection but did not aid message reception. Egan *et al.* (1954) found that selective bandwidth restriction and attenuation both aided competing message reception. The limitations and precautions are that neither method of actually decreasing the information passing capability of a channel in the clear can be so severe as to decrease appreciably the word intelligibility. Within this limitation, however, any alteration that gives competing messages a "distinctive sound" aids in their reception.

V. AIDS FOR SELECTIVE LISTENING

A. Spatial and Spectral Source Separation

In another "basic" experiment, Spieth and Webster (1955) set out to find the frequency limits beyond which restricting the bandwidth no longer increased proficiency in selective listening to one, two, or more simultaneous or overlapping voice messages. Pairs of messages of the type "Burbank (or North Island) Tower, this is Cowboy 29, with Zulu, Metro, Over" were recorded by seven male talkers. There were two addresses in each pair of messages; four possible spondaic word IDs with 99 possible digits, and two, from a set of 26 possible, International Civil Aeronautics Organization phonetic alphabet words. Nine normal hearing listeners wrote down the message response (C29, ZM) to the "tower" they were preassigned to guard. The results, in terms of percentage of correct words and digits received, showed that "differential filtering almost always improved performance—whether it was the desired message that was filtered or—one or more of the competing messages . . . and the degree of filtering was relatively uncritical. High-pass cutoffs of 565, 800, or 1130 cps [Hz] were about equally effective and . . . better than—280. . . . Low-pass cutoffs of 1600, 1130, and 800 cps [Hz] also improved performance."

B. Simplifying Response Complexity

Webster and Solomon (1955) hypothesized that increasing the complexity (density or degree of overlap) of competing input stimuli, the complexity of the physical listening conditions, and/or the complexity of the listener's response would decrease response accuracy in an additive fashion. They had three groups of 12 males listen to sequences of two, three, or four competing (simultaneous or overlapping) messages. There were four physical listening conditions: spatial separation (channels split, channels together) and spectral separation (filters in, filters out), in all combinations. Filtering consisted of one broadband channel, and one band-passed (565–1600 Hz) which occurred together in the "split channel/filter" condition, as did the high-pass (1600 Hz) and low-pass (800 Hz) channels.

The response complexities included responding to one or two of the two-, three-, or four-message sets. The messages were the same ones used by Spieth and Webster (1955) augmented by a third and fourth message of the same type but with different addresses. The response always included a repeat of the "correct" or assigned message ID plus the message content. However, one group wrote their responses (same procedure as Spieth and Webster, 1955), a second group spoke the answer, while the third group wrote down a transposed answer for the message content. If they heard Alpha (A), Bravo (B), they wrote C, D, i.e., two letters on in the alphabet.

The results showed (1) *more than* twice as many errors when responding to two versus one message of the set, (2) an increase of 10% in errors for either speaking or transposing the (written) response, (3) about a 5% increase in accuracy by inserting the channel filters (spectral separation) when all four channels occurred together (in both earphones, diotic), (4) a 6 or 7% increase in accuracy by spatially separating two (unfiltered) channels into each earphone (dichotic), and (5) an additional accuracy increase of 1 or 2% if both spatial and spectral separation were used at the same time.

There were definite interactions between stimulus, response, and physical listening complexities. Responding to one message from sets of two, three, or four simultaneous message sets always gave less accurate results than when the sets overlapped but were not simultaneous. The accuracy was less than 35% when neither spatial nor spectral separation was used and three or four messages occurred simultaneously, but increased to above 70% when there were but two simultaneous messages. When both spatial and spectral separation were used, responding to one of four simultaneous messages was still somewhat difficult (47% correct) but scores of one of three or two were relatively high and were very dependent on type of response, transposing being most difficult (60 and 70% correct), speaking next most difficult (70 and 80%), and writing the easiest (75 and 90%). Scores on overlapping, as opposed to simultaneous, messages were always higher increasing from 47 to 86% for four-message sets, from 68 to 90% for sets of three, and from 80 to 94% for message pairs.

Spoken responses were less accurate than transposed responses if at least one irrelevant message followed the relevant one, i.e., if the listener had to speak in the presence of an incoming, though irrelevant, message. Even the listener's instructions showed effects of irrelevant messages. To wit, the stimuli were presented such that when asked to guard two channels and only two messages completed, only one assigned message actually occurred, yet more errors were made by those responding to the one while guarding for a second, than by those responding to the one while not guarding for a second even though it never occurred.

There was no way of equating the relative difficulty of increasing complexities in stimuli, listening conditions, or responses but some generalities seem evident. Answering two of three- or four-message sets as opposed to answering one of two-, three-, or four-message sets, or answering simultaneous sets as opposed to overlapping sets caused about equal increases in errors (a decrease of about 25% in correct responses); answering by speech or transposition instead of a simple written response decreased correct responses about 10%; the use of either spectral or spatial listening aids were about equally effective (increasing correct responses by between 5 and 6%) and were not additive (using both increased correct responses only 1 or 2% over using either alone).

The results are conclusive in showing that listening to and/or processing messages in sequence instead of at the same time is far and away the best aid in the handling of competing incoming information. Simplifying the response and/or using listening aids help but cannot relieve an overloaded human perceptual system in any major way.

Webster and Sharpe (1955) carried out the obvious concluding set of experiments on the message sets used by Spieth and Webster (1955) and Webster and Solomon (1955). If messages could not be handled efficiently, if they overlap or compete with each other, how much better could they be handled if they were purposely made sequential. Webster and Sharpe had both experienced and inexperienced listeners answer one, two, three, or four of the same two-, three-, or four-message sets cited earlier under one of two conditions. In the first instance, messages on one channel were preprogrammed as before (Spieth and Webster, 1955; Webster and Solomon, 1955) and signal lights indicated when messages were available to be heard on the other three channels. The listeners played back these latter three messages when they were ready for them. In the second instance, all four channels were played back in sequence whenever the listeners wanted to hear them. As might be expected the results in terms of correctly heard (and verbally repeated back) message elements increased substantially when sequenced. When responding to one (two, three, or four) message under the best listening conditions, the listeners in the Webster and Solomon experiment obtained 83% correct scores (in 30 min, the preprogrammed time). When able to "sequence" messages on three of the four channels, Webster and Sharpe listeners obtained scores of 86% (in 30 min). When allowed to sequence messages on all four channels, average scores rose to 98% (in 21 min). When sequencing, listeners could answer two, three, or four messages almost as easily (accurately) as answering one. In terms of information rates, listeners transmitted (handled) between 1.1 and 1.4 bits per second in answering one message (and even less when answering two) when the messages could not be sequenced (Webster and Solomon, 1955). On the other hand, Webster and Sharpe's listeners transmitted

2 bits per second when answering one message and 2.85, 3.7, and 4.2 bits per second when answering two, three, or four messages.

With the conclusion of the Webster and Sharpe (1955) experiment, the limitations of a human processer of speech (voice) input information in terms of handling time overloads were pretty well in focus. And the physical aids that could help a person process competing (overlapping and/or simultaneous) messages were pretty well defined. Anything that caused a message to differ from competing messages aided in its reception. Cherry (1953) had shown context to be important. The actual or apparent location of the message source was found to be very effective by Broadbent (1952b, 1954) and Poulton (1953). Webster and Thompson (1953a) and Spieth *et al.* (1954) found both message location (spatial cues) and relative onset time to be advantageous. Broadbent (1952b) found the use of different voices to be important and Speith *et al.* (1954), Egan *et al.* (1954), Spieth and Webster (1955), and Webster and Solomon (1955) found that filters in the channels were also effective. Egan *et al.* (1954) also found that making channels differ in intensity aided in differential reception (even if the desired message was somewhat less intense than its competition). The amount of information (in bits/second) was found to influence competing message reception by Webster and Thompson (1953a). Broadbent (1956) found the influence of nonverbal competing tasks and Webster and Solomon (1955) found the negative effects of response complexity.

C. Application of Results

Concurrent with these laboratory experiments, Beitscher and Webster (1956) made some systematic field observations and collected data for laboratory evaluations. With a survey team in a specially equipped USN airplane they visited and ran plane-to-tower and tower-to-plane intelligibility tests at 15 control towers. Two talkers, one in the aircraft and one in the tower, read the same words (Haagen, 1945) used in the original air control tower laboratory study while the aircraft flew in a 20-mile radius circle around the 15 towers. The intelligibility of the recordings of these words was determined by five listeners back in the laboratory. The percentage of words heard correctly from tower-to-plane varied from 90 to 38 (average 73.7) and from plane-to-tower from 63 to 3 (average 44.4). "The correlation among towers between hearing and being heard was fairly high." On approaching and leaving each tower, contacts were systematically established. The average contact range was 50 miles and on departure communications were often maintained to distances in excess of 100 miles. At the conclusion of this phase of laboratory and survey studies, a team of human engineers worked with installation engineers in redesigning (and moving) the control tower at NAS North Island and the en route traffic control installation at NAS Miramar.

D. Feasibility of Sequencing Messages

With a team applying the results of the past experiments, the researchers continued the obvious task of seeking better solutions to the competing message problem. The experimental results from various laboratories in the United States and United Kingdom showed that the best way to aid an operator processing competing speech messages was to simplify the response and to sequence (preferably self-pace) the information input. Reducing the message information rate and using spatial and spectral channeling aids while maintaining an adequate speech-to-noise differential and speech bandwidth improved message reception but not to the same degree as decreasing the information input per unit time. This must have been the reasoning, at least tacitly, of Carson and Sanderson (1945) who had used the newly developed technique of magnetic recording to develop a fixed-delay message storage device. This radio repeat unit was installed in the combat information center (CIC) of certain World War II aircraft carriers. When the author asked about its use and advantages in 1963 on an information gathering trip abroad USS ORISKANY, CVA-34, it was found that the personnel had never used it, and, in fact, did not know what it was, how it worked, or what its function was. Since the existence of this fixed-delay device was known in 1955, an experiment was designed to test the concept of its use. It was hypothesized that it would be of no value. Simple logic plus the results from Webster and Sharpe (1955) indicated that what was needed was a sequencing or variable-delay message storage device. Therefore, an elaborate game-type verbal message input situation was designed that was meant to simulate certain aspects of information processing centers such as air control towers and combat information centers. Operators were then tested on message transcription errors and number of message repeats (Bertsch *et al.*, 1956) and on problem solving (Thompson *et al.*, 1958) using simulations of fixed and variable-delay devices and a control case of a no-message storage device.

The speech information game was played on a plotting board made up of four quadrants each with ten rows (A to J) and ten columns (1–10) (see Fig. 5). A plotter–listener–decision maker needed four pieces of information each from a different but specific and unique source (talker) to fully specify one of four geometric figures (target), in one of four colors (speed), in one of 100 grid intersections (location) in one of four quadrants (altitude). Each incoming message contained three pieces of information, one of which was always the quadrant. The remaining two concerned row and arrow direction, column and color, shape and direction, and shape and color. From this information, the operator was trained to synthesize and surmise that the red object in column 6, the upward pointing arrow in row G, the red circle, and the circle with an upward pointing arrow were in fact the one and only solution for an upward pointing, red, circle at the intersection of column 6 and row G. The message format was typical of the formats used in the previous studies reported here and typical of military mes-

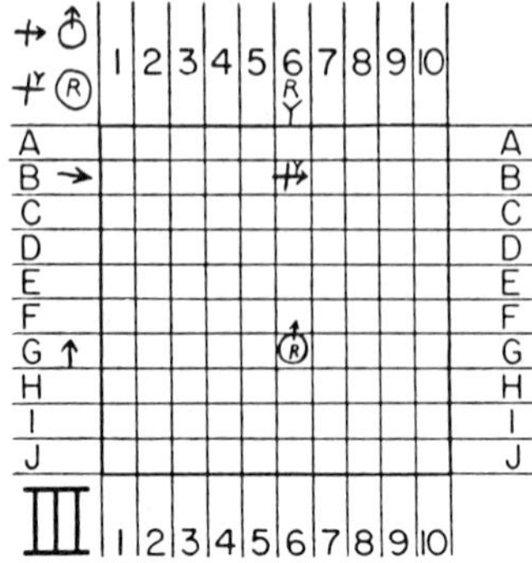

Figure 5 Quadrant (position) III of the operator's four-quadrant plotting board showing the necessary partial information and complete solution for two objects. In this problem the operator plotted in the margins (1) row and direction information from Moat, (2) column and color information from Stick, (3) shape and direction information from Taxi, and (4) shape and color information from Rabbit. Interlocking information indicates that the Circle which is Red and pointed North should be in cell G-6, while the East-directed, yellow, Plus should be in cell B-6. A single quadrant might have from zero to four objects and each object could have any of four shapes, colors, or directions, and be in any one of the 400 cells (100 cells, four quadrants). The total number of objects ranged from six to eight over the six problems. (From Thompson *et al.*, *J. Speech Hear. Res.* **1**, 145, 1958).

sages, for example, address (Whidbey), ID (this is Moat), message (quadrant 3, column 6, red), sign off (over). Three other messages from three other specific IDs completed the necessary sequence. Messages of this type were in no specific order, and certainly did not specify one object completely before partial information about other objects came in. Average message duration was 4.5 sec.

There were six basic experimental problems with from six to eight objects in each. Over the six problems there were 180 relevant messages and 33 duds (to or from irrelevant addresses). Many messages overlapped each other but some came in isolation as long as 20 sec after other messages.

In Bertsch *et al.* (1956), the results from six operators (who transcribed the messages but did not solve the problem) indicated that the "variable-delay" scheme was superior for all criteria (fewer errors, fewer repeats, less time per repeat), primarily because the variable-delay eliminated all overlapping messages." The fixed-delay scheme did reduce the number of messages repeated on the communication channel at least for the condition where the operator did not have to solve the problem. The results of Thompson *et al.* (1958) for eight operators who were required to solve the problem showed a slight decrease of channel usage due to repeats using the fixed-delay scheme but the overall advantages of the variable-delay (sequencing) scheme were overwhelming. "As compared to the no-storage (control) condition, the readout-on-demand storage conditions—cut—the errors (by about one-half), the—repeats—by—three-fourths, and the time to—solve the problem (by one-half). Performance under the fixed-storage condition was essentially the same as—no-storage—.'' Slower operators in particular benefited from readout-on-demand. The most proficient operators ''by great concentration and effort'' finished the problem with no-storage as fast as with readout-on-demand but on questionnaires state ''that intensification or extension of their task would have resulted in saturation and probable breakdown in performance.''

E. Sequencing Device and Visual/Data Transmissions

The advantages of sequencing information input are intuitely obvious and the experiments of Webster and Sharpe (1955), Bertsch *et al.* (1956), and Thompson *et al.* (1958) merely showed the magnitudes and limitations of the obvious. None of this would be of any practical value unless a message sequencing storage device could be designed. The principle of such a device was shown in Fig. 1 of Bertsch *et al.* (1956) and a patent on it was issued in 1962.[1] This solution to the problem was never incorporated into any military system. Rather parts of the problem were solved by fast visual readouts (on demand) of targets found and tracked on radar scopes in combat information centers (CICs) by such systems as the Navy Tactical Display System (NTDS) which came into use in the 1960s. NTDS had very complex visual and data readout and transmission capabilities among various consoles doing various aspects of target detection, classification, and weapon assignment. The voice intercom among elements of the system was relegated to secondary importance and was very elemental. As soon as NTDS began handling target information at higher rates, more people asked, by voice, for updates and tentative recommendations based on the upgraded information. These command and staff type people often did not have, or did not have time to properly use, the visual/data terminal consoles and, as is human nature in any case, asked for the information over voice circuits. So although one phase of the information load/competing message problem was solved at the input end of the chain a new link was added to the output or final decision stage and voice message channels were again overloaded, overlapping and in need of engineering decisions and redesign based on the competing message research of the 1950s at government laboratories in the United States and the United Kingdom.

F. Peripheral versus Central Masking of Speech

With the experience gained from these studies and the assignment of the problem of designing a radio to be used by the plane directors on the flight deck

---

[1]U.S. Patent 3,041,417. Readout on Demand Tape Storage Device. J. Stroud, J. C. Webster, F. Steiner, and S. Sessions. 26 June 1962.

of aircraft carriers the research emphasis changed from the central aspects of speech masking to the peripheral effects: Webster *et al.* (1957) studied the relative efficiencies of picking up speech from various anatomical locations. Klumpp and Webster (1958) evaluated and summarized many of the acoustical aspects of speech communication systems to be used in high noise levels.Klumpp and Webster (1961) studied the intelligibility of time-compressed speech and Thompson *et al.* (1961) studied the effects of "liveness" on speech intelligibility. The general conclusions were maximize the speech-to-noise differential and do not overprocess the speech signal, and eliminate noise by mouth and ear noise shields, pick the speech up in front of the mouth, and do not time-compress or add liveness to speech. A summary of these and other studies by Webster (1965) showed the state-of-the-art limitations on speech communications by ambient noise. Some general conclusions were that face-to-face communications (at 1.5 feet) were limited to levels less than about 95 dB(A) at which point (normal hearing) people should wear hearing protection; the use of interior communication devices (telephones, intercoms) should be avoided at noise levels above 76 dB(A); and all "noise-proofing techniques" should be employed when communicating in levels in excess of 106 dB(A).

One study by Webster and Klumpp (1962) does bear more directly on the subject matter of this article. They studied the effects on voice level of ambient noise and of additional talkers. They had one, two, or four pairs of talkers read and verify phonetically balanced monosyllabic words in ambient noise levels of quiet (less than or equal to 55 dB), 65, 75, and 85 dB. The pairs were instructed to maintain word intelligibilities of 95% and did manage an average of 94% with no scores below 84%. The results were that "the speech level . . . increased about 5 dB for an additional 10 dB noise or for each doubling of the number of talking pairs." In general, errors increased as the number of talkers increased but not until the ambient noise reached 85 dB.

VI. AUDITORY SELECTIVE ATTENTION RESEARCH
AFTER 1958

Broadbent (1958) summarized most of the studies reviewed above and the similar work done at the Applied Psychology Unit (APU) in Cambridge, England. He concluded that the human perceptual system was a limited capacity system. To keep from overloading this system, Broadbent proposed a filter theory. The perceptual filter was based on some physical characteristic of the desired or selected message. In summarizing his 1958 filter theory Broadbent (1971) states, "a listener can give efficient response to all stimuli possessing some common feature, provided that he is allowed to reject those . . . which do not." The rejected stimuli "must be discarded before they have been fully processed . . . the physical cue separating relevant from irrelevant must act by assisting the discarding (answering one of two) because it is less helpful when discarding is impossible (answering both of two).''

Since under certain circumstances responses from more than one overlapping message are possible, Broadbent postulated there must be a buffer stage early in the perceptual mechanism where simultaneous processing and temporary storage (S) is carried out. This is followed by a stage where successive processing only is carried out, a perceptual (P) store. He suggests that the filter lies between S and P and that ''there is a limit to the speed (it) can change the basis . . . for selection.'' A limited quantity of information to the nonresponding ear goes into the buffer store (S) but is lost after a short time.

The selection or rejection of a message by the filter based on physical differences was easily accommodated by the theory. Selection based on message content was not so easily accommodated. The next logical steps were to see how the theory might be modified or broadened to account for content.

VII. SINGLE-SYLLABLE MESSAGES

A year after Broadbent's 1958 book the present author, on a sabbatical at Broadbent's Applied Psychology Unit, ran an experiment to evaluate the differences between physical characteristics and message content and prosody on the simplest of all messages, one-syllable messages. At the time, I thought that any aspect of a message that made it different from another would aid in selecting it and rejecting the other. In some unspecific way this included content even though I appreciated that it would take more time to select or reject a message on the basis of content than on a physical characteristic. That is, more of the message would have to be perceived before a decision could be made. However, in the most elemental of messages, one or the other of two steady-state vowels, the message content could theoretically be ascertained as rapidly as the physical difference in location (left ear/right ear) or vocal timbre (male/female speaker). Only the prosodic feature of rising or falling inflection would require hearing the message to the end before channeling the desired message through the ''select'' or the ''reject'' filter. The rate of stimulus presentation in terms of bits per second was a parameter in the experiment so that relative speed and accuracy of using physical cues, content, or prosodic features as the filter selector could be evaluated. In this experiment (Webster, 1961) the competing stimuli consisted of single sounds each encoded with four bits of information, either the vowel /a/ (*father*) or /i/ (*even*), spoken by a male or a female, with a rising or falling inflection on track 1 or track 2 of a tape recorder such that on (earphone) playback it would sound in the left or right ear. Four balanced sets of sounds were recorded such that in any pair of simultaneous sounds (1) one was in the left ear while the other was in the right, or (2) one was /a/, the other /i/, or (3) one was spoken by a male, the other by a female, or (4) one had a rising, the other a falling, inflection. Subjects were alternately asked to concentrate on the sound (1) in the left (or right) ear, (2) /a/ or /i/, (3) spoken by the male (or female), or (4) with the rising (or falling) inflection. In all cases the subject was to list the other three elements in the sound. For example, the sound in the left ear may have been /i/ spoken by a male with a falling inflection (while that in the right ear may have been /i/ spoken by a female with a falling inflection).

Webster (1961) showed that fewer errors were made if the physical cues, ear of reception (left/right) or vocal timbre (male/female), were used as the selection criteria, than if message content (/a/, /i/) was used, but the difference was not pronounced. If inflection were the selection criterion many errors were made. Decision time was ruled out as the reason for inflection being the most difficult by adding the consonants /k/ and /t/ before and after the vowel. It made no difference whether the initial or the final consonant was used as the selection criterion. The data also showed (Fig. 3 of Webster, 1961) that on the average, listeners made fewer errors when asked to monitor the right ear message than when asked to monitor the left ear message. However no notice was made of this "right ear advantage" at the time. In summary, for these elemental messages, content was almost as efficient as physical cues for selecting one message and rejecting another.

VIII. SHADOWING EXPERIMENTS

All experiments in the 1950s except for Cherry's (1953) used the paradigm of having the listener respond to the specific message with a given address, from a given source, in a given voice, etc. The messages and the responses were relatively short. The relevant message could and often did change, in localization or voice, with each succeeding message (set). This represents typical listening situations in information, command, and control centers and in fact at cocktail parties or church fetes. There are other applied problems in selective attention where a "shadowing" response is required to a continual usually low information content stimulus. Shadowing, the verbative repeat of running speech, is the first perceptual task for navy sound-powered telephone talkers, court stenographic reporters, interpretors for the deaf, or real-time foreign language translators. Anyone listening to instantaneous translations of scientific papers or to navy telephone talkers can appreciate that in the words of Cherry (1953) "he may have very little idea of what the message that he has repeated is all about, especially if the subject matter is difficult." Nevertheless Cherry (1953) was the first one to use shadowing as the response method for the study of auditory selective attention and in the 1960s the shadowing response was used quite extensively.

IX. BILINGUAL SELECTIVE ATTENTION

Treisman (1964a,b), using the shadowing paradigm, utilized foreign languages as one method of controlling the meaningfulness of the content of the irrelevant message. If English prose were being shadowed Treisman (1964a) found that Anglisized Czech nonsense, English prose, and a second-order approximation of English were equally and more interfering than English digits. Treisman (1964b) later added French, German, and Italian as well as technical and reversed English to the Czech Anglisized nonsense as irrelevant content against English prose. She also used subjects who varied in their knowledge of the foreign languages. She found that the most interfering context was the same English prose, equally and next most interfering were technical English and a foreign language well known by the subjects, next most interfering were reversed English, Angelisized Czech, and a foreign language for which the listeners had a moderate proficiency, and least interfering was a foreign language unknown by the listeners.

There were significant differences in the interfering aspects of the foreign language depending on the degrees of proficiency of fluency. It would appear from these results that a selective attention task using messages in two different languages might be a method of determining the relative degree of bilingualism. Gat and Keith (1978) showed that in a straightforward speech discrimination test where noise, not interfering speech, is the problem linguistic experience also affects the scores. In their case native Americans heard more monosyllabic words in progressive levels of noise than did a group of six foreign students who had been in the United States between 3 and 4 years. This group in turn obtained higher speech discrimination scores than did a group of foreign students with less than 1 year in United States. These two studies show that if the scores on the competing message bilingual test are too high, the usual method of increasing the difficulty by increasing the background noise level should increase the differential between those who are maximally and minimally proficient in a nonnative language.

X. PILOT TRIAL OF A BILINGUAL COMPETING MESSAGE TEST

A competing message test using the 1950 response method of making the select/reject choice on each pair of short items was designed on a National

Academy Science exchange with the USSR and Czechoslovakian Academies in the academic year 1980/81. The scripts were designed such that any two of the languages English, Russian, Serbo-Crotian, German, or Czech could be paired against each other. Four equivalent forms of the test were recorded in English/Russian and English/Czech. Although four different types of sentence materials had been constructed in English, due to time restraints, only the mathematical type statements to be described were used for the pilot tests.

A. Test Construction

The easiest ensemble of spoken words to discriminate in most languages are numerals; therefore, a numeral test was constructed in English that would lend itself to adaptation in other languages. The framework is a set of sentences stating simple arithmetic truths. For example, "Twenty less four equals sixteen" $(20-4=16)$. A multiple choice answer sheet of five columns would contain

$$
\begin{array}{llll}
\text{12 plus} & 0 = & 1 & 16 \\
\text{17 and} & 4 = & 8 & 23 \\
\text{20 minus} & 7 = & 9 & 24 \\
\text{70 less} & 11 = & 13 & 31
\end{array}
$$

with instructions to select or mark through the numbers and word actually heard.

Seven other statements, eight in all, could be generated using this same answer foil, i.e.,

$$12 \text{ or } 20 \text{ plus or minus } 4 \text{ or } 11.$$

By using all possible problem sets 32 statements can be generated, i.e., 12 or 20 plus or minus 4 or 11; 12 or 20 plus or minus 0 or 7; 17 or 70 plus or minus 4 or 11; and 17 or 70 plus or minus 0 or 7. To accommodate all four sets of problems three additional answer sets must also be generated. These 32 problems can be doubled to 64 by using both "plus" and "and" for $(+)$ and "minus" and "less" for $(-)$. And by using four different double columns of problem sets, 256 equally probable statements can be generated.

The choice of these double columns of problem sets is unique to each different language and should be chosen to make the numerals maximally confusable. In English the spoken numerals 30–13, 40–14, . . . 90–19 differ only by the addition of one phoneme /n/ to the last syllable, i.e. /-i/ vs /-in/. In addition the numerals 15 and 16 and 50 and 60 sound very much alike because they have the same medial sound, /I/.

Similarly in English, single digit confusions exist between the monosyllables five and nine, and two and three, and among the two/three syllable numerals, zero, seven, and eleven. These number pairs should therefore appear in opposition to each other to maximize confusabilities. The English version of the test therefore includes the following problem sets:

12	0	13	1	15	2	18	1
17	4	14	8	16	3	19	5
20	7	30	9	50	10	80	6
70	11	40	11	60	12	90	9

In Russian, preliminary experiments and a priori analyses of vowel and multiple syllable stress confusions indicated that confusions existed between 0 and 2, 14 and 18, 20 and 30, 50 and 60, 19 and 90, and among the numerals 12, 13, 15, 16, 17, and among 5, 6, 8, and 10. Therefore these four problem ensembles were generated:

12	1	12	6	19	5	20	0
13	3	14	8	70	6	30	2
15	5	17	10	80	9	50	4
16	7	18	12	90	10	60	11

In German the logic of making numerals from 13 to 19 and 30, 40, 50, . . . 90 is very similar to English. The numerals 13 to 19 are made by appending "zehn" and the decades 30 to 90 are made by appending "zig." Obviously dreizehn and dreizig are confusable in the same manner as thirteen and thirty. In German 2 and 3 (zwei and drei) are confusable as 2 and 3 are in English and are possibly confusable with 1 (eins). Other possible confusions are 0 and 9 (null and neun), 6 and 10 (sechs and zehn), 2 and 12 (zwei and zwölf), 1 and 11 (eins and elf), and 10, 11, and 12 (zehn, elf, and zwölf). To maximize these confusions the following problem sets were chosen:

12	2	13	3	15	1	18	0
17	6	14	4	16	2	19	8
20	10	30	5	50	3	80	9
70	12	40	7	60	11	90	10

In Serbo-Croatian the number sets 1 and 11, and 2, 12, 20; 3, 13, 30; . . . 9, 19, 90 are confusable, so the following problem sets were generated:

12	1	13	3	15	5	18	8
17	2	14	4	16	6	19	9
20	11	30	13	50	15	80	18
70	12	40	14	60	16	90	19

And in the Czech language the following problem sets were chosen:

10	1	11	2	15	4	19	7
20	9	12	3	16	12	70	8
30	10	13	5	50	13	80	17
40	11	14	6	60	14	90	18

The problem and answer formats just described were designed to be, and were, used in two manners: in a competing message sequence as a possible test of bilingual proficiency, and in a noncompeting sequence as a classification or profiling test of numeral discrimination for the severely/profoundly deaf. In the competing message sequence the messages were combined as follows:

Twenty less four equals sixteen.
Fünfzehn und drei ist achtzehn.

or

Neunzig weniger acht ist acht und neunzig.
Forty plus eleven equals twenty nine.

Note that the second pair is false arithmetically as indeed half of the statements were constructed to be, since this is a hearing or language test not an intelligence test. In the recording of the test 16 pairs of messages were used on each equivalent form. Four talkers were used, two males and two females; two were native talkers of English who could also speak fluent German (Russian, Serbo-Crotian, Czech) and two native talkers of German, . . . who also spoke English. Half of the time the English message was the first of the pair, half of the time it was the second, half were spoken by males, half by females. Within each pair one was on channel (track) one and the other on two. Therefore on playback one could be heard from the left and the other from the right. Since in every pair one message is English and one is not, a noncompeting numeral test in a single language can be made by a simple rerecording process.

B. Trials of Russian and Serbo-Crotian Noncompeting Test

The actual recording of this test in an institute not specifically set up for psychoacoustic testing is not easy. In the USSR time ran out before the competing message sequence was in good enough shape to administer. So a simplified form was administered to two groups of students at a school for the deaf. The test was administered over a classroom auditory trainer (earphones) individually adjusted to their preferred listening level. Twenty people were tested in the age range 16 to 18.

Since multiple-choice tests are not common in USSR schools the answer format was difficult for the students to understand. To get them acquainted with the test many pretest trials were run. The first was to play a series of 16 noncompeting messages half of which were in Russian and half in English and their initial response was to answer the question, "Is it in the Russian language or is it not?" As a group they scored just above the chance level; only a very few could make that judgment. On the next hearing they heard only the Russian language numerals and were asked to identify the talker's voice as male or female. They performed considerably better. Many identified the male voice as female (and vice versa) but were consistent. In general they could make the voice quality distinction. They were then asked to identify the last numeral (the answer) on the multiple-choice answer format and with much coaching learned to cope. Finally those who could hear well enough and could cope with the multiple-choice format (18 of 20) took the complete 16-item Russian numeral test.

Records were made available of their pure tone audiograms and a consensus of three teachers' ratings of their ability to comprehend spoken language. Pearson product–moment correlations were run between the numeral word discrimination scores and their average hearing level for the frequencies 500, 1000, and 2000 Hz ($r = 0.47$) and between word score and teacher evaluation ($r = 0.67$). These correlations are in the expected range. It is more important to note that these severely to profoundly deaf students did hear enough of these numerals to make this, or a modified version of this, test useful as a classification or profiling test. The genesis of this numeral test was a simpler version used by Webster and O'Shea (1980) to categorize American hearing-impaired college students who could not achieve above chance scores on sentence or multiple-choice modified rhyme test (MRT) words. The Russian language version of this more sophisticated numeral test appears to work on the Russian students.

A Serbo-Crotian version of this test given to three groups in a school for the deaf in Belgrade gave very similar results. The multiple-choice format for each numeral and operation word in the arithmetic statement is difficult for these students. But if used as a power test at three levels of difficulty it adequately profiles deaf late-teen-age deaf students. The basic procedure was (1) identify the male/female voice, if successful, (2) write down, then mark through on a multiple-choice format, the "answer" (last numeral) only, if successful, (3) respond to all four elements in the statement. Scores, or lack of them at these stages, agree very well with teacher evaluation of the students' auditory language receptive abilities and to a somewhat lesser extent with scholastic standing in classroom subjects.

C. Trial of Czech/English Competing Message Form

In Czechoslovakia the facilities and appropriate personnel of the Prague Broadcasting Station were made available and a very adequate version of the competing message bilingual numeral test was recorded. Pilot tests were given to nine technical/scientific associates at the Institute of Experimental Psychology in Bratislava. Previously made arrangements to give the test to the 1981 contingent of English-speaking students learning Czech at Charles University were canceled when a new director was appointed. So the only results are from the not too well controlled pilot study (the order effects were not counterbalanced).

A general outline of the parameters built into the design was discussed earlier. In a relatively simple rearrangement of the messages on the two tracks the following message pair sequences could be and were generated: Two equivalent forms of English/Czech (E/C) bilingual messages, one by the native Czech-speaking couple and one by the native English-speaking couple; and one set of English/English (E/E) messages and one set of Czech/Czech (C/C) messages still balanced on an item-by-item basis by male/female.

The Bratislava trial was meant to be preliminary and the relative difficulty of the task was not known. Therefore the order of giving the sequence of such tests was chosen to enhance the learning of the routine, namely, from what was thought to be the easiest to the most difficult task. Whatever learning took place was not counterbalanced among subjects. The order of presentation was (1) listen to pairs of Czech/English messages. Answer only the Czech one; (2) listen again and answer the English one; (3) this time answer the first (and on the next run the second) message of the pair; (4) listen to pairs of Czech/Czech messages, answer the message coming from the loudspeaker to your left (next run right); (5) listen to pairs of English/English messages and answer those from your left (right).

Two, three, or four listeners were tested in groups. They sat about 2 m from two loudspeakers that were roughly 3 m apart in a relatively small semi-sound-treated room (4 × 5 × 3 m). The listening level was adjusted to meet a consensus [70±3 dB(A) in a room noise level of 50±1 dB(A)]. Instructions were re-recorded in Slovak (as opposed to the Czech instructions originally recorded in Prague) even though the messages were in Czech which did not seem to bother them. Adequate time was given to reinterpret the instructions by stopping for questions before the test sequences of 16 items.

Responses were scored by number of correct binary decisions. Referring back to the answer format in Section X,A note that the first numeral is one of four that could be marked so a correct response was worth two points (bits). Similarly the operator word could be one of four, worth 2 points. The second number was worth 2, and the nominal answer being a choice of one in eight was worth 4 points. The total correct at this point could be 10. Subjects were also asked to identify the message as to time of arrival (first or second) worth one point, and source (left or right) worth one point. (If they were instructed to answer the first or the left they got a point by choosing the correct message.) Finally, after two subjects were run and it became evident the scores were very high, the nine subjects whose results will be discussed were asked to judge whether the statement was arithmetically true or false. A totally correct answer was worth 14 points. If they chose not to judge true/false they could score only 12 points per item or get a maximum score of 86%.

The results are shown in Table II. They are arbitrarily ranked by the score on the English message from the English/Czech script. Although no statistical significance can be shown because of the small number of subjects some trends are

TABLE II

INDIVIDUAL SCORES IN PERCENTAGE RANK ORDERED BY ENGLISH SCORE
ON ENGLISH/CZECH (EC) SCRIPT, COLUMN 1

Column number		1	2	3	4	5	6
Type script		EC	EE	CE	CC	CE	—
Test order		2	5	3	4	1	Av
Decision ques.		E	L,R	1,2	L,R	C	—
	1	98	96	99	95	99	97.4
	2	96	88	98	97	94	94.6
	3	93	91	100	93	99	95.2
	4	89	91	86	87	98	92.2
Mean 1–4		94.0	91.5	96.8	94.5	97.5	94.9
	5	80	76	86	87	98	85.4
	6	70	85	77	96	94	84.4
	7	61	63	71	90	87	74.4
	8	51	64	76	78	94	72.6
Mean 5–8		65.5	72.0	77.5	87.8	93.3	79.2
	9	46	29	60	73	77	57.0
Mean 1–9		76.0	75.9	84.1	89.1	93.3	83.7
		76.0			91.2		

evident: when all the messages to be answered are in a nonnative language (English), columns 1 and 2, the average score is much lower (76.0) than when the messages are in a native language (Czech), columns 4 and 5 (91.2); when half are in each language the average score is half-way in between.

There appears to be two groups of people: those who score well above the mean English language score (subjects 1 to 4 whose scores indicate they are very proficient in English), and those at or below the mean. For the group very proficient in both languages the differences among any scores across the five columns are minimal. The real differences in scores could be masked by truncation which in any retesting would be reduced by adding a steady background noise. One subject, subject 9, found the selective attention task very difficult and scored very badly on everything, especially on competing English messages.

Of the remaining four subjects (5–8) two questions can be asked. Do Czech messages interfere with English messages (column 1) more than English messages interfere with English messages (column 2)? On the average the answer is yes (65.5 vs 72.0). The second question is do Czech messages interfere with Czech messages (column 4) more than English messages interfere with Czech messages (column 5)? Again, yes (87.8 vs 93.3). For these people their native language, Czech, is their dominant language and it interferes with itself or a nonnative language (English) more than the nonnative language does. These people who already have a good, but not excellent, command of a second language would function better in that language in situations in which their primary language is not spoken, that is where it does not compete for their attention. Their own language may function in the same fashion that Moray (1959) found for one's own name. If it is the irrelevant message it will be noticed. Broadbent (1971) says "the selection of one . . . shuts out most of the information on the other . . . if some does break through, the items are not random; but are . . . of certain kinds." If the results of this study could be verified on a larger sample it could almost certainly be generalized that your own native language is the kind of nonrandom content that makes it difficult to attend to another moderately well-learned language.

References

Beitscher, H. R., and Webster, J. C. (1956). Intelligibility of UHF and VHF transmissions at fifteen representative air control towers. *J. Acoust. Soc. Am.* **28**, 561–564.

Bertsch, W. F., Webster, J. C., Klumpp, R. G., and Thompson, P. O. (1956). Effects of two message storage schemes upon communications within a small problem solving group. *J. Acoust. Soc. Am.* **28**, 550–553.

Black, J. W. (1957). Multiple choice intelligibility tests. *J. Speech Hear. Disorders* **22**, 213–235.

Botsford, J. H. (1969). Using sound levels to gauge human response to noise. *Sound Vibr.* **3**(10), 16–28.

Broadbent, D. E. (1952a). Listening to one of two synchronous messages. *J. Exp. Psychol.* **44**, 51–55.

Broadbent, D. E. (1952b). Failures of attention in selective listening. *J. Exp. Psychol.* **44**, 428–433.

Broadbent, D. E. (1954). The role of auditory localization in attention and memory span. *J. Exp. Psychol.* **47**, 191–196.

Broadbent, D. E. (1956). Listening between and during practiced auditory distraction. *Br. J. Psychol.* **47**, 51–60.

Broadbent, D. E. (1958). "Perception and Communication." Pergamon, Oxford.

Broadbent, D. E. (1971). "Decision and Stress." Academic Press, New York.

Carson, R. H., and Sanderson, A. E. (1945). "The Radio Repeat Unit, an Application of Magnetic Reading." (OSRD Rep. 6070), Washington, D.C.

Cherry, E. C. (1953). Some experiments on the recognition of speech, with one and with two ears. *J. Acoust. Soc. Am.* **25**, 975–979.

Egan, J., Carterette, E. C., and Thwing, E. J. (1954). Some factors affecting multichannel listening. *J. Acoust. Soc. Am.* **26**, 774–782.

Garner, W. R. (1972). The acquisition and application of knowledge: A symbiotic relation. *Am. J. Psychol.* **27**, 941–946.

Gat, I. B., and Keith, R. W. (1978). An effect of linguistic experience. *Audiology* **17**, 339–345.

Gulian, E. (1973). Psychological consequences of exposure to noise, facts, and explanations. *Proc. Int. Congr. Noise Public Health Problem, May, Dubrovnik.* Available as U.S. Environmental Protection Agency Rep. 550/9-73-008 from U.S. Govt. Printing Office,Washington, D.C.

Haagen, C. H. (1945). "Intelligibility Measurement: Twenty-four Word Multiple Choice Tests" (OSRD Rep. 5567). Psychological Corp., New York.

Karlin, J. E., Abrams, M. H., Sanford, F. H., and Curtis, J. F. (1944). "Auditory Tests of the Ability to Hear Speech in Noise" (OSRD Rep. 3516). Harvard Univ., Cambridge, Massachusetts.

Klumpp, R. G., and Webster, J. C. (1958). Acoustical aspects of a speech communications systems designed for operation in high level noise. *J. Aud. Eng. Soc.* **6,** 179–183.

Klumpp, R. G., and Webster, J. C. (1961). Intelligibility of time-compressed speech. *J. Acoust. Soc. Am.* **33,** 265–267.

Klumpp, R. G., and Webster, J. C. (1963). Physical measurements of equally speech interfering noises. *J. Acoust. Soc. Am.* **35,** 1328–1338.

Moray, N. (1959). Attention in dichotic listening: Affective cues and the influence of instruction. *Q. J. Exp. Psychol.* **11,** 56–60.

Poulton, E. C. (1953). Two channel listening. *J. Exp. Psychol.* **46,** 91–96.

Spieth, W., and Webster, J. C. (1955). Listening to differentially filtered competing voice messages. *J. Acoust. Soc. Am.* **27,** 866–871.

Spieth, W., Curtis, J. F., and Webster, J. C. (1954). Cues that aid in listening to one of two simultaneous voice message. *J. Acoust. Soc. Am.* **26,** 391–396.

Thompson, P. O., Webster, J. C., Klumpp, R. G., and Bertsch, W. F. (1958). Two voice-message storage schemes. *J. Speech Hear. Res.* **1,** 142–154.

Thompson, P. O., Webster, J. C., and Gales, R. S. (1961). Liveness effects on the intelligibility of noise-masked speech. *J. Acoust. Soc. Am.* **33,** 604–605.

Treisman, A. M. (1964a). Effect of irrelevant material on efficiency of selective listening. *Am. J. Psychol.* **77,** 533–546.

Treisman, A. M. (1964b). Verbal cues, language, and meaning in selective attention. *Am. J. Psychol.* **77,** 206–219.

Webster, J. C. (1961). Information in simple multidimensional speech messages. *J. Acoust. Soc. Am.* **33,** 940–944.

Webster, J. C. (1965). Speech communications as limited by ambient noise. *J. Acoust. Soc. Am.* **37,** 692–699.

Webster, J. C. (1975). Psychoacoustic problems with noise control. *Conv. Audio Eng. Soc., 51st, Los Angeles* (Preprint).

Webster, J. C., and Klumpp, R. G. (1962). Effects of ambient noise and nearby talkers on a face-to-face communication task. *J. Acoust. Soc. Am.* **34,** 936–941.

Webster, J. C., and Klumpp, R. G. (1963). Articulation index and average curve-fitting methods of predicting speech interference. *J. Acoust. Soc. Am.* **35,** 1339–1344.

Webster, J. C., and Klumpp, R. G. (1965). "Speech Interfering Aspects of Navy Noises" (NEL Rep. 1314). Navy Electronics Laboratory, San Diego, California.

Webster, J. C., and O'Shea, N. P. (1980). Current developments in auditory speech discrimination tests for the profoundly hearing impaired at NTID. *Am. Ann. Deaf* **125,** 350–359.

Webster, J. C., and Sharpe, L. (1955). Improvements in message reception resulting from "sequencing" competing messages. *J. Acoust. Soc. Am.* **27,** 1194–1198.

Webster, J. C., and Solomon, L. N. (1955). Effects of response complexity upon listening to competing messages. *J. Acoust. Soc. Am.* **27,** 1199–1203.

Webster, J. C., and Thompson, P. O. (1953a). "Factors affecting Speech Intelligibility in Aircraft Control Towers" (NEL Rep. 357). Navy Electronics Laboratory, San Diego, California.

Webster, J. C., and Thompson, P. O. (1953b). Some audio considerations in air control towers. *J. Audio Eng.* **1,** 171–175.

Webster, J. C., and Thompson, P. O. (1954). Responding to both of two overlapping messages. *J. Acoust. Soc. Am.* **26,** 396–402.

Webster, J. C., Thompson, P. O., Snidecor, J. C., and Washburn, D. D. (1957). Speech pickup from various anatomical locations. *In* "A Decade of Basic and Applied Science in the Navy," pp. 213–218. U.S. Govt. Printing Office, Washington, D.C.

Young, R. W. (1964). Single-number criteria for room noise. *J. Acoust. Soc. Am.* **36,** 289–295.

IHC–TM Connect–Disconnect and Mechanical Interaction among IHCs, OHCs, and TM

Hewitt D. Crane

Sensory Sciences Research Center
SRI International
Menlo Park, California

HEARING RESEARCH AND THEORY, VOLUME 2

I. INTRODUCTION

How are we to reconcile these observations regarding the advanced mammalian auditory system?

1. The inner hair cells (IHCs) are disconnected from or only loosely coupled to the tectorial membrane (TM).
2. The majority of afferents innervate the IHCs.
3. The outer hair cells (OHCs) are firmly connected to the TM.
4. The majority of efferents terminate on the OHCs.
5. The main consequence of efferent excitation is afferent inhibition.
6. The maximum amplitude of the cochlear traveling wave at threshold is subangstrom.
7. The dynamic range of the auditory system is greater than 120 dB.

The first item is probably the most controversial, although evidence in its favor continues to accumulate (e.g., Kimura, 1966; Lim, 1972; Hoshino and Kodama, 1977).

For some time, the author has been developing a connect–disconnect model of IHC–TM interaction that is based on the assumption that the IHCs and TM are functionally disconnected. The model was motivated, first, by the growing number of indications that the IHCs, in contrast to the OHCs, seem to be disconnected from the TM, and second, by a type of mechanical impacting device developed by the author whose novel properties seemed applicable to an IHC–TM ''impact'' scheme. The basic notions behind these impacting devices are summarized in Section III.

Five previous papers (Crane, 1966, 1972, 1982a,b; Crane and Bell, 1976) have demonstrated that a connect–disconnect model of IHC–TM interaction is consistent with a broad range of psychophysical data. The present article pulls together the previous material and some new material in an attempt to explicate a model that makes sense of the entire set of observations noted above.

In all previous papers, a great simplification was made by ignoring the viscoelastic medium in which IHC–TM interaction occurs. Furthermore, ''connect'' and ''disconnect'' are macroscopic notions, whereas the deflection magnitudes of the BM at and even slightly above threshold are atomic and subatomic in magnitude. Clearly a more microscopic description of IHC–TM interaction is necessary. Section V brings together material that may bear on the nature of IHC–TM interaction. This literature currently exists only in the form of relatively isolated references. By bringing them together in one place, in an attempt to explore a connect–disconnect model in greater detail, we may see how these otherwise isolated references contribute to an integrated picture.

In all of the author's previous papers, except for the last, the focus was solely on IHC–TM interaction. The presence of OHCs was completely ignored. However, the OHC system represents a huge anatomical and physiological investment, and one might reasonably expect it to play a major role in cochlear function. A potentially interesting clue seemed to lie in a number of reports indicating that the OHCs exhibit large changes in size following intense auditory excitation. Given the relative orientation of the IHCs and OHCs and the prominent radial fiber system of the TM, it became intriguing to speculate that a change in OHC size might reflect itself in a change in IHC–TM spacing. That thought, in turn, led to a speculation that the (evolutionary) advantage of IHC–TM disconnect might be the achievement of wide dynamic range. However, such an achievement would require a means for dynamically controlling IHC–TM spacing. It was next speculated (Crane, 1982b) that such spacing control is achieved via the OHCs, under control of the efferent system, and that the entire network forms a slow-speed mechanical servo system distributed along the length of the cochlea. Sections VIII through X review some of the relevant literature and explore this notion in some detail.

Having extended the IHC–TM connect–disconnect model to include the potential for slow-speed mechanical interaction among the IHCs and OHCs, it is a direct step to envision the same mechanism playing a role at auditory frequencies as well, as discussed in Section VI. In particular, it is speculated that mechanical interaction among the IHCs and OHCs leads to motion magnification and a reduction in auditory threshold. Although the notion of IHC–OHC mechanical interaction at auditory frequencies actually followed the notion of slow-speed mechanical interaction, it seemed more logical in this treatment to present the former notion first.

Finally, it is shown that an extended connect–disconnect model, which includes the effects of IHC–OHC interaction, is also consistent with other familiar notions in the literature: second-filter phenomena (Section VII), nonlinear phase relations (Section XI), and two-tone suppression (Section XI).

II. BACKGROUND

With the IHCs disconnected from the TM, we could model their interaction as shown in Fig. 1. The stereocilia, represented by the single stereocilium, S, are connected to an IHC body represented simply by a spring (K_{HC}), which in turn is

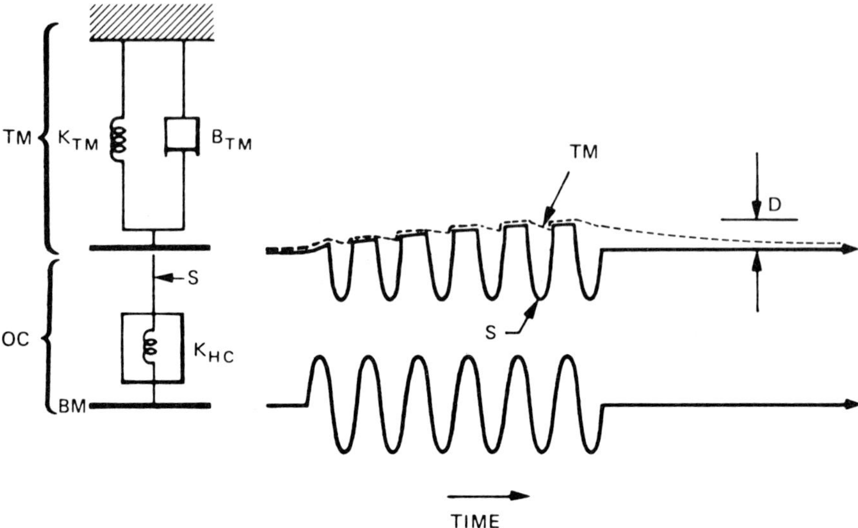

Figure 1 Modeling of impact between an IHC and the TM: S, stereocilium; K_{TM} and B_{TM}, spring and viscosity components of TM; K_{HC}, spring component of hair cell; D, steady-state separation; OC, organ of Corti; BM, basilar membrane.

connected to the basilar membrane (BM). The viscoelastic TM is modeled by a spring (K_{TM}) and dashpot (B_{TM}). At rest, it is assumed that the lower surface of the TM is in light contact with the stereocilium. In response to a sinusoidal input, the stereocilium would contact the TM during each upward half cycle of motion, and the TM and IHC would begin to separate, reaching a steady-state value, *D*, after some time interval. When excitation ceases, the separation would reduce toward zero. The rate and extent of separation and recovery depend on the mechanical properties of the stereocilia, the TM, the hair cells, and the fluid. The increase in separation during acoustic excitation would result in decreased impact strength and, therefore, would represent a component of afferent adaptation. The separation remaining after termination of the excitation would account for a short period of increased threshold and reduced spontaneous firing.

To model the entire cochlea would require a line of impacting IHC elements of the type shown in Fig. 1. In response to a steady tone, waves increase in amplitude as they propagate along the cochlear partition. According to the model, during each upward-directed half cycle, the IHCs would sequentially impact the TM with increasing strength along the cochlear partition, up to the characteristic place position, and with rapidly decreasing strength beyond that point. During each subsequent half cycle, the IHCs would pull away from the TM with corresponding amplitude distribution. In steady state, an IHC–TM separation would develop along the cochlea at each location that is proportional to the amplitude of the traveling-wave envelope at that point. It is predicted, therefore, that in steady state a plot of separation as a function of distance along the cochlea would have a shape similar to that of one side of the traveling-wave envelope.

The previous papers noted above have demonstrated how this sort of IHC–TM connect–disconnect can explain phenomena such as adaptation, fatigue, the masking of a high-frequency tone by a low-frequency tone, pitch shifts associated with such masking as well as with fatigue, the generation of the $2f_1-f_2$ combination tone (especially its constant intensity relation to the primaries), and, in conjunction with OHCs, the achievement of extended dynamic range under efferent control.

III. MECHANICAL IMPACTING DEVICES

The idea of a connect–disconnect mechanism evolved initially from a study of ways to abstract the envelope of an amplitude-modulated (a-m) wave with non-linear mechanical elements (Crane, 1966). In one arrangement, two mechanical elements were simply pressed against each other, as suggested in Fig. 2a. One element was driven by the a-m wave and the other served as a follower. In this configuration, the two elements could push but not pull on each other, and at any moment the two elements were either in contact (pressing against each other) or disconnected. During excitation the two elements separated automatically, the average separation depending upon the amplitude of excitation, the magnitude of the force holding the two elements together, and the time constant of the follower element. Such a mechanism has characteristics analogous to those of an envelope-follower, electronic-diode circuit. As more and more articles appeared in the auditory literature claiming that the IHCs were not firmly connected to the TM, it was suggestive that a similar disconnect mechanism might be at work. Of special interest in an envelope-follower mechanism are the noncritical nature of the contact force in the rest state and the one-sided nature of the contact, or excitation, which also seems typical of neural excitation in the cochlea.

Another configuration that was studied involved the generation of subharmonics. Whereas harmonics are easy to produce and require heroic efforts to avoid, subharmonic generation is generally much more difficult. It turns out, however, that subharmonic generation is easily achieved in an impact configuration (Crane, 1966). As suggested in Fig. 2b, the follower system is simply tuned to the desired subharmonic frequency and energy is transferred to it from the driver on every impact cycle. It is intuitively self-evident that a generator in this form can function properly, once started, if the driver and follower elements are correctly spaced. But we sought a mechanism that would self-start, and, because the motions involved were very tiny, we were concerned about being able to adjust and maintain the proper spacing. The answer both to proper spacing and self-starting turned out to be very simple. It was enough just to press the driver

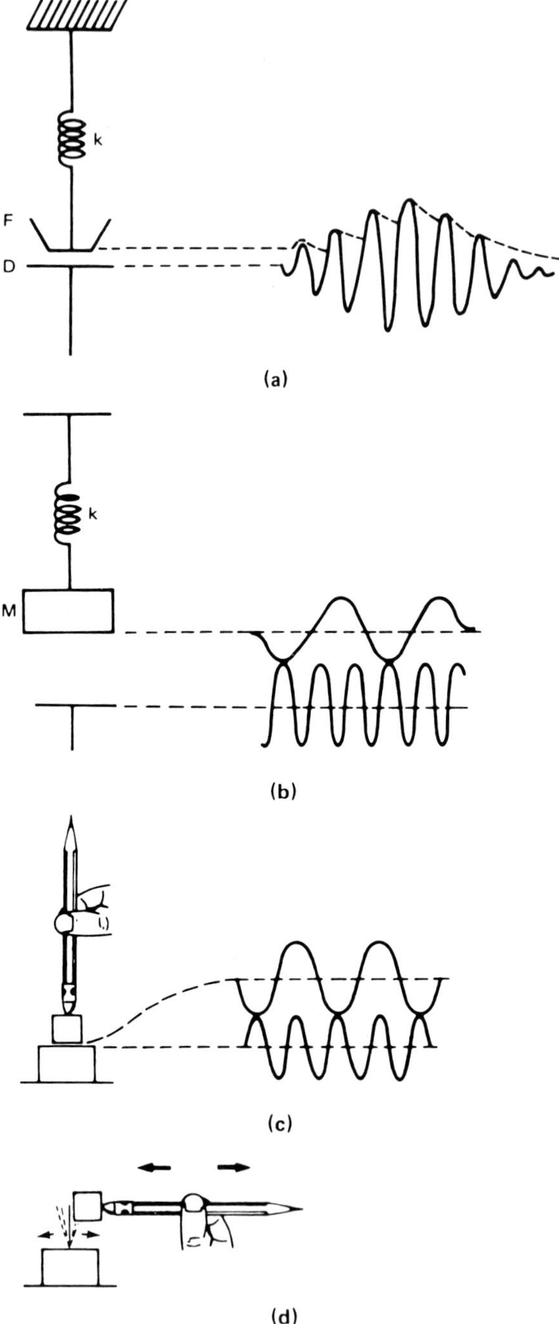

Figure 2 (a) Mechanical demodulator—driver element D can push but not pull on follower element F; (b) subharmonic generator; (c) automatic spacing—driver and follower elements are pressed together in the rest state and separate automatically during excitation; (d) rotating the direction of connect–disconnect by 90°.

and follower elements together with the proper compliance elements—e.g., the rubber end of a pencil—as illustrated in Fig. 2c. When the driver was energized, the follower element would begin to oscillate and would automatically space itself the proper distance away. Thus, even when dealing with tiny crystals operating in the megacycle range and with micron and submicron amplitudes of oscillation, spacing was not a problem because of this automatic spacing property. Shortly after this study was completed, Dallos (1966) reported subharmonics in the cochlea at very high acoustic levels. It might be that this sort of mechanism underlies his observations.

The idea of automatic spacing is basically behind the notion of Fig. 1 also. It is assumed that in the rest state the two "elements" (i.e., the BM–IHC–stereocilia system and the TM) are simply pressed together and that during excitation they separate by an amount dependent on the level of excitation. Questions for ultimate modeling are How, and by how much, are the IHCs and TM pressed together in the rest state? How much do they separate during excitation?

IV. MAGNITUDE AND DIRECTION OF CONNECT–DISCONNECT

Extrapolating from measurements made at high sound levels, von Békésy (1960) suggested that the threshold of a mid-range tone corresponds to a BM displacement on the order of 0.01 Å. Controversy remains on whether the magnitude at threshold is actually that small, although it seems clear that it is at least of atomic dimensions.

The amplitude of vibration increases 10-fold for every 20 dB increase in SL (or SPL). Given a 0.01 to 1.0 Å estimate at threshold, and that the amplitude of vibration might be decreased by up to 20 dB or so by the gain control mechanism of the middle ear, the amplitude of vibration at 120 dB would be on the order of 1 μm. A connect–disconnect mechanism, whether composed of mechanical or IHC–TM "devices," seems intuitively plausible at the micron level, which is huge compared with atomic dimensions. It is intuitively clear also that at this level of vibration, a change in separation of even a few tenths of a micron would lead to a large change in contact strength and contact duration each cycle. Given that it is the magnitude and duration of IHC–TM contact that control IHC excitation, such a change in spacing would lead to a correspondingly large change in afferent excitation. In Section X, we will speculate that control of afferent excitation, by means of IHC–TM spacing contol, is a primary function of the efferent system.

But what are we to say about a connect–disconnect mechanism at the angstrom level of excitation, i.e., near the threshold of auditory perception? The mechanism of Fig. 2 suggests a perfect state of separation between the two impacting surfaces alternating with a perfect state of connection. However, similar effects would be obtained if the two states were not so pure—e.g., if the two surfaces were coupled by a spring constant of one magnitude during separation and of another magnitude when pressed together. Similar mechanical effects, in other words, although weaker, may be obtained even when the connect and disconnect states are not pure. That would seem to be a way to characterize the effects when the amplitude of auditory vibration is of atomic dimensions: short-range, atomic field effects would become effective and the connect and disconnect states would no longer be so distinct. In that case, we may expect that the mechanical effects of connect–disconnect would hold over most of the auditory range but suddenly weaken when the amplitude of vibration reaches atomic dimensions.

It is commonly accepted that bending of the IHC stereocilia is involved in afferent excitation. A number of authors have pointed out, however, that the energy required for such bending is not compatible with the energy available at threshold levels of vibration. They suggest that molecular mechanisms of excitation are more appropriate; Naftalin (1977), for instance, analyzes several possible molecular mechanisms involving stereocilia–TM interaction. It is beyond the scope of this article to explore such mechanisms. However, we might note that even atomic or molecular size changes in IHC–TM separation could be effective in modulating field effects and therefore also effective in modulating afferent excitation, assuming excitation mechanisms of atomic or molecular scale.

In sum, we might expect that the space modulation caused by IHC–TM connect–disconnect would be effective in afferent control down to acoustic threshold levels whereas the mechanical effects of connect–disconnect may be significantly weakened at or slightly above threshold.

In addition to suggesting pure states of contact and separation, the mechanisms of Fig. 2 also suggests that the relevant direction of connect–disconnect is along the axis of vibration. However, the configuration is easily changed so that the relevant direction may be altered—e.g., by 90°, as suggested in Fig. 2d. This may be relevant because a number of experiments have suggested that the direction of IHC motion that causes afferent excitation may be primarily orthogonal to the axes of the stereocilia. Later we will point out that the extension of the TM known as Hensen's stripe provides a configuration similar to that of Fig. 2d and permits connect–disconnect action along an axis parallel to the TM.

The following section explores the anatomical relationship between the IHCs and TM in greater detail.

V. IHC–TM RELATIONSHIP

If IHC–TM contact underlies afferent excitation, then a low acoustic threshold requires that the TM and IHC stereocilia be in very close contact in the rest state.

This section explores briefly ways in which the TM and IHC stereocilia may be pressed together in the rest state and ways to characterize the nature of that state.

A. Contact Mechanisms

Figure 3 is a schematic of a mammalian organ of Corti drawn from samples prepared so as to minimize shrinkage of the TM. One gets the impression from such a drawing that the TM, which is bonded to all three rows of OHCs, simply presses against the IHC stereocilia and perhaps no other mechanism is required. On the other hand, Lim (1977, p. 404) notes that

> On the basis of SEM [scanning electron microscope] observations the presence of trabeculae-like structures along Hensen's stripe, which are suspected to be anchored to the inner hair cell region, has been reported.

These very tiny but stiff trabeculae, which are not always seen, apparently bridge from the TM to the IHCs in the region of Hensen's stripe and could be involved in adjusting IHC–TM spacing or preventing the TM and IHCs from moving too far apart. Or, as Lim (1980, p. 1692) suggests, they may be only "developmental remnants" without real function in adult animals.

In postulating rest–state mechanisms, it should be kept in mind that many elements may be at work. For instance, Flock (1980) has shown that actin filaments are present in the stereocilia of cochlear hair cells. Slepecky *et al.* (1980, p. 418) note a striated body that exists in the infracuticular plate region of IHCs (but not OHCs) and that

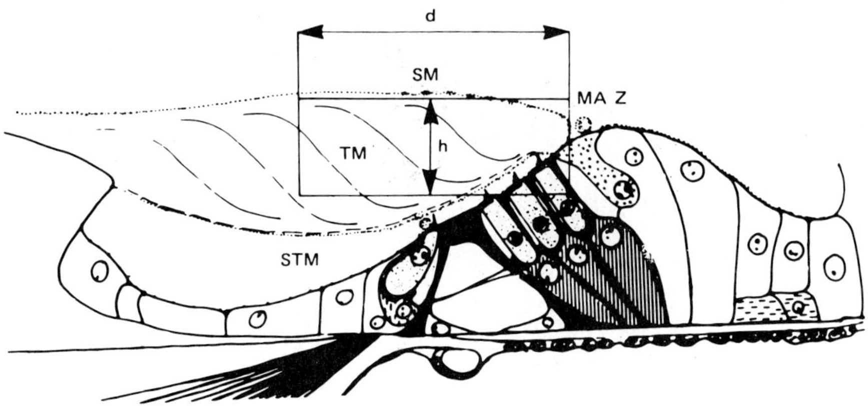

Figure 3 Schematic drawing of a mammalian organ of Corti with a well-preserved tectorial membrane (TM). *d*, diameter; SM, scala media; MA Z, marginal zone; h, height; STM, subtectorial membrane space. (From Kronester-Frei, 1979.)

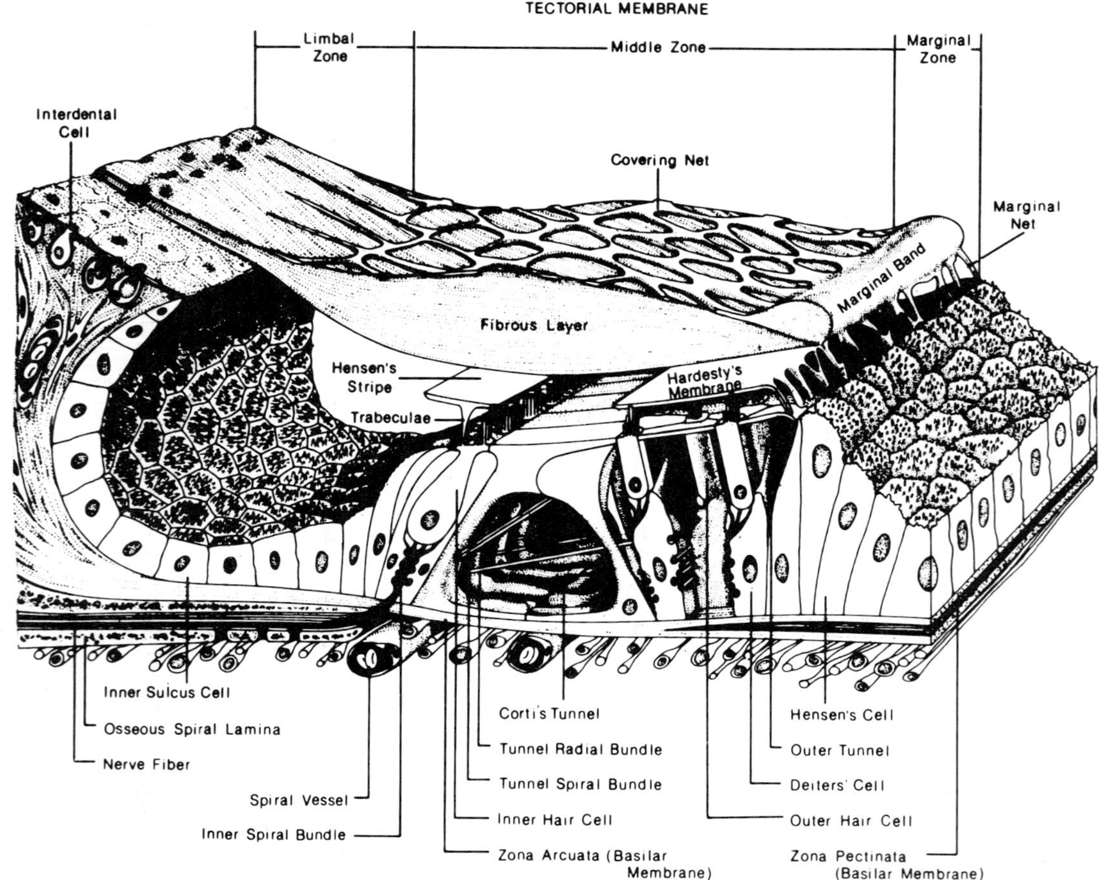

Figure 4   Schematic drawing of organ of Corti. (Reprinted from Lim, 1980.)

> Although we have no anatomical evidence for the shortening of stereocilia in the cochlear sensory cells [due to actin], there is some evidence that [a] circumferential contraction may occur [via the striated body].

Such a contraction could be involved in adjusting the vertical height of the IHCs and therefore could also be effective in IHC–TM spacing control.

In these discussions, it is important to realize that anatomical references are often highly oversimplified. The tectorial membrane, for instance, is made up of many different tissues. Figure 4, from Lim (1980), shows a relatively detailed schematic of the relationships among the various components of the tectorial membrane and organ of Corti.

B. IHC–TM Separation

The implication of Fig. 1 is that separation is taken up mainly by yielding of the viscoelastic TM. However, mechanisms within the cell body might also be involved. For instance, Hudspeth (1981, p. 94) notes that

> the relationship between displacement of the hair bundle's distal tip and the cellular response is remarkably steep [which] indicates a remarkable sensitivity [but small dynamic range]. The hair cell can, however, extend its effective operating range by an adaptation process that shifts the displacement-response curve along the displacement axis as a function of time following a static displacement.

If the stereocilia of the cochlear IHCs could adjust their average position during excitation, it would be equivalent to changing IHC–TM spacing, in the sense of Fig. 1. The implication might be that the cuticular plate, which contains the stereocilia, can rotate to some extent within the cell body. If that were the case, then following excitation both the TM and cuticular plate would relax back toward their rest–state condition. Equilibrium would be reached when the stereocilia touch the TM and the restoring forces are balanced. If the spontaneous firing rate at each position is determined by the equilibrium contact pressure, then its high variability might be indicative of variable equilibrium pressure from point to point along the cochlea.

Subtectorial fluid flow could also be a source of IHC–TM separation. For instance, Steele (1973) calculates that acoustic excitation would cause a rectified (i.e., DC) component of flow of endolymph from the inner sulcus, between the TM and reticular layers, and into the scala media. Such a flow would be in a direction to move the IHC stereocilia away from Hensen's stripe and therefore increase IHC–TM spacing. The magnitude of flow would depend on the level of excitation, and the magnitude of IHC–TM separation due to this component would therefore be graded along the cochlea. Steele suggests that this DC component of flow would probably occur only at high acoustic levels, but that is the range in which it would be of most interest as a mechanism for achieving extended dynamic range (see Section VIII). Subtectorial fluid flow is still questionable. Lawrence and Burgio (1980), for instance, find that in the normal cochlea the TM is tightly sealed to the Hensen's cells and endolymph cannot flow into the subtectorial space; but the seal can apparently be easily broken by mechanical damage or ionic changes in the fluids caused by experimental manipulation.

In addition to local flow within the scala media, other kinds of flow are also possible within the cochlea. For instance, Legouix and Pierson (1973, p. 18) report that, with intense sounds, a differential pressure develops between scala vestibuli (SV) and scala tympani (ST) with a resulting upward displacement of the cochlear partition. In particular, there is

> an outward flow of perilymph through small holes drilled in the wall of scala vestibuli. . . . In scala tympani the fluid pressure seemed to be decreased in such a way that, after a hole was made in the wall of scala tympani, air was often aspirated and tended to replace the fluid.

Following the end of the tone, the fluids flow back slowly and the cochlear partition resumes its original position. These studies were done with guinea pigs; the fluid flow as well as the deflection of the cochlear partition were observed directly under a low-power microscope. The authors also note that, following termination of an intense tone that is added to a sustained medium-level tone, the cochlear microphonic (CM) response to the sustained tone is greatly decreased for several seconds to several tens of seconds. During the recovery period, the CM response can be returned to normal instantly, simply by introducing an excess pressure in SV, which pushes the cochlear partition back to its normal position; if the excess pressure is removed, the normal CM recovery phase is resumed. Another observation of interest is that there is also a large decrease in action potential (AP) following the end of an intense tone, and that both the AP and CM responses to the sustained tone recover with the same time constant, suggesting that both responses may be controlled by the same mechanism.

The extended model of Section VI suggests that an upward movement of the BM may tend to *increase* rather than decrease IHC–TM separation and therefore reduce IHC–TM contact. This increased separation would reduce afferent excitation and therefore could explain the decreased magnitude of AP, noted above, for some period following termination of the intense tone. In line with the recent report of Pierson and Moller (1980), that the normal CM may be composed of contributions from both the IHCs and OHCs, it is possible that the reduced CM might also be due, in part, to the decreased IHC excitation following an intense tone.

Leguoix and Pierson (1973, p. 21) suggest that deflection of the cochlear partition might serve as a protective mechanism "since the vibratory movements [as reflected by the decrease in CM] are probably decreased" by these deflections. According to the model developed here, we would suggest that any protective mechanism would more likely be reflected in decreased IHC–TM impact strength. In any case, if this fluid-flow mechanism leads to an increase in IHC–TM separation during intense tones, it would also contribute to the achievement of extended dynamic range (see Section VIII).

C. Sensitization

A connect–disconnect model would suggest that an increase in average IHC–TM separation along the cochlea would cause an increase in acoustic threshold because a larger amplitude of vibration would then be required to cause

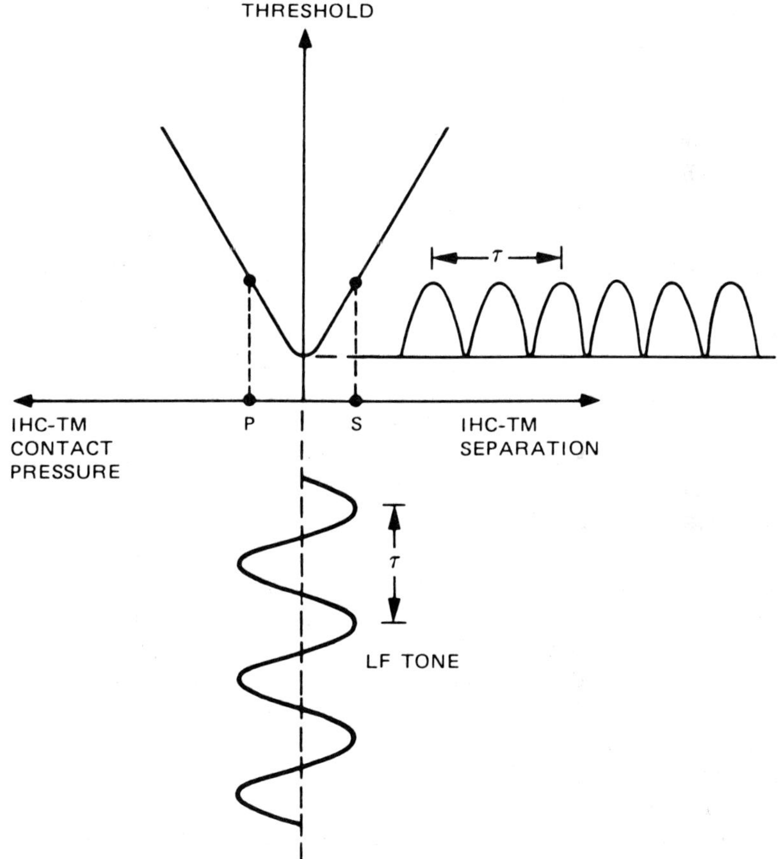

Figure 5 Even-valued function of threshold as a function of IHC–TM spacing. If the rest state corresponds to the minimum point, as illustrated, the threshold increases for either direction of spacing change. If the rest state is shifted to one side or the other of the minimum (i.e., to point P or point S), the threshold will decrease (sensitization) for small motions in the direction opposite to the shift.

IHC–TM contact. We would expect that an increase in average IHC–TM contact pressure would similarly cause an increase in acoustic threshold, because the increased IHC excitation would result in an increased background noise level (spontaneous firing rate). In other words, the model predicts an increase in threshold both with increased IHC–TM separation and with increased IHC–TM contact pressure, as suggested in Fig. 5. Zwicker (1977) shows that there are, in fact, two increases in the threshold of a short high-frequency (HF) tone burst as its phase position is varied through one period of a simultaneous low-frequency (LF) tone. Crane (1982a) suggests that the LF tone synchronously alters the threshold in the basal region of the cochlea according to a curve of the form shown in Fig. 5, and that the two maxima of threshold shift are related to these two mechanisms: increased IHC–TM separation and increased IHC–TM excitation.

If the IHC–TM rest state were precisely represented by the minimum position in Fig. 5, there would be a threshold increase for BM motion in either direction. However, the results of Deatherage and Henderson (1967) and Zwicker (1977) suggest that the rest state is not at the minimum point. Both papers show that at some particular phase of the LF tone the threshold for the HF tone burst is even less than if the LF tone were not present. Deatherage and Henderson called this phenomenon ''sensitization,'' referring to the fact that the threshold in the presence of the second tone is actually less than the unmasked threshold. This result suggests that the resting state is displaced from the minimum (e.g., to some point P or point S in the figure) and that at the proper phasing, the IHC–TM spacing is brought nearer to the minimum threshold point. A basic question is which direction of displacement properly defines the rest state: a rest-state pressure, denoted by point P, or a rest-state separation, denoted by point S?

Crane (1982a) concludes that point S properly describes the rest state *if* Zwicker's assumptions regarding BM phasing with respect to LF input tones are correct, and if one makes the common assumption that IHC excitation corresponds with upward (SV-directed) BM motion. However, in Section VI we will argue that at low frequencies, IHC–TM contact may more likely correspond with downward (ST-directed) BM motion. This result would reverse the conclusion and argue for point P of Fig. 5 (i.e., a static pressure) as the proper description of the rest state. In that case, we would expect a decrease in firing rate (below the spontaneous rate) for a small decrease in contact pressure and an increase in firing rate for a small increase in contact pressure. Schmiedt (1980), recording from Mongolian gerbils and using a very-low-frequency (10 Hz) triangular pressure wave (which results in trapezoidal BM motion) reports just such a result; in particular he reports a significant decrease in firing rate (below spontaneous) during SV displacement of the BM and an increase during ST displacement. (We disagree with his interpretation, however, that the response to a test tone during the ST phase, because of the increased firing rate, is more sensitive than during the SV phase. According to our model, the higher firing rate during the ST phase would correlate with an increase in threshold to a test tone and the response would therefore be *less* sensitive.) In any case, as discussed in Crane (1982a), the nature of the rest state is still not clear. The discussion of the next section, for instance, lends some credence to point S as representing the rest state. This uncertainty suggests that although sensitization seems convincingly demonstrated, further research is necessary to describe the exact rest–state condition.

D. Brownian Motion

Harris (1968) analyzes the expected level of Brownian motion in the cochlea and compares it with the actual auditory threshold. His conclusion is that if the hair cells are tightly coupled to the TM so that they are forced to vibrate in synchronism, the magnitude of vibration caused by thermal excitation is about 20 dB below the actual auditory threshold and is therefore insignificant. With very weak coupling to the TM, however, the hair cells can vibrate independently, and Harris calculates that the thermal motion would then be about 30 dB above the actual auditory threshold. He concludes from these extremal calculations (Harris, 1968, p. 176) that

> it is necessary to assume that the stereocilia are attached to the tectorial membrane and that the hair-cell bodies are imbedded in the organ of Corti with some degree of rigidity.

An additional parameter offered by a connect–disconnect model is the potential for variable IHC–TM coupling. In particular, as the IHCs and TM are pressed together, we would expect from Harris' argument that increased system coupling might at first cause a decrease in the (spontaneous) firing rate before it increases with increasing contact pressure. This perspective would suggest that the rest state might properly be described by point S in Fig. 5, and that the dip in threshold for operating points slightly to the left of point S (i.e., sensitization) is due to increased system coupling and therefore decreased noise level.

The next section explores the potential for variable IHC–TM coupling from yet another perspective.

E. Static Bonding: Dynamic Release

Over the years an increasing number of authors have referred to the presence of mucopolysaccharides in the vestibular and cochlear ducts. Malcolm (1974, p. 769), for instance, notes that certain

> properties of the vestibular apparatus can be explained if one considers the gel often seen in the inner ear. Vilstrup and Jensen [1960] reported on a mucopolysaccharide in the vestibular apparatus which they believed was either hyaluronic acid or chondroitin sulphate.
>
> Von Békésy often noticed that the scala media of the guinea pig was filled with a gel when it

> was carefully opened. The present author has found that the ampulla of the frog is filled with a gel . . . [and that] the gel is quite flexible, and can be moved back and forth through the ampulla. If the motion is made just a little too vigorously, the plug of gel seems to suddenly disappear, as if it turned to liquid in one quick stroke.

Malcolm notes that in concentrations greater than 0.1%, mucopolysaccharides form a thixotropic material. A thixotropic material has the property of being solid at rest but fluid under shear motion (Wilkinson, 1960). The presence of such a material in the scala media suggests other possibilities for the nature of IHC–TM interaction. It has been noted, for instance, that the various rows of stereocilia may be bound together by mucopolysaccharides (e.g., Kimura, 1966; Lim, 1972; Ross, 1974; Flock, 1977). Taber (1979) suggests that this bonding may make the stereocilia array on each hair cell stiffer. But the presence of thixotropic material in the scala media suggests not only that the stereocilia may be bound to each other but also that the interaction between the IHC stereocilia and the TM may be mediated by this form of material. In that case, the IHC stereocilia and TM may not have to be in actual contact in the rest state or during excitation, because the space between would be filled with a firm gel. However, the gel may soften or liquefy in the vicinity of the stereocilia during acoustic stimulation; in that case, the magnitude of the local "pocket" so formed would depend on the magnitude and frequency of the acoustic excitation. Thus, it may be necessary to distinguish between the nature of the bonding in the static and dynamic cases. If the stereocilia are embedded in a thixotropic material, they might appear to be tightly bound to each other and to the TM in the rest state. However, if the material liquefies during motion, they would become more and more separated during excitation. This type of variable pocket-forming mechanism was suggested by Crane (1972) as a possible explanation for the normalizing type of "essential" nonlinearity that seems necessary to account for the constant intensity relation between the $2f_1 - f_2$ combination tone and the f_1, f_2 primaries.

Materials with thixotropic properties are found throughout the body (Wainwright *et al.*, 1976, pp. 119–123). However, their properties have been studied and are understood mainly in connection with macroscopic motions. The nature and magnitude of the softening or liquefication that may occur with angstrom and subangstrom motions is not known. A plot of viscosity versus shear rate for a tpyical thixotropic material shows a relatively constant viscosity up to some critical level of shear rate, beyond which the viscosity can decrease abruptly. Below the critical shear rate, new entanglements (of the macromolecules) are created as rapidly as old ones are released. Beyond the critical rate, entanglements are released faster than new ones can be formed and the material becomes more liquid. D. B. Cotts (personal communication) suggests that some materials can show significant thixotropic effects at extremely low shear rates not because of entanglement effects but because of the making and breaking of weak chemical bonds or cross-links such as hydrogen bonds. If this were the case with the thixotropic materials in the cochlea, there might be significant softening or liquefying effects even with very small motions.

Research is showing that a gel is an intermediate state between a liquid and solid, with unusual properties. For instance, Tanaka (1981) notes that a gel can release interstitial fluids and change volume reversibly by factors greater than 100 : 1. He notes also (p. 19) that the change in state can be rapid, at least for small volumes:

> [The time to reach a new equilibrium volume] is proportional to the cross-sectional area of the gel. A column of gel one micron in diameter . . . would shrink or swell in about a millisecond.

Tanaka *et al*. (1982) note that the large, reversible volume changes can occur as a result of very tiny changes in electric field.

We might also note these observations of Naftalin *et al*. (1964, p. 1064):

> The usual histological picture . . . shows a retracted tectorial membrane occupying perhaps a tenth part of the [scala media]. In the fresh specimen the relative volumes of the jelly and of endolymph seem to be the reverse. . . .

and (p. 1065) that

> the jelly [i.e. the TM] quickly retracts and becomes a friable whitish fibre after a few moments on a glass slide [after the TM has been surgically removed].

Naftalin *et al*. also note that the TM is much larger in the apical turns than in the basal end. (No mention is made about where along the cochlea the sketch of Fig. 3 derives.)

Given that the explanation of afferent excitation and neural tuning remains stalled at the mechanical–neural interface, it seems critical that major research be focused on understanding these cochlea fluids and gels. Bits and pieces of ideas exist; for example, the fact that stereocilia membranes carry a surface charge has been suggested by Flock *et al*. (1977). Might this charge electrostatically bind the thixotropic material and might it be these bonds that break at low shear rates? And might this making and breaking of electrical bonds be involved in the mechanism of resistance change?

The presence of thixotropic materials in the scala media can possibly also explain the conflict that still exists regarding how tightly the IHCs are connected to the TM. Some experimenters report that the connection must be firm because they find broken tips of IHC stereocilia bound to the TM when they separate the organ of Corti and the TM, while others report clean separation. The difference in results might simply depend on the ''rate'' at which the organ of Corti is pulled from the TM. A clean separation might be achieved every time if the separation were made during acoustic stimulation, which would ensure liquefaction or softening (i.e., dynamic disconnect) if thixotropic properties indeed govern the binding mechanism. Stereocilia and hair-cell binding by a gel-like material might also significantly affect the rest-state noise level caused by Brownian motion.

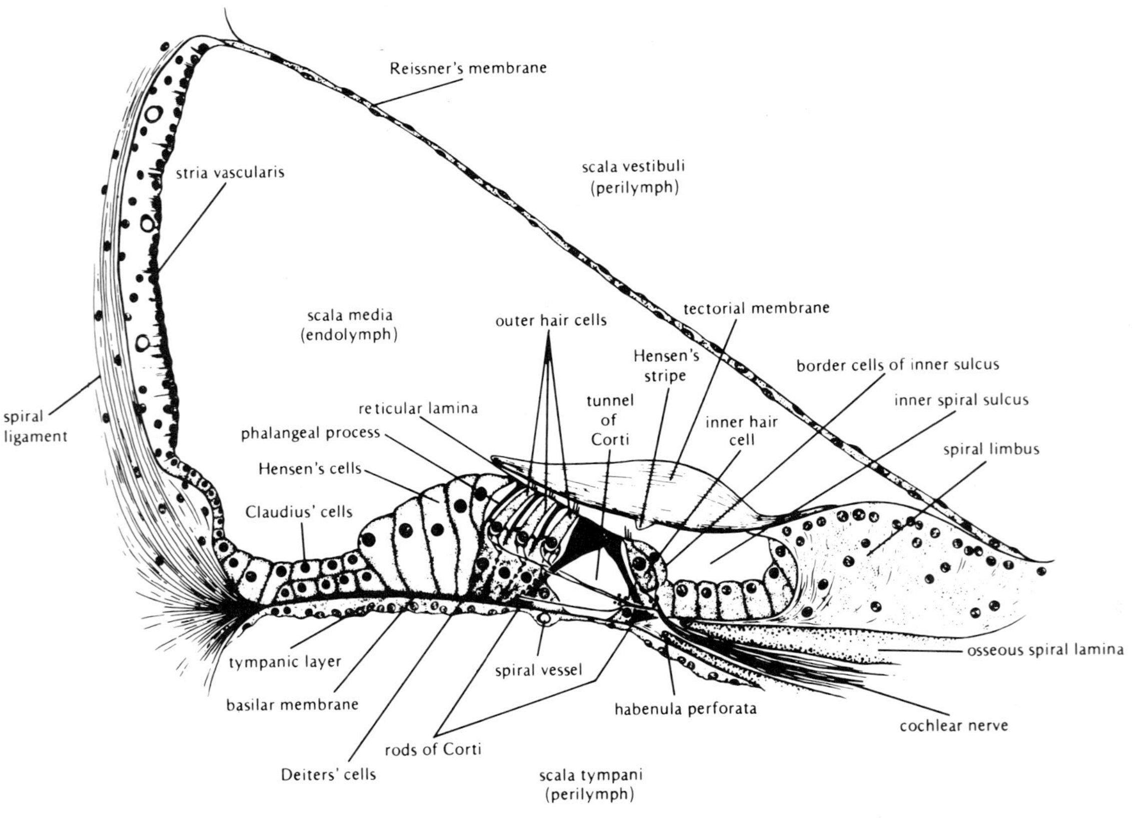

Figure 6 Cross-sectional sketch of organ of Corti. (Reprinted from Yost and Nielsen, 1977.)

VI. MECHANICAL INTERACTION BETWEEN IHCs, OHCs, AND TM

Figure 6, from Yost and Nielsen (1977), shows in the vicinity of the IHCs an extension of the TM known as Hensen's stripe. Figure 8 of Lim (1972) shows a similar form of stripe. (Such a stripe was indicated schematically in Fig. 4.) The illustrations suggest that the sloping side of the stripe facing the IHCs tends to match the stepped rows of stereocilia. In that case, vibration of the BM would tend to cause both lateral and axial components of contact between the TM and the IHC stereocilia, as suggested in Fig. 7a. In other words, the presence of a Hensen's stripe allows for lateral as well as axial modes of impact. The exact mechanical situation is unclear, however, because of reported variation in the form of Hensen's stripe not only between species but also between turns of the cochlea and even between animals of the same species. Assuming a stripe of the form illustrated in Fig. 7a, IHC–TM contact could occur if the IHC moved upward—i.e., toward SV—or if the TM moved downward—i.e., toward ST.

A. Phase Opposition between the IHC and TM Components of Motion

The notion that both IHC and TM motion can alter IHC–TM spacing brings us to a further development of the model. Let us define the TM movement in the vicinity of the IHCs that results from radially adjacent OHC movement as the "TM component" of motion. In view of the radial fiber system in the TM (Iurato, 1967), and because the OHCs and TM are firmly bonded, any OHC movement would likely cause a corresponding TM movement. The radial structure of the TM is also emphasized by Naftalin (1977, p. 359), who notes that the embryological TM is formed in the radial direction and the individual sections are later fused longitudinally. The essence of the arrangement illustrated in Fig. 7a is that an upward movement of the TM would have an *opposite* polarity of effect, regarding IHC–TM contact or separation, from an upward movement of the IHCs.

Let us assume that an upward movement of the BM causes an upward motion of both the IHCs and OHCs and, further, that the upward OHC motion results, in turn, in a corresponding upward movement of the TM. In that case, either IHC or OHC movement could dominate IHC (afferent) excitation, but with opposite polarity effects, depending on the relative magnitude of the two components. With a small TM component, IHC movement would dominate and we would expect afferent excitation during downward (ST-directed) movement of the BM.

It is not yet clear how to model OHC–IHC mechanical coupling quantitatively in a radial direction. The strength of the radial TM fibers, the properties of the TM gel, and the mechanical impedances offered by the surrounding scala media

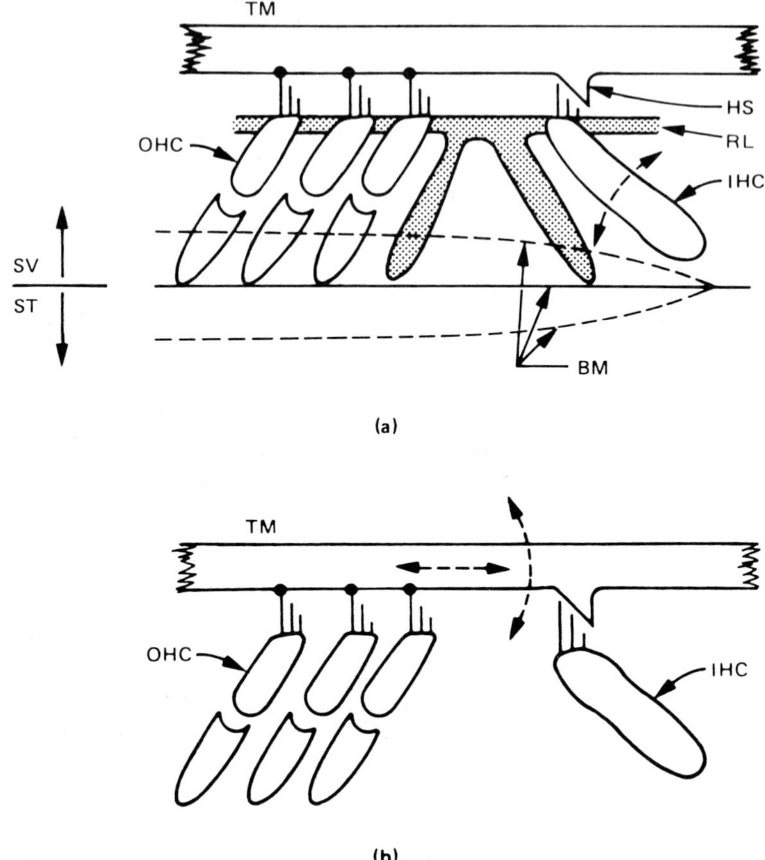

Figure 7 Schematic drawing of the mechanical relationship between IHCs, OHCs, and TM. (a) Upward BM movement would tend to rotate IHC stereocilia into contact with Hensen's stripe (HS); (b) mechanical resonance of OHC stereocilia and TM would cause sharply tuned and amplified radial motion of OHCs (straight dashed line) or transverse motion (curved dashed line): SV, scala vestibuli; ST, scala tympani; TM, tectorial membrane; RL, reticular lamina.

and inner spiral sulcus fluids are basically unknown. [The elements of such an analysis are illustrated by Zwislocki and Kletsky (1979) who attempt to model the effects of radial shear between the tectorial and reticular membranes.] Nevertheless, the configuration of Fig. 7a is interesting because it allows for a mechanical explanation of either ST- or SV-directed BM motion as the cause of afferent excitation, depending on the relative magnitudes of IHC and TM motion. This is of interest because of increasing evidence, noted below, that at low frequencies afferent excitation correlates with ST-directed BM motion (at least in the apical region of the cochlea), which is contrary to the commonly held belief that afferent excitation generally correlates with SV-directed BM motion. If that indeed is the case, then it is necessary to explain a transition from ST-directed excitation at low acoustic frequencies (corresponding to maximum excitation in the apical region of the cochlea) to SV-directed BM excitation at higher frequencies (corresponding to maximum excitation toward the basal region).

To explore the extent to which the phase-opposition mechanism of Fig. 7a might underlie such a transition, we make the further assumptions that (1) there is a transmission delay in the TM component of motion relative to OHC motion, and (2) OHC motion is larger than IHC motion. The first assumption seems reasonable in view of the viscoelastic properties of the TM. The second assumption seems reasonable on anatomical grounds, because the OHCs are set well out on the BM as compared with the IHCs. Furthermore, Zwislocki (1980) speculates that the stereocilia and TM form a sharply tuned system and that the magnitude of lateral stereocilia motion may be significantly larger than the magnitude of the (vertical) BM motion. This result would lend further credence to the second assumption if it were shown that it is mainly the OHCs, which are firmly bonded to the TM, that undergo such highly tuned motion. In suggesting this mechanism, Zwislocki is primarily interested in identifying a sharpening or second-filter mechanism. In addition, a high-Q lateral motion of the OHCs, coupled with lateral *mechanical* interaction of the IHCs and OHCs, as suggested by the horizontal dashed line in Fig. 7b, would result in an increase in auditory sensitivity. That is, a small (vertical) BM motion would be amplified into a larger TM component of motion, which could dominate IHC–TM connect–disconnect and therefore significantly lower the threshold of afferent excitation. Loss of this amplification mechanism could offer a partial explanation for the large increase in afferent threshold with kanamycin poisoning of the OHCs (Ryan and Dallos, 1975). (See ''Note,'' p. 167.)

We might add one additional consideration. If the IHCs as well as the OHCs were firmly bonded to the TM, then primary interest would be with lateral-motion mechanisms (i.e., relative shear). With IHC–TM disconnect, however, a vertical rocking motion of the OHC stereocilia–TM system, as suggested by the curved dashed line in Fig. 7b, would be of as much interest as a radial motion (suggested by the straight dashed line) as far as enhancing afferent excitation.

Given the two assumptions noted above, we could expect that the TM component might be larger than the IHC component and would dominate, causing ST-directed excitation. In fact, Konishi and Nielsen (1978) obstructed the helicotrema in guinea pigs and manipulated the ST pressure directly at the round window. For low frequencies of excitation, they report (p. 297):

> The principal findings were that the majority of the auditory nerve fibers were excited by the motion of the basilar membrane . . . toward the scala tympani and that the spontaneous activity was decreased by motion in the opposite direction.

Because of the viscoelastic elements present, it is also likely that, relative to OHC motion, the amplitude of the TM component of motion would be frequency dependent. It is not clear a priori whether to expect an increasing or decreasing function of frequency, for that would depend on how the TM is supported as well as the nature of the interaction between the radial TM fibers and the surrounding gel structure. To correlate with OHC dominance at low frequencies and IHC dominance at high frequencies, we would predict a decreasing function (i.e., increasing attenuation with increasing frequency). However, if attenuation of the TM component were the sole effect of increasing acoustic frequency, we would expect zero excitation (i.e., exact cancellation of the IHC and TM components) at some intermediate frequency. However, this is unlikely because of phase shift. For instance, even if the IHC and TM components were identical in amplitude, the net amplitude of IHC–TM variation with a 90° phase shift between the two components would be larger than either component (zero phase here implies that the TM and the IHC stereocilia would be moving in the same direction); with 180° phase shift, the TM component would directly add to, rather than subtract from, the IHC component. There are a number of possible sources of mechanical delay and phase shift along the pathway involving the cell bodies, stereocilia, and TM. The TM itself is often described as a gel. One special property of gels is their unusually low acoustic velocity. For instance, Naftalin (1970) notes that the velocity of sound in a solution of 10% gelatine is 5 m/sec (Table 17-1, p. 209) although the

> . . . wavelength [velocity] might be even smaller in the tectorial membrane because of its ordered structure as opposed to the random arrangement in gelatine.

At one-tenth the velocity in gelatine (i.e., at 0.5 m/sec) the propagation delay along the approximately 50 μm that separate the IHCs and the center of the OHC rows would be about 100 msec, which represents 90° at 2.5 kHz.

B. Experimental Data on Phase Opposition

The notion that there may be a polarity, or phase, opposition between the IHCs and OHCs, with regard to afferent excitation, was explored in a model by Zwislocki (1977). The type of data on which he based his model is shown in Fig. 8. A triangular sound pressure wave, Fig. 8a, causes a traveling wave of trapezoidal displacement along the cochlear partition, as evidenced by the averaged round-window CM (Fig. 8b). Figure 8c shows a typical post-stimulus time (PST) histogram response from a LF fiber (<2 kHz) in normal gerbils. For these fibers, the firing rate during SV displacement is below the spontaneous level and during ST displacement is above the spontaneous level; this could be explained by a larger TM than IHC component of motion, as noted earlier. Also note the transient responses during the transitions; according to our model, these could be

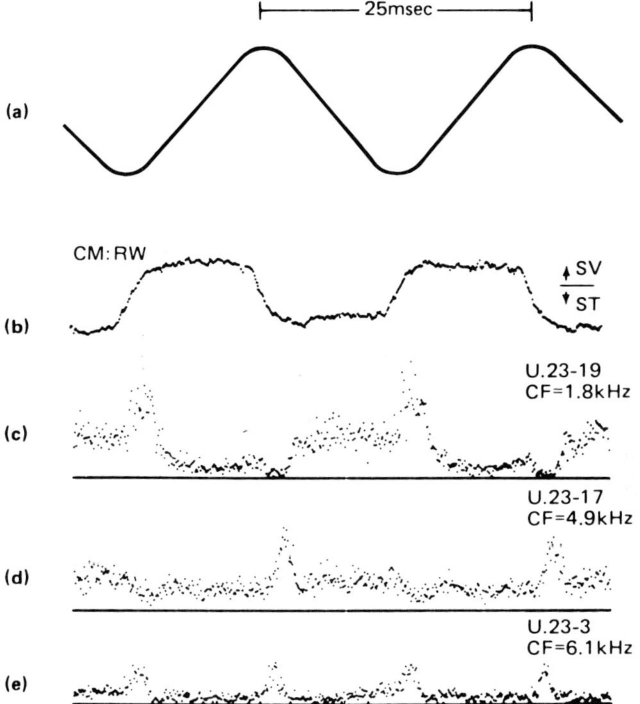

Figure 8   (a) Triangular pressure input waveform leads (b) to a trapezoidal CM: (c,d,e) are PST histograms for different CF fibers. (These records are adapted from Sokolich *et al.*, 1976.)

explained by a short delay in the mechanical transmission from the OHCs via the TM to the region of the IHCs. Thus, during an ST-to-SV movement of the BM, the afferent firing rate would transiently increase before decreasing, because the IHCs would move upward, causing increased excitation, before the TM in the neighborhood of the IHCs could begin to move upward by an even larger amount as a result of OHC movement. Conversely, during an SV-to-ST movement of the BM, the firing rate would transiently decrease before increasing, because the IHCs would move downward, causing decreased excitation, before the TM in the neighborhood of the IHCs could begin to move downward.

Figure 8d and e shows different forms of response for the same LF input signal but from medium-frequency and high-frequency fibers. It is tempting to try to alter our model to account for such variation in response along the cochlea; however, that is probably premature. Furthermore, there might be variations in the exact form of response among different animals. For instance, Fig. 9, from Sellick and Russell (1980), shows for the same form of input signal an intracellular recording from an IHC of the basal turn (i.e., a *high-frequency* fiber) in

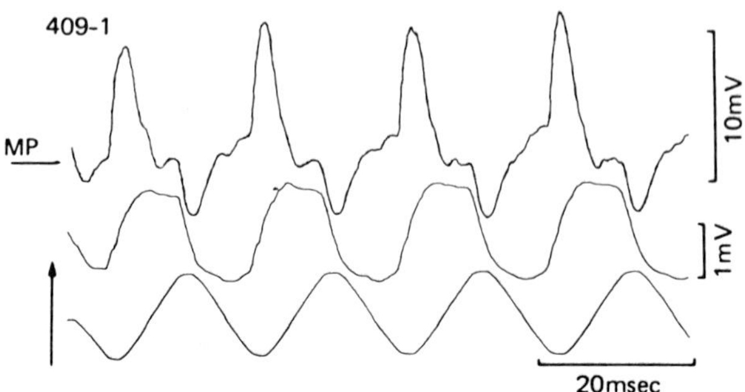

Figure 9   Receptor potential recorded intracellularly from IHCs in the basal turn of the guinea pig cochlea in response to a 52-Hz triangular acoustic stimulus at 100 dB SPL: upper trace, receptor potential; middle trace, CM recorded adjacent to intracellular recording site; lower trace, sound pressure recorded at tympanic membrane. MP indicates membrane potential. Arrow in bottom trace indicates direction of rarefaction. (Figure and caption adapted from Sellick and Russell, 1980.)

guinea pigs, which has almost exactly the same form as the firing histogram shown in Fig. 8c for a low-frequency fiber in Mongolian gerbils.

In any case, based on this type of data, Zwislocki (1977, p. 126) concluded that

> The complex response patterns [to triangular pressure waveforms] could only be explained by assuming that they resulted from two displacement components of opposite polarity, which tended to cancel each other but were not exactly matched in amplitude and latency.

Zwislocki suggests that the phenomenon is probably caused by some sort of direct (''private line'') neural interaction between the OHCs and IHCs, and that the two components have different relative strengths in the basal and apical regions. However, it is not clear that the physiology is appropriate to a neural inhibitory action of the OHCs on the IHCs. What is appealing about the mechanical coupling mechanism of Fig. 7a is that the OHCs and IHCs are equally potent with respect to afferent excitation, the net effect depending simply on the relative strengths and latencies of their motion.

C. Other Modes

In the previous section, we assumed that an upward movement of the OHCs results in an upward movement of the attached section of TM. However, other modes are possible. Steele (1976) analyzes three deflection modes of the arch in the organ of Corti: a stationary mode, arch rotation, and vertical arch vibration without rotation. We do not know which type of deflection model is correct, although each implies different motions for the adjacent IHCs. Also, the mode might vary along the cochlea, being different in the basal, middle, and apical turns. For instance, with a relatively stationary arch, and with the three rows of OHCs firmly bonded to the TM, the impression from Fig. 3 is that an upward BM motion might well create a downward pivoting of the TM. The IHC component of motion would then be zero, and the TM component of motion would be reversed in polarity compared with the mode discussed in the previous section.

Our inability to quantify these modes, or even to predict which is more likely, emphasizes the premature nature of the model. At this stage, perhaps the strongest statement that can be made regarding the immediate issues is that the potential exists for explaining a wide range of data. For instance, it is possible that there is even a shift in these arch modes along the cochlea or that at a given point along the cochlea the mode may depend on frequency. This result, and the possibility of attenuation of the TM component with frequency, as discussed in the previous section, could both underlie shifts between IHC and OHC dominance along the cochlea.

VII. SECOND FILTER

There have been extensive efforts to identify a second filter in the cochlea (e.g., Evans and Wilson, 1973; Zwislocki and Kletsky, 1979). By "second filter" is meant a mechanism by which the broadly tuned traveling wave is transformed into sharp neural tuning curves. The model developed here offers other second-filter mechanisms.

Zwislocki (1980) suggests that radial TM motion, represented by the horizontal dashed line of Fig. 7b, may be highly tuned and therefore could result in neural tuning that is much sharper than the mechanical tuning of the BM. A rocking motion of the TM, represented by the curved dashed line of Fig. 7b, could yield similar results. Second, assuming that afferent excitation is caused by some form of IHC–TM contact and that the contact pressure depends on both IHC and TM motion, the net excitation will depend on both the relative *phase* and *direction* of the OHC contribution at the location of the IHCs. The phase of the IHC and TM components can differ because the IHC and OHC motions can be out of phase (e.g., caused by radial-wave modes) or because of phase shift in the transmission path via the TM. Regarding directional effects, von Békésy (1960, p. 497) noted a radical shift in the direction of hair cell vibration along the cochlea: a vertical motion at the maximum position, a radial motion on the stapes side of the maximum, and a longitudinal motion on the helicotrema side of the maximum. Maximum IHC–TM excitation would occur when the IHC and TM components of motion at the IHC location were along the same direction of motion and 180° out of phase. If that were the condition at the maximum, or place, position, any relative phase or directional shifts between the IHCs and OHCs on either side of the maximum would reduce the net excitation and result in sharpening of the neural response curve relative to the mechanical traveling wave. Zwislocki and Sokolich (1974) also suggested that a phasing relationship might underlie the second-filter effect but in the realm of neural rather than mechanical OHC–IHC interaction.

If OHC–IHC interaction is the basis of the second-filter mechanism, we might expect a significant change in neural tuning curves following kanamycin destruction of OHCs. Although there is general agreement about a large increase in threshold, it is still controversial whether there is a significant change in tuning characteristics. Evans and Harrison (1975) claim a loss in tuning sharpness, whereas Dallos *et al.* (1977) report little change. Further data will be necessary to resolve this issue.

VIII. VARIABLE IHC–TM SPACING AND DYNAMIC RANGE

Techniques for measuring tiny motions obviously require parameters that are sensitive to such motions. One common measurement technique depends on variation in spacing between two closely spaced surfaces, as in a capacitive microphone. Another technique depends on variation in the phase of a tone or wave, as in interferometry or Mössbauer techniques. With the development of a closely spaced TM and hair-cell layer, evolution seems to have adapted the former technique in achieving extreme sensitivity to motion in the inner ear. However, given this counterposed set of hair cells and TM, a logical question is how the sensory receptors (hair cells) should interact with the TM. Specifically, should they be firmly attached or only in loose contact?

The auditory system has an amplitude range greater than six orders of magnitude (i.e., greater than 120 dB). What is astonishing is not that the eardrum, middle ear bones, or cochlear duct can handle that large a range but that the afferent system does not saturate. Plots of single-fiber firing rate as a function of the level of an input tone indeed do saturate, in a range of 20–50 dB (e.g., Kiang, 1965, p. 82); in fact, the average firing rate often declines with further increases in level. However, average firing rate per se is *not* the sole feature of interest. At least in the frequency range where firing is synchronized with the acoustic signal, the preservation of timing and synchronization is of as great interest as average rate; indeed, timing and synchronization of firing are well preserved over a wide dynamic range (Kiang, 1965; Johnson, 1980). In thinking about mechanism, therefore, it is as important to focus on methods for preserving timing relations as on average firing rate.

Large dynamic range in the visual system is accounted for by an adjustable pupil, automatic gain control in the neural circuitry (e.g., by means of lateral inhibition), and bleaching of the receptor photopigments. Like the pupil of the eye, the stapedius muscle of the middle ear accounts for a small amount of dynamic range. There likely are similar gain-control circuits in the auditory neural circuitry. Whether there are processes in the IHCs that are triggered by mechanical rather than by electromagnetic energy and that would correspond to optical bleaching is an open question; an example of such a process might be a reversible loss of stereocilia stiffness with intense sounds—for example, Engstrom and Engstrom (1978) note such a softening, at least for OHC stereocilia; Naftalin (1977, pp. 367–368) discusses the possibility from a molecular perspective.

IHC disconnect can also contribute to wide dynamic range. In Fig. 1, a small input signal above threshold will cause IHC excitation. If the stimulus amplitude were suddenly increased by a factor of 10^6 (i.e., 120 dB)[1] the hair-cell output would saturate (as happens in the visual system when entering a bright room after the eyes have become dark adapted). But as the spacing between the IHCs and TM increased, the magnitude of impact and presumably also the average firing rate would decrease, although timing would be preserved. The question is, how is IHC–TM spacing controlled? Is it simply passive in the sense of Fig. 1 and in the sense of the self setting feature noted in connection with the subharmonic generator of Section IV, or is there also an active process of control? Section X will explore the notion that the efferent system represents an active process of IHC–TM spacing control that extends dynamic range at both high and low acoustic frequencies. Specifically, it is postulated that IHC–TM spacing is controlled by the OHCs changing the position of the TM. In terms of this postulated system, the answer to the question—Should the hair cells be firmly attached to the TM or only in loose contact?—is that the IHCs should be decoupled, to extend the dynamic range, and the OHCs should be firmly coupled, to control the position of the TM.

IX. EFFERENT SYSTEM

There is still confusion regarding the role of the efferent system. Capps and Ades (1968) suggest that it might improve frequency selectivity, De Reuck and Knight (1968) offer that it might stabilize the endocochlear potential (EP), Dewson (1968) submits that it might improve signal-to-noise ratio, and others propose that it is a peripheral gating mechanism (Klinke and Galley, 1974, p. 344). Still others have suggested that it might be an evolutionary holdover without any modern function. To such a proposition, Davis (1973, p. 261) replies that

---

[1] A million-fold increase in an initial stimulus drawn as ½ in. high would result in a stimulus approximately 10 miles high!

it is biologically ridiculous that such a phylogenetically old and anatomically prominent system has no really significant function.

Searching for a suggestion, he asks:

Does it provide some missing metabolite that is needed to sustain the function of the external hair cells? . . . I submit that one thing that such large [efferent] structures with many mitochondria can be counted on to have is a high metabolic rate.

Crane (1982b) has proposed that the efferent system controls IHC–TM spacing at high acoustic levels. The "high metabolic rate" noted by Davis may be important in this proposed function. This section reviews some of the basic properties of the efferent system, and the following section discusses the proposed efferent control system.

Efferent fibers innervate the IHCs and the OHCs via the inner spiral bundle and tunnel radial fibers, respectively. Mainly, the latter terminate directly on the OHCs and the former on the dendrites of the first-order neurons that innervate the IHCs. The efferents enter the cochlea via the olivocochlear bundle (OCB), which has both crossed and uncrossed components (i.e., fibers that derive from both the contralateral and ipsilateral superior olivary regions of the brainstem). Until recently it was thought that the OHCs were innervated almost solely by the crossed bundle and the IHCs by the uncrossed bundle (e.g., Yost and Neilsen, 1977, pp. 73–77). More recently, Warr (1978) has shown that the division may not be quite as simple; he finds in cats that about 70% of the efferent fibers that innervate the OHCs derive from crossed fibers and about 30% from uncrossed fibers. About 85% of the fibers that innervate the IHCs derive from uncrossed fibers and 15% from crossed fibers. Furthermore, the cells of origin of the various fibers in the olivocochlear regions differ considerably.

Fex (1974, p. 615) notes that

it is a great advantage that all the efferent cochlear actions are in a sense unambiguous. Efferent stimulation always inhibits.

Although the crossed efferents innervate mainly the OHCs, stimulation of the crossed efferents during auditory stimulation nevertheless inhibits afferent output, which derives mainly from the IHCs. A puzzle, as yet unsolved, is how the OHCs inhibit the IHCs. Some of the possibilities that have been considered include

1. Changes of polarization at the OHCs may cause a change in current flow and therefore excitation at the IHCs (Geisler, 1974b).
2. Spiral OHC afferents, although not numerous, may directly excite radial IHC afferents in the region of the habenula perforata (Lynn and Sayers, 1970). Efferent inhibition of the OHC afferents would remove a component of afferent excitation and therefore appear inhibitory.

3. Some fibers of the crossed efferent bundle might directly inhibit the afferent fibers under the IHCs.

Section X speculates on another method of inhibitory control: change of IHC–TM spacing caused by movement of the OHCs under efferent control.

The following observations are from the survey article by Klinke and Galley (1974).

Regarding normal sound stimulation (pp. 326–327):

the discharge [pattern] of efferent fibers is very regular [and] only a few were spontaneously active. . . . Many of the efferent fibers could be activated by sound stimuli; this required a relatively high sound pressure level, generally above 60 dB SPL. Only in rare cases was it possible to activate efferent fibers with sounds of 15 to 25 dB SPL. . . . Often it was possible, as for afferent units, to measure characteristic frequency and tuning curves. The tuning curves . . . are substantially flatter than for afferent fibers.

Regarding electrical excitation of the crossed olivocochlear bundle (COCB) (pp. 330, 331);

[Electrical] stimulation of the COCB produces, after 15 to 30 ms, a reduction in amplitude of the CAP [compound action potential] induced by a click or tone burst. . . . The effect is fully developed about 50 ms after the start of COCB stimulation. . . . After termination of COCB stimulation, the inhibition dies away again in the course of 100 to 150 ms.

For some fibers spontaneous activity can be inhibited [by electrical stimulation of the COCB], especially for those units with CF between 6 and 12 kHz. But in every case the inhibition is weak, whereas sound-evoked activity in the frequency range from 6 to 10 kHz and at low sound pressure levels can be very strongly inhibited, in some circumstances to a degree corresponding to a reduction of the sound pressure up to 25 dB.

Wiederhold and Kiang (1970, p. 962) note that

The effect of COCB [electrical] stimulation is dependent on the level of acoustic stimulation, being least at extremes of low and high levels and maximal at an intermediate level.

These results suggest that under normal physiological conditions, the efferent system may be activated only at high levels (>50 dB) and that the efferent fibers are frequency sensitive. Electrical stimulation experiments show that the efferent system has a relatively long course of onset and an even longer course of recovery, and that for a given level of electrical stimulation, tones of intermediate intensity level are most strongly inhibited and there is relatively little effect on spontaneous firing.

X. EFFERENT CONTROL OF OHCs

We will explore here the possibility of an active system for controlling IHC–TM spacing and thus excitation level. The reason an active system seems appropriate is as follows: IHC–TM connect–disconnect is inherently a nonlinear process. Nonetheless, to the extent that the basic components, or parameters, of Fig. 1 are linear, separation will increase linearly with excitation (i.e., a 1000-fold increase in excitation would lead to a 1000-fold increase in separation as well as a 1000-fold increase in impact strength). In other words, afferent excitation would still tend to increase linearly with excitation. Overdriving and saturation would be prevented only if the basic parameters changed appropriately with level so that impact became weaker, or if IHC–TM spacing increased faster than a linear function of acoustic input level. However, there is no way at present to predict or quantify such parameter changes. One method for achieving a faster-than-linear increase in IHC–TM spacing is by an active feedback process as described here.

A. OHC Control of IHC–TM Spacing

As noted earlier, physiological studies suggest that the efferent system is normally effective only at relatively high acoustic levels (>50 dB SPL), and that its primary measurable effect is inhibition. The primary task, then, is to determine what effect the efferent system has on the OHCs that could result in IHC (afferent) inhibition.

We noted in connection with Fig. 7 that acoustic motion of the OHCs may be transmitted to the region of the IHCs by means of the TM. It is interesting to note also that the long axes of the OHC bodies are basically orthogonal to the sloped stereocilia of the IHCs. We can thus also conceive of a (slow-speed) system in which any change in size or form of OHCs is transmitted to the region of adjacent IHCs: an expansion or outward axial motion of the OHCs leading to an increase in adjacent IHC–TM spacing, a contraction or downward axial motion leading to a reduction in adjacent IHC–TM spacing.

The structural arrangement is also suggestive, inasmuch as the efferent endings on the OHCs are especially large and numerous and cover a large portion of the lower end of the OHC body. Thus, one might expect a relatively large neurotransmitter discharge as a result of efferent excitation. Although it is generally assumed that neurotransmitter discharge is associated primarily with postsynaptic polarization and depolarization, a growing body of data leads one to question whether the combination of neurotransmitter discharge and acoustic vibration might not have some other role as well in the OHCs—namely, a change in size or form, or both, which would alter IHC–TM spacing, as noted above.

At this stage, it is not clear exactly how such physical changes might occur. However, regardless of the exact mechanism of IHC excitation, very small changes can have profound effects. As noted in Section IV, if the effective amplitude of BM motion near and just above threshold is indeed in the angstrom range, then a change in IHC–TM spacing of even a small fraction of a micron would cause a large change in excitation level. The apical ends of the OHCs terminate in openings in the reticular lamina that are on the order of 5 μm in diameter, as illustrated in Fig. 10a. Given a relatively rigid, radial-fiber system in the TM, any mechanism that moved the OHC stereocilia, and therefore the TM, by an amount as small as even 0.1 μm could thus cause a significant change in IHC–TM spacing. At the same time, this magnitude of deflection would represent only a very tiny movement, or deflection, of the upper surface of the OHC relative to the size of the reticular lamina opening. Furthermore, the stereocilia are embedded in a cuticular plate, which apparently can pivot as a whole. An upward rotation of the stereocilia, as illustrated in Fig. 10b, would cause both a lift and translation of the TM. In the presence of a Hensen's stripe, the translation component would be as effective as the lift component in altering IHC–TM spacing.

Given a mechanism that alters OHC size or shape (see below) we could visualize the efferent system operating as follows. Each (radial) efferent fiber is controlled by some measure of the firing pattern of radially adjacent afferent fibers. When that measure passes some threshold (presumably corresponding to acoustic levels >50 dB), these efferent fibers are stimulated and cause the nearby IHC–TM spacing to increase in the way suggested above. The increased spacing would prevent overdriving and thereby stabilize the afferent firing pattern. The speed of any such control system would depend on the rate of chemical transfer and subsequent removal as well as on the mechanical time constants. In the previous section, it was noted that the inhibition effect caused by electrical stimulation of the COCB is not fully developed until about 50 msec. After termination of stimulation, the inhibition effect dies away in 100 to 150 msec. These would seem to be quite long delay times if the effects were purely electrical or neural and would be more understandable if chemical transfer and mechanical time constants were also involved, as speculated here.

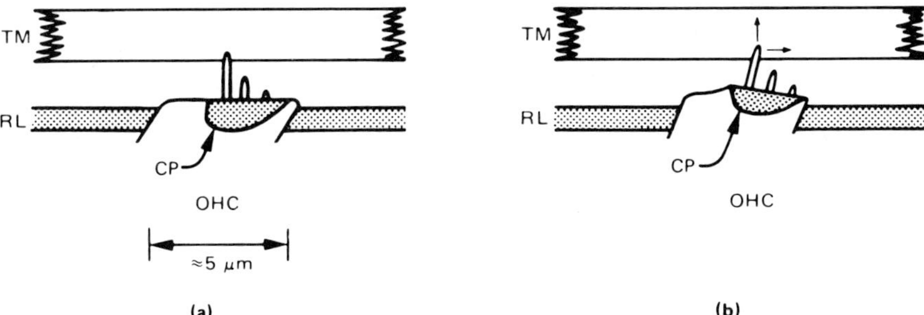

Figure 10   (a) Enlarged schematic drawing of the apical end of an OHC. (b) Rotation of the CP would cause both a lift and translation of the TM both of which would cause an increase in IHC–TM spacing: RL, reticular lamina; CP, cuticular plate; TM, tectorial membrane; OHC, outer hair cell.

The following sections review certain OHC anatomical and physiological data that seem important to understand even if the conjecture derived here (primarily from such data) should prove wrong.

B. Shape and Size Change of the OHCs

Ward (1963, p. 279) notes a report by Wustenfeld that

> with exposure to high-frequency tones, nuclei of hair cells in the basal region swelled to many times their normal volume, and similarly for cells in the apical region following exposure to low-frequency tones. *This was true only for the outer hair cells . . . .;* nuclei of the inner hair cells remained nearly unchanged [emphasis added].

Vinnikov and Titova (1964, p. 76) also note

> changes in shape, or rounding of the cell, vacuolation of the cytoplasm, and swelling or, conversely, compression of the *nuclei of individual outer hair cells,* arising after exposure to sound lasting 15 to 20 minutes. . . . So far as the inner hair cells are concerned, vacuolation of their cytoplasm was also observed, although the shape of their body and nucleus was changed to a lesser degree [emphasis added].

Bruns (1976, p. 88) working with the horseshoe bat, notes that

> Exposing the ear to continuous, intense pure tone stimulation results in a reversible metabolic change in the stimulated hair cells. . . . Among other effects the high metabolic activity shows up in swelling and characteristic staining of the *nuclei of the OHC.* This phenomenon was first investigated by Neubert and Wustenfeld, who investigated the distribution of swollen nuclei in the cochlea of the guinea pig after pure tone exposure and so mapped the frequency response of the BM [emphasis added].

Bruns (1976, p. 91) reports changes in nuclear volume up to 600%.

Although the structural relationship among the OHCs, IHCs, and TM makes the notion of IHC–TM spacing control via OHC motion or change in shape appealing, all of the measurements thus far noted are in connection with high-intensity tones of long duration. For evaluating the postulated mechanism, it would be necessary to determine how graded these effects are with acoustic level, and how rapid the "reversible metabolic change" is that leads to swelling of the OHC nucleus. Of course, there may be multiple time constants involved; very slow changes may, for instance, be associated with long-term temporary threshold shift (TTS). Also, it is not clear whether any of the reported OHC size change is caused by the acoustic vibration itself or by the efferent neurotransmitter discharge. A way to test this would be to repeat the intense sound experiments with the olivocochlear bundle inactivated, so that there would be no simultaneous neurotransmitter discharge, and to establish an extended electrical excitation of the efferent bundle but without simultaneous acoustic stimulation.

In any case, one indication that OHC function differs from IHC function is that only the former swells with acoustic stimulation. This difference may be due either to a difference in cell type, to the fact that the IHCs experience less acoustic vibration (lying at the edge of the BM), or to the fact that only the OHCs receive direct efferent excitation.

C. Differential Excitation of the OHC Rows

If all of the OHC rows are excited equally by the efferent system, the TM would tend to be moved parallel to itself, according to our postulated mechanism. It would be of even greater interest if the innermost row of OHCs received more excitation than the outermost row, in which case there could be a pivoting action and magnification of any spacing effects at the IHCs. Ishii and Balogh (1968) and Klinke and Galley (1974) note such a difference in efferent innervation. Specifically, Klinke and Galley (p. 320) note that

> The OHCs of the basal turn exhibit the most dense efferent innervation, and among them those of the first (inner) row are especially well supplied.

Bruns (1976, p. 91) notes not only extreme swelling of OHC nuclei, as noted in the previous section, but also that

> The three rows of OHC show different responses to sound exposure. The [number of cells showing] swollen nuclei as well as the diameter of the OHC-nuclei decrease strongly from OHC_1 to OHC_2 and less from OHC_2 to OHC_3. [The subscripts refer to row number from inner to outer.]

Unless it can be demonstrated that the different OHC rows receive differential vibratory excitation in response to acoustic input, it seems reasonable to assume that differential swelling between rows correlates with the differential efferent excitation between rows.

Note that if the outermost row of OHCs received the greater excitation and therefore experienced the greater swelling, the pivoting action of the TM would be reversed. An upward motion of the OHCs would cause a downward motion of the TM (i.e., a reduction in IHC–TM spacing and presumably increased afferent firing).

D. Differential Excitation between the Basal and Apical Regions

The advantage of greater efferent innervation in the basal end as compared with the apical end of the cochlea might depend on the difference between a frequency coding scheme based on synchrony of firing at low frequencies (i.e., at the apical end) and a spatial coding scheme based mainly on the position of maximum firing at high frequencies (at the basal end). Saturation of average firing rate would be serious in the latter case, although possibly of only minor consequence in the former case. If anything, synchrony is likely to be improved with a faster-than-linear increase in IHC–TM separation, because the percentage dwell time per cycle of acoustic vibration would decrease with level. Thus, we would expect synchrony to be preserved with an IHC–TM spacing-control mechanism, or even to increase with level (i.e., interval histograms may even become more sharply peaked with level for a pure tone).

According to this argument, the efferent system would have to be more finely tuned and sensitive for high acoustic frequencies, which might account for the greater efferent innervation in the basal region. In fact, merely preserving synchrony might not require very fine control. Perhaps the main reason for IHC–TM spacing control in the apical end is to prevent general overdriving of the hair cells or damage to the cilia at high sound levels.

The need for finer control in the basal region at least correlates, then, with the finding of more extensive efferent innervation in that region.

E. Implied Size Change of OHCs

It was noted in Section IV that stereocilia movements at 120 dB SPL might be on the order of 1 μm for a mid-range tone. Thus a change in IHC–TM spacing of that order of magnitude would represent a very large shift in peripheral excitation caused even by a 120-dB tone. Let us assume further that a typical OHC is on the order of 5 μm in diameter and 20 μm long, and that for simplicity of computation the cylindrical body of the cell is inelastic so that any volume change is reflected in a change in cell length. Recall that Bruns (1976) reported changes in nucleus volume up to 600%. If a normal nucleus is approximately 4 μm in diameter, a change in nuclear volume of just 100% would represent an elongation of almost 1 μm (i.e., just about the right amount). This would represent a volume change in the cell of a few percent.

There are two basic mechanisms of volume change. The first involves a flow of material. Klinke and Galley (1974, p. 320) note that "The granulated efferent nerve endings . . . contain numerous synaptic vesicles about 300 Å in diameter." The efferent endings are generally shown as covering a major portion of the lower end of an OHC. Just a single layer of such vesicles transferred from all of these endings to a single OHC might itself result in a "lift effect" on the order of 0.1 μm. But the combination of acoustic excitation and efferent excitation may stimulate a more general inflow of materials in addition to the neurotransmitter. In this regard, note that whereas the IHCs are closely surrounded with supporting cells, the OHCs are surrounded with endolymph, which would make such exchange easy and rapid.

The second mechanism does not necessarily involve flow. In Section V we noted that a column of gel 1 μm in diameter might experience a large change in volume in a millisecond or so, and that the speed varies with cross-sectional area.

Thus, a plug 3 μm in diameter might experience such a change in about 10 msec. In general, we might ask whether the "high metabolic rate" that Davis predicts would accompany the dense mitochondria located near the efferent endings of the OHCs is the basis for these sorts of reversible changes. Bruns also referred to the large volume changes in terms of a reversible metabolic change.

Many other possible effects may be involved, and it is difficult to do much more quantitative prediction. For instance, it is not clear just how far the cuticular plate can move relative to the reticular lamina. Neither is it clear how much the supporting Deiters cell would compress in response to an OHC enlargement rather than the upper surface of the OHC move upward; we estimated the volume change of the nucleus, but there might be changes in other parts of the cell as well.

Relative to the speed of OHC volume change, we have been assuming here a relatively slow mechanism. Wilson (1980) speculates on a rapid volume change in the hair cells (a "volumetric vibration") in synchronism with acoustic excitation as the mechanism of the cochlear echo effect. Although he proposes no particular mechanism for such change, he notes (p. 530) that

> simple calculation reveals that 20 dB SPL in the ear canal would require less than 0.01 percent volume change over a 1-mm segment of hair cells, which seems not unreasonable considering the large ionic changes occurring.

Rapid volume change, if true, would also affect the nature of IHC–OHC interaction, as discussed in Section VI.

F. Source of Efferent Signals

Although afferent fibers generally have irregular firing patterns and a wide range of spontaneous firing rates, it was noted in Section IX that efferent fibers generally are not spontaneously active and, when activated, have very regular firing patterns. It was also noted that tuning curves can be derived for efferent fibers, although they are generally flatter than neural tuning curves.

Extending dynamic range through the mechanism postulated here requires that regions with high acoustic activity along the cochlea receive the greatest increase in IHC–TM spacing. We would thus suppose that efferent fibers are tonotopically arrayed so that a fiber of a certain best frequency would innervate OHCs at locations corresponding to that frequency. If the typical form of neural fan-out and convergence found throughout the nervous system holds here also, it is even more likely that afferent activity from each IHC would contribute efferent excitation to a band of radically adjacent OHCs and that each OHC would receive efferent excitation from a band of radically adjacent IHCs. In that case, the magnitude of efferent inhibition at any point along the cochlea would depend on some measure of the afferent activity at that point as well as at neighboring points. The net result would be a form of lateral inhibition that, in the visual system, leads to image sharpening and Mach bands (Ratliff, 1965) and which here, too, could lead to sharpening of the neural tuning curves, although only at acoustic levels high enough to activate the efferent system.

In the basal region, efferent signals presumably would depend mainly on some measure of total firing rate, whereas in the apical region they might depend as well, or primarily, on some measure of synchronous firing. Geisler (1974a), without speculating on a mechanism, also suggests that the efferent system could lead to extended dynamic range if it could control average firing rate.

Apart from afferent control from the same-ear, experimental results suggest that efferent control also derives from the contralateral ear. Afferent activity at any point along the cochlea of one ear presumably affects IHC–TM spacing, according to this model, at the corresponding location in the other cochlea.

G. OHC Afferents

A small percentage of afferent fibers innervate the OHCs, although their role is not clear. Spoendlin (1979, p. 381) notes that

> There is evidence that the [OHC afferents] are not effectively connected to the central nervous system, have no functional interconnections to other neurons and their functional significance in the adult animal is only rudimentary.

Morest (1981, p. 100), however, states that

> Although it has been suggested that OHCs do not communicate with the CNS, there is no compelling evidence for this view. Indeed our own studies suggest the opposite and offer some insight into inner and outer hair cell representation in the cochlear nucleus.

Lynn and Sayers(1970) suggest that the OHC afferents add their excitation to the IHC afferents at the habenula perforata. It is clearly unsettled just what the role of the OHC afferents is.

Following the line of argument being developed here, we would simply note that another possibility is that the OHC afferents are part of the servo-control system (for instance, reporting back the state of OHC responses to efferent excitation); the speed of a servo system can generally be increased if ''position'' information is available from the mechanism under control. Another possibility is that the OHC afferents reflect a crude estimate of the acoustic level at the OHCs and that they, rather than the IHC afferents, are the source of efferent excitation. Not enough is known about the elements of the proposed system to speculate further at this time. However, the ability to record from OHC afferents may be important in trying to prove the existence of a servo system of the sort proposed here and trying to determine the role that OHC afferents might play in such a system.

H. Latency Shift

The model suggests that a certain level of efferent excitation at some region of the cochlea will create a corresponding increase in IHC–TM spacing in that region. Such an effect should have measurable consequences. For instance, in terms of Fig. 1, when a tone is suddenly turned on we would expect a difference in latency, depending on whether the IHC–TM system is in its rest state or separated. Dayal (1968) tested the effect of efferent excitation on latency. His stimulus was a single half cycle of a 2000-Hz tone repeated every 2.5 sec. The situation is sketched in Fig. 11. He reports that with electrical stimulation of the efferent system, the latency of the action potential (AP) was increased in the range of 60–100 μsec. From Fig. 11, we see that that range of latency change is just about what we would predict from variable IHC–TM spacing when the half-cycle tone arrives. Sohmer (1966) reported similar results.

I. Effects at Zero Acoustic Input

During normal operation, we would expect the level of efferent excitation to vary with acoustic level. Research experiments, however, often involve testing the effect of a given level of electrical stimulation of the efferent system by using acoustic stimuli of different levels. In that case, we would expect that some level of IHC–TM separation would be created by the given level of efferent excitation. This induced separation would have the greatest effect at low acoustic levels, where the amplitude of motion is small, and progressively less effect at high acoustic levels, where the amplitude of motion is large. In general, these results are found, except that there is only a very small effect at zero acoustic level. That is, electrical excitation of the efferent system seems to have little effect on the spontaneous firing rate, although it has clearly been demonstrated that the spon-taneous firing rate can reduce to zero at certain instances during acoustic excita-

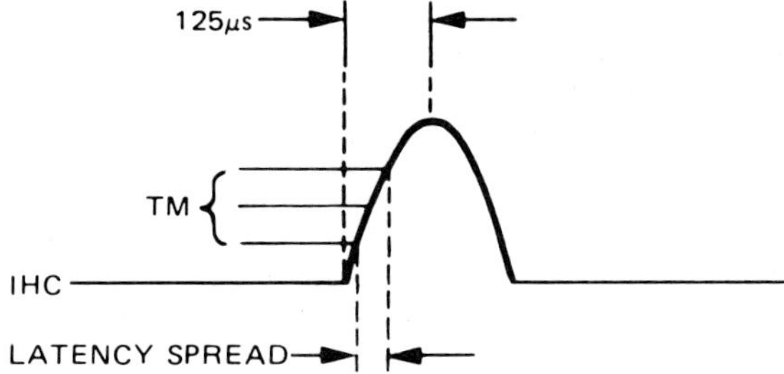

Figure 11   Variable latency for a stimulus consisting of a single half-cycle of a 2000-Hz tone, for different amounts of IHC–TM separation.

tion (e.g., Brugge *et al.*, 1970; Lynn and Sayers, 1970). Possibly the difference in results depends on the postulated difference between the static and dynamic bonding states (Section V). If during acoustic stimulation each stereocilium is surrounded by a liquid pocket, then OHC movement due to efferent excitation could result in variable IHC–TM spacing. If, however, the stereocilia remain tightly bonded to the TM during zero acoustic excitation, then any movement of the OHCs might be taken up in other parts of the mechanical "circuit," and there may be little effect on IHC–TM contact force and therefore on the spontaneous firing rate also.

XI. NONLINEAR PHASE AND TWO-TONE SUPPRESSION

IHC–TM connect– disconnect is an inherently nonlinear mechanism. To the extent that lossy (i.e., viscoelastic) elements are coupled to the traveling-wave structure during the connect phase, then IHC–TM connect–disconnect represents a nonlinear damping mechanism along the length of the cochlea. In addition to its nonlinearity, the magnitude of the damping is also variable, depending at each point on the state of IHC–TM separation. With large separation, a traveling wave would not "feel" the presence of the IHCs and would experience minimum damping. Since wave velocity is generally affected by damping, we would also expect variable velocity, or phase, depending on the state of separation. In other words, we could expect a change in damping and velocity as a result of any process that affects IHC–TM spacing.

Given such a distributed nonlinearity along the length of the cochlea, one is tempted to test it as a source of all manner of nonlinear phenomena, such as combination tones, echo effect (Kemp, 1978), two-tone suppression, or variable phase delay as a function of level. However, quantitative prediction requires much more data on the IHC–TM connect–disconnect mechanism and on the tissue and fluid properties of the scala media than is currently available. We will conclude with a few brief observations on nonlinear phase effects and two-tone suppression.

Goldstein *et al.* (1978, p. 483), using a cancellation method, developed an extensive set of data on the effect of varying the level of various input tones on the phase of primary and secondary $2f_1 - f_2$ combination tones. They note that

> the psychophysical cancellation phase can be greatly modified through a nonlinear interaction from primary tones higher in frequency. . . . A simple rule allows us to comprehend the otherwise bewildering character of the CT [combination tone] phase data. . . . A tone of higher frequency and amplitude advances the cochlear transmission phases (i.e. decreases delay) of its neighboring stimulus tones at the rate of $5°–12°$ per decibel increase in the intensity of the higher-frequency tone.

According to our model, tones of higher frequency would create spatiotemporal patterns of IHC–TM separation that the lower frequency tones would have to pass through. In general, the effect of the higher frequency tones would be to increase the average IHC–TM separation in these regions. Apart from reducing the damping, increased average separation would also increase propagation velocity through the region (i.e., would decrease delays, as noted).

Goldstein *et al.* also note a difference in phase functions in their neural data from anesthetized cats and their psychophysical data. To the extent that our postulated variable nonlinear damping mechanism is correct, we would expect differences among species, depending on the exact nature of the IHC–TM separation mechanism, or, even with nominally similar mechanisms, on the effects of anesthesia on this nonlinear component.

Kim *et al.* (1980), p. 1704) postulate a nonlinear BM damping model that results in qualitative agreement with their two-tone suppression data. The nonlinear model suggested here might be a realization of such a mechanism. They note also that

> both neurally observed and acoustically observed distortion products are reversibly reduced by exposing the ear for 1 or 2 min to a fatiguing tone at SPL of 80 to 90 dB at a frequency near or slightly below the primary frequencies.

To the extent that an intense tone of long duration results in a temporary IHC–TM separation, the reduction of distortion products with fatigue is qualitatively what our model would predict. If the temporary separation were larger than the amplitude of the propagating wave, the nonlinear mechanism would not be engaged at all.

Finally, we should note that IHC–TM connect–disconnect can be a source of *two* types of nonlinearity—a nonlinearity in the mechanical propagation system and a nonlinearity in the neural excitation mechanism at each point along the cochlea. Variable IHC–TM separation in response to one tone, at any given location, would represent a continuously variable threshold, in the sense of Fig. 5, to a second tone at the same location. This neural aspect of the mechanism could also be important in explaining aspects of nonlinear phenomena.

XII. DISCUSSION

There remain at least three fundamental gaps in our understanding of cochlear function:

1. It is becoming more generally accepted that the IHCs are disconnected from the TM, although there is no satisfactory theory of IHC–TM interaction.
2. The OHCs affect IHC excitation, but the mechanism is not understood.

3. There is no consensus regarding the primary role, if any, of the efferent system.

As noted in Section I, the notion of IHC–TM connect–disconnect resulted from a study some years ago of ways to abstract the envelope of an amplitude-modulated wave with nonlinear mechanical elements. The goal was achieved with a system in which two mechanical elements were simply pressed against each other, one serving as the driver and the other as the follower. During excitation, the two elements separate by a distance determined by the level of excitation. With increasing reference to the fact that the IHCs seemed disconnected from the TM, it became appealing to think that a similar mechanism might be involved in the cochlea: basically, that the BM–IHC–stereocilia system and the TM are simply pressed together in the rest state and that they separate during excitation. Crane (1966) showed that an IHC–TM connect–disconnect mechanism in the presence of viscoelastic materials could explain phenomena such as adaptation, fatigue, pitch shifts associated with fatigue, and the amplitude modulation of a high-frequency tone in the presence of a low-frequency tone. A connect–disconnect mechanism could also explain nonlinear mechanical effects at low acoustic levels—for example, generation of the $2f_1-f_2$ tone when the two primaries are only 20–30 dB above threshold (Crane, 1972). We might note that saturation and trigonometric nonlinearities, which are typically used in modeling, are relatively weak nonlinearities as compared with connect–disconnect.

Connect–disconnect thus became an interesting mechanism against which to test psychophysical and electrophysiological data. Unfortunately, it is not clear what ''connect'' and ''disconnect'' mean when the physical motions involved are atomic in size. Clearly a more microscopic theory is ultimately necessary. Sections IV and V discuss IHC–TM interaction from a more detailed perspective. A clear outcome of this discussion is the need for coordinated research into the kinds of viscoelastic, thixotropic, and gel-like materials that are present in the cochlea. Understanding the properties of such materials will likely be important for ultimately understanding IHC–TM interaction, afferent excitation, nonlinear effects, and how the efferent control system operates.

It is generally found that OHC excitation can affect IHC excitation in several ways: altered threshold sensitivity, alteration of neural tuning curves (second filter), and afferent inhibition at high acoustic levels as a result of efferent activation. Models based on electrical, neural, and chemical effects have been proposed. The goal of Sections VI through X was to show that these effects can also be modeled in the mechanical domain based on appropriate mechanical interaction of the IHCs, OHCs, and TM. The exact nature of the interaction cannot be predicted at this time, however, because the exact modes of IHC and OHC motion are unknown. Nevertheless, the potential exists for mechanical explanations for a wide range of psychophysical results: for example, the basic polarity opposition of the OHCs and IHCs in connection with afferent excitation.

From the perspective of parsimony, it is interesting that a relatively simple mechanical extension of the model derived directly from the inferred anatomy can serve also as a model for the efferent system function. Progressing from a basic IHC–TM connect–disconnect mechanism through an extension to include the potential effects of OHC interaction, it is a relatively straightforward step to predicting a possible role for, and mechanism of, efferent function. A potential advantage of IHC–TM disconnect is the realization of extended dynamic range. However, achieving extended range through this mechanism would almost necessarily require some kind of servo system for controlling IHC–TM spacing. It is proposed that the efferent system controls this servo system, for the purpose of extended dynamic range, and that the mechanism of the servo system is physical movement and/or change in shape of the OHCs. This model is explored in Section X. Although there is currently no proof of such a mechanism, many points come together from the literature to offer elements of support.

This idea first took form with reports in the literature of large reversible changes in the volume of OHCs, especially in the nuclei, in the presence of intense sounds of extended duration. Also intriguing is the relative orientation of the OHCs with respect to the IHC stereocilia. Most anatomical cross sections show the long axes of the OHCs as basically orthogonal to the stepped face of IHC stereocilia, which in turn seems to match the sloping face of Hensen's stripe (at least the way it is anatomically depicted in a number of sources). Thus, any changes in OHC length would tend to change IHC–TM spacing directly at radially opposite locations. This latter conclusion is based on the assumption that the OHCs can move the TM, which seems reasonable on the generally accepted basis that the OHCs and TM are firmly bonded and that there is a relatively strong radial fiber system in the tectorial membrane. The next data came from the observation that efferent innervation is graded among the OHC rows, being greatest in the innermost row, less in the second row, and least in the outermost row. If the function of efferent excitation is to expand the size of the OHCs, the greater activity in the innermost as compared with the outermost row would cause a pivoting action and desirable mechanical amplification of TM motion.

It is intriguing to note that efferent innervation is also graded along the cochlea, being greatest in the basal region and least in the apex. This too seems reasonable, based on the expected difference in coding scheme in the two regions. In the apex, frequency coding likely involves timing and synchronization of firing. However, it is generally assumed that synchronization is not involved in the basal end, but that coding there depends rather on the spatial form of the excitation envelope. In terms of average firing rate, afferent fibers typically saturate in a range as small as 20–40 dB, although synchronization is preserved over a very wide dynamic range. On this basis, the presumption is made that efferent control, for the purposes of achieving wide dynamic range, would be more critical in the basal than in the apical end of the cochlea, which at least correlates with the grading of innervation found along the cochlea.

Proof of this proposed control system ultimately comes down to whether the reported changes in OHC size, following intense excitation, are merely side effects or a telltale of a primary mechanism. A number of points come together here, too, to suggest the worth of pursuing the idea further. First, the changes in size required may even be less than those already reported: according to this model, a fraction of a micron of movement should cause a huge reduction in excitation caused by a tone even at the discomfort level (120 dB). Second, there are basically two different possibilities for size change, one based on a flow of material and the other on state changes. With regard to the former, it is often pointed out that the efferent endings of the OHCs are unusually large and cover a large area of the cell. Thus, we might expect a large neurotransmitter flow, which might itself contribute to a significant volume change. If such a flow is only a trigger for even greater flow, it is intriguing also that the OHCs are completely surrounded by fluid, in contrast to the IHCs, which are closely constrained within supporting cells. A fluid surround would facilitate the easy and rapid flow of material into and out of the OHCs. Finally, regarding the mechanism of state change, recent research shows that gel-like materials of the sort that exist throughout the body (e.g., in the vitreous of the eye as well as in the cochlea) can exhibit large, rapid, and reversible changes in volume.

The auditory system, like the nervous system as a whole, is so complex that one can find instances and evidence to support almost any theory. Evidential support becomes more difficult, however, as the theory becomes more comprehensive, for then many more pieces must fit together. Although a number of pieces seem to fit, notions such as IHC–TM connect–disconnect and the adjustment of IHC–TM spacing by OHC movement in a distributed system are so highly speculative that it is necessary to resist the temptation to weave intricate tales based on them. What the author has tried to do here is to present a skeletal discussion of these thoughts, focusing mainly on the mechanical aspects, in the hope that others will eventually be able to show which elements might be relevant to the auditory process and which not.

XIII. SUMMARY

A number of speculations are introduced to try to account for these well-known facts regarding the auditory system: OHC–TM connect, IHC–TM disconnect, afferent innervation mainly of the IHCs, efferent innervation mainly of the OHCs, wide dynamic range, and extremely low amplitude threshold. It is speculated that

1. IHC–TM disconnect is a mechanism for extending the dynamic range.
2. A distributed mechanical servo system controls IHC–TM spacing along the cochlea, as part of the dynamic range mechanism.
3. Movement and shape change of the OHCs, under efferent control, is an element of the closed-loop servo system.
4. The OHCs control IHC–TM spacing by means of the radial fibers of the TM.
5. Movement of the OHCs also affects IHC–TM spacing over the range of auditory frequencies. The opposing effects of IHC and OHC movement may correlate with Zwislocki's polarity–opposition mechanism as well as provide a mechanism of threshold reduction.
6. Variable phase difference between the IHC and OHC components along the cochlea may be the basis of a second-filter mechanism.
7. The rest state of the IHCs and TM is mediated by thixotropic materials, which are solid or gel-like at rest (i.e., with zero or low acoustic input) but tend to soften and liquefy during motion, resulting in a tight IHC–TM bond in the static state but IHC–TM release during motion.
8. A static-bonding/dynamic-release property could explain phenomena such as the lack of inhibition of spontaneous firing during efferent excitation, as well as why some researchers find clean IHC–TM separation while others find broken stereocilia tips attached to the TM (this may depend on the manner, or rate, at which the TM is pulled from the organ of Corti).
9. IHC–TM connect–disconnect represents a variable, nonlinear mechanism distributed along the entire length of the cochlear partition. It is suggested that this mechanism may underlie phenomena such as two-tone suppression and the variation in propagation phase of one tone in the presence of a second tone.

Note

Recent thought regarding the possibility of an active mechanical process underlying the sharply tuned, 40–50 dB "tip" of the mechanical traveling wave is summarized in a recent article by Davis (1983). It is generally believed that the OHCs are essential for the postulated cochlear amplifier (CA) mechanism, although both the form of the mechanism and the manner in which the enhanced mechanical activity couples to the IHCs remain unspecified. It was suggested in connection with Fig. 7 that a passive, high-Q, OHC–TM resonance could increase IHC excitation by *direct mechanical coupling*. If an active mechanical process involving the OHCs is also present, the amplified motion at the OHCs could increase IHC excitation by means of the same mechanical coupling path. Furthermore, if IHC–TM interaction is involved in the CA mechanism itself, variable IHC–TM spacing (an inherent component of a connect–disconnect mechanism) could explain phenomena such as the apparent inactivation of the CA mechanism in the 40–50 dB range or following exposure to a loud tone, resulting in temporary threshold shift (TTS).

Acknowledgments

The author wishes to express sincere thanks to Dr. Earl Schubert for his continual support, important leads to the literature, and very helpful ideas through many drafts of this article.

References

Brugge, J. F., Anderson, D. J., Hind, J. E., and Rose, J. E. (1970). Time structure of discharges in single auditory nerve fibers of the squirrel monkey in response to complex periodic sounds. *J. Neurophysiol.* **32,** 386–401.

Bruns, V. (1976). Pheripheral auditory tuning for fine frequency analysis by the CF-FM bat, rhinolophus ferrumequinun. *J. Comp. Physiol. A* **106,** 87–97.

Capps, M. J., and Ades, H. W. (1968). Auditory frequency discrimination after transection of the olivocochlear bundle in squirrel monkeys. *Exp. Neurol.* **21,** 147–158.

Crane, H. D. (1966). Mechanical impact: A model for auditory excitation and fatigue. *J. Acoust. Soc. Am.* **40,** 1147–1159.

Crane, H. D. (1972). Mechanical impact and fatigue in relation to nonlinear combination tones in the cochlea. *J. Acoust. Soc. Am.* **51,** 508–514.

Crane, H. D. (1982a). IHC–TM connect-disconnect in relation to sensitization and masking of a HF-tone burst by a LF tone, IV. *J. Acoust. Soc. Am.* **71,** 1183–1193.

Crane, H. D. (1982b). IHC–TM connect–disconnect and efferent control, V. *J. Acoust. Soc. Am.* **72,** 93–101.

Crane, H. D., and Bell, D. W. (1976). Phase effect of an input f_2-f_1 tone on the level of the $2f_1-f_2$ combination tone. *J. Acoust. Soc. Am.* **59,** 123–128.

Dallos, P. (1966). On the generation of odd-fractional harmonics. *J. Acoust. Soc. Am.* **40,** 1381–1391.

Dallos, P., Ryan, A., Harris, D., McGee, T., and Ozdamar, O. (1977). Cochlear frequency selectivity in the presence of hair cell damage. *In* "Psychophysics and Physiology of Hearing" (E. F. Evans and J. P. Wilson, eds.). Academic Press, New York.

Davis, H. (1973). The cocktail hour before the serious banquet. *In* "Basic Mechanisms in Hearing" (A. R. Moller, ed.). Academic Press, New York.

Davis, H. (1983). An active process in cochlear mechanics. *Hear. Res.* **9,** 79–90.

Dayal, V. S. (1968). The effects of olivocochlear bundle stimulation on latency of action potential. *Laryngoscope* **78,** 1590–1596.

Deatherage, B. H., and Henderson, D. (1967). Auditory sensitization. *J. Acoust. Soc. AM.* **42,** 438–440.

De Reuck, A. V. S., and Knight, J. (1968). General discussion on efferent innervation. *In* "Hearing Mechanisms in Vertebrates" (A. V. S. De Reuck and J. Knight), pp. 298–309. Churchill, London.

Dewson, J. H. (1968). Efferent olivocochlear bundle: Some relationships to stimulus discrimination in noise. *J. Neurophysiol.* **31,** 122–130.

Engstrom, H., and Engstrom, B. (1978). Structural changes in the cochlear following overstimulation by noise. *Trans. Congr. Scand. Oto-Laryngol. Soc. 20th, Oslo, June 19–21.*

Evans, E. F., and Harrison, R. V. (1975). Correlation between cochlear outer hair cell damage and deterioration of cochlear nerve tuning properties in the guinea pig. *Physiol. Soc. Nov.,* 43–44.

Evans, E. F., and Wilson, J. P. (1973). The frequency selectivity of the cochlea. *In* "Brain Mechanisms in Hearing" (A. R. Moller, ed.). Academic Press, New York.

Evans, E. F., and Wilson, J. P. (1973). The frequency selectivity of the cochlea. *In* "Brain Mechanisms in Hearing" (A. R. Moller, ed.). Academic Press, New York.

Fex, J. (1974). Neural excitatory processes of the inner ear. *In* "Handbook of Sensory Physiology, Vol. 5: The Auditory System," Part 1, pp. 585–646. Springer-Verlag, Berlin and New York.

Flock, A. (1977). Physiological properties of sensory hairs in the ear. *In* "Psychophysics and Physiology of Hearing" (E. F. Evans and J. P. Wilson, eds.). Academic Press, New York.

Flock, A. (1980). Contractile proteins in hair cells. *Hear. Res.* **2,** 411–412.

Flock, A., Flock, B., and Murray, E. (1977). Studies on the sensory hairs of receptor cells in the inner ear. *Acta Oto-Laryngol.* **83,** 85–91.

Geisler, C. D. (1974a). Hypothesis on the function of the crossed olivocochlear bundle. *J. Acoust. Soc. Am.* **56,** 1908–1909.

Geisler, C. D. (1974b). Model of crossed olivocochlear bundle effects. *J. Acoust. Soc. Am.* **56,** 1910–1912.

Goldstein, J. L., Buchsbaum, G., and Furst, M. (1978). Compatibility between psychophysical and physiological measurements of aural combination tones. *J. Acoust. Soc. Am.* **63,** 474–485.

Harris, G. G. (1968). Brownian motion in the cochlear partition. *J. Acoust. Soc. Am.* **44,** 176–186.

Hoshino, T., and Kodama, A. (1977). The contact between the cochlear sensory hair cells and the tectorial membrane. *In* "Scanning Electron Microscopy," Vol. II, pp. 409–414. IIT Research Institute, Chicago, Illinois.

Hudspeth, A. J. (1981). Signal transduction in hair cells. *Midwinter Res. Meet. 4th, St. Petersburg Beach, Florida, Jan. 19–21,* pp. 94–95. (Abstr.)

Ishii, D., and Balogh, K., Jr. (1968). Distribution of efferent nerve endings in the organ of corti. *Acta Oto-Laryngol.* **66,** 282–288.

Iurato, S. (1967). "Submicroscopic Structure of the Inner Ear." Pergamon, Oxford.

Johnson, D. H. (1980). The relationship between spike rate and synchrony in responses of auditory-nerve fibers to single tones. *J. Acoust. Soc. Am.* **68,** 1115–1122.

Kemp, D. T. (1978). Stimulated acoustic emissions from within the human auditory system. *J. Acoust. Soc. Am.* **64,** 1386–1391.

Kiang, N. Y-S. (1965). "Discharge Patterns of Single Fibers in the Cat's Auditory Nerve." Research Monograph No. 35. M.I.T. Press, Cambridge, Massachusetts.

Kim, D. O., Molnar, C. E., and Matthews, J. W. (1980). Cochlear mechanics: Nonlinear behavior in two-tone responses as reflected in cochlear-nerve-fiber responses and in ear-canal sound pressure. *J. Acoust. Soc. Am.* **67,** 1704–1721.

Kimura, R. S. (1966). Hairs of the cochlear sensory cells and their attachment to the tectorial membrane. *Acta Oto-Laryngol.* **61,** 55–72.

Klinke, R., and Galley, N. (1974). Efferent innervation of vestibular and auditory receptors. *Physiol. Rev.* **54,** 316–357.

Konishi, T., and Nielsen, D. W. (1978). The temporal relationship between basilar membrane motion and nerve pulse initiation in auditory nerve fibers of guinea pigs. *Jpn. J. Physiol.* **28,** 291–307.

Kronester-Frei, A. (1979). Effect of changes in endolymphatic ion concentrations on the tectorial membrane. *Hear. Res.* **1,** 81–94.

Lawrence, M., and Burgio, P. A. (1980). Attachment of the tectorial membrane revealed by scanning electron microscope. *Ann. Otol.* **89,** 325–330.

Legouix, J. P., and Pierson, A. (1973). Mechanism of the short-term poststimulatory depression of the cochlear microphonics (hysteresis). *J. Acoust. Soc. Am.* **54,** 16–21.

Lim, D. J. (1972). Fine morphology of the tectorial membrane. *Arch. Otolaryngol.* **96,** 199–215.

Lim, D. J. (1977). Current review of SEM techniques for inner ear sensory organs. *In* "Scanning Electron Microscopy," Vol. II, pp. 401–408. ITT Research Institute, Chicago, Illinois.

Lim, D. J. (1980). Cochlear anatomy related to cochlear micromechanics. A review. *J. Acoust. Soc. Am.* **67**, 1686–1695.

Lynn, P. A., and Sayers, B. M. (1970). Cochlea innervation, signal processing, and their relation to auditory time-intensity effects. *J. Acoust. Soc. Am.* **47**, 525–533.

Malcolm, R. (1974). A mechanism by which the hair cells of the inner ear transduce mechanical energy into a modulated train of action potentials. *J. Gen. Physiol.* **63**, 757–772.

Morest, D. K. (1981). Representation of the cochlea in the cochlear nucleus. *Midwinter Res. Meet., 4th, St. Petersburg Beach, Florida. Jan. 19–21* pp. 100–102. (Abstr.)

Naftalin, L. (1970). Biochemistry and biophysics of the tectorial membrane. *In* "Biochemical Mechanisms in Hearing and Deafness" (M. M. Paparella, ed.). Thomas, Springfield, Illinois.

Naftalin, L. (1977). The peripheral hearing mechanism: New biophysical concepts for transduction of the acoustic signal to an electrochemical event. *Physiol. Chem. Phys.* **9**, 337–382.

Naftalin, L., Harrison, M. S., and Stephens, A. (1964). The character of the tectorial membrane. *Laryngol. Otol.* **Dec.**, 1061–1078.

Pierson, M., and Moller, A. (1980). Effect of modulation of basilar membrane position on the cochlear microphonic. *Hear. Res.* **2**, 151–162.

Ratliff, F. (1965). "Mach Bands: Quantitative Studies on Neural Networks in the Retina." Holden-Day, San Francisco, California.

Ross, M. D. (1974). Tectorial membrane of the rat. *Am. J. Anat.* **139**, 449–482.

Ryan, A., and Dallos, P. (1975). Effects of absence of cochlear outer hair cells on behavioral auditory threshold. *Nature (London)* **253**, 44–45.

Schmiedt, R. A. (1980). Low-frequency biasing of the basilar membrane and its effect on some responses of auditory-nerve fibers. *Meet. Acoust. Soc. Am., 99th, Atlanta, April 21–25.*

Sellick, P. M., and Russell, I. J. (1980). The responses of inner hair cells to basilar membrane velocity during low-frequency auditory stimulation in the guinea pig cochlea. *Hear. Res.* **2**, 439–445.

Slepecky, N., Hamernik, R. P., and Henderson, D. (1980). A reexamination of a hair cell organelle in the cuticular plate region and its possible relation to active processes in the cochlea. *Hear. Res.* **2**, 413–421.

Sohmer, H. (1966). A comparison of the efferent effects of the homolateral and contralateral olivo-cochlear bundles. *Acta Oto-Laryngol* **62**, 74–87.

Sokolich, W. G., Hamernik, R. P., Zwislocki, J. J., and Schmiedt, R. A. (1976). Inferred response polarities of cochlear hair cells. *J. Acoust. Soc. Am.* **59**, 4, 963–974.

Spoendlin, H. (1979). Neural connections of the outer haircell system. *Acta Oto-Laryngol.* **87**, 381–387.

Steele, C. R. (1973). A possibility for sub-tectorial membrane fluid motion. *In* "Basic Mechanisms in Hearing" (A. Moller, ed.). Academic Press, New York.

Steele, C. R. (1976). Cochlear mechanics. *In* "Handbook of Sensory Physiology, Vol. 5: The Auditory System," Part 3, pp. 443–478. Springer-Verlag, Berlin and New York.

Taber, L. A. (1979). "An Analytic Study of Realistic Cochlear Models Including Three-Dimensional Fluid Motion." Ph.D. thesis, Stanford University, Stanford, California, Dept. of Aeronautics and Astronautics.

Tanaka, T. (1981). Gel collapse in phase transition. *Phys. Today Jan.*, 18–20.

Tanaka, T., Nishio, I., Sun, Shao-Tang, and Ueno-Nishio, S. (1982). Collapse of Gels in an Electric Field. *Science.* **218**, 467–469.

Vilstrup, T., and Jensen, C. E. (1960). On the chemistry of human cupulae. *Acta Oto-Laryngol.* **52**, 383.

Vinnikov, Y. A., and Titova, L. K. (1964). "The Organ of Corti" (H. Davis, trans.). Consultants Bureau Enterprises, New York.

von Békésy, G. (1960). "Experiments in Hearing." McGraw-Hill, New York.

Wainwright, S. A., Biggs, W. D., Currey, J. D., and Gosline, J. M. (1976). "Mechanical Design in Organisms." Wiley, New York.

Ward, W. D. (1963). Auditory fatigue and masking. *In* "Modern Developments in Audiology" (J. Jerger, ed.). Academic Press, New York.

Warr, W. B. (1978). The olivocochlear bundle: Its origins and terminations in the cat. *In* "Evoked Electrical Activity in the Auditory Nervous System" (R. F. Naunton, ed.). Academic Press, New York.

Wiederhold, M. L., and Kiang, N. Y. S. (1970). Effects of electric stimulation of the crossed olivocochlear bundle on single auditory-nerve fibers in the cat. *J. Acoust. Soc. Am.* **48,** 950–965.

Wilkinson, W. L. (1960). "Non-Newtonian Fluids." Pergamon, Oxford.

Wilson, J. P. (1980). Model for cochlear echoes and tinnitus based on observed electrical correlate. *Hear. Res.* **2,** 527–532.

Yost, W., and Nielsen, D. W. (1977). "Fundamentals of Hearing." Holt, New York.

Zwicker, E. (1977). Masking-period patterns produced by very-low frequency maskers and their possible relation to basilar-membrane displacement. *J. Acoust. Soc. Am.* **61,** 1031–1040.

Zwislocki, J. J. (1974). A possible neuro-mechanical sound analysis in the cochlea. *Acustica* **31,** 354–359.

Zwislocki, J. J. (1977). Further indirect evidence for interaction between cochlear inner and outer hair cells. *In* "Psychophysics and Physiology of Hearing" (E. E. Evans and J. P. Wilson, eds.). Academic Press, New York.

Zwislocki, J. J. (1980). Theory of cochlear mechanics. *Hear. Res.* **2,** 171–182.

Zwislocki, J. J., and Kletsky, E. J. (1979). Tectorial membrane: A possible effect on frequency analysis in the cochlea. *Science* **204,** 639–641.

Zwislocki, J. J., and Sokolich, W. G. (1974). Neuro-mechanical frequency analysis in the cochlea. *In* "Facts and Models in Hearing" (E. Zwicker and E. Terhaedt, eds.). Springer-Verlag, Berlin and New York.

Physiological Bases of Sensorineural Hearing Loss

Richard Salvi, Don Henderson, and Roger Hamernik

Callier Center for Communication Disorders
University of Texas at Dallas
Dallas, Texas

I. INTRODUCTION

Sensorineural hearing loss (SNHL) is the most common form of hearing impairment in the adult population. Clinically, the diagnosis of SNHL is relatively straightforward with the principal symptoms being high frequency loss of sensitivity, no difference in air and bone-conducted thresholds, abnormal growth of loudness (recruitment), subjective tinnitus, poor speech discrimination, and a general reduction in both temporal and frequency resolution.

The clinical procedures for diagnosing SNHL have developed much faster than our understanding of the underlying histopathologies and pathophysiology of SNHL. Our lack of understanding of the neural mechanisms involved with SNHL becomes more apparent when we move from diagnosis to remediation. Clinicians rapidly learn that simple knowledge of the degree of pure tone hearing loss does not necessarily allow one to predict either a patient's competence on speech discrimination tasks or how much a listener's performance will improve with a hearing aid. Recent laboratory studies have confirmed the clinician's dilemma. Patients with essentially the same hearing loss may perform much differently on complex listening tasks such as forward masking or gap detection (Wightman, 1981).

Anatomists and physiologists are just beginning to piece together the pattern of morphological and physiological changes associated with SNHL. Conventional wisdom about the relationship between the degree of hearing loss and the pattern of hair cell loss in the cochlea is much too simple. Several studies have reported instances in which listeners have permanent losses in sensitivity but have no recognizable pathology in the cochlea (Lindquest *et al.*, 1954; Hunter-Duvar and Elliot, 1972; Salvi *et al.*, 1981). Conversely, other studies have reported normal hearing in experimental animals with large lesions of cochlear hair cells (Ades *et al.*, 1974; Henderson *et al.*, 1974; Hunter-Duvar and Bredberg, 1974; Dolan *et al.*, 1975).

Studies on the physiological basis of SNHL have generally focused on changes in the cochlear microphonic, the whole nerve action potential, and, recently, the firing patterns of individual VIIIth nerve fibers. The changes that occur in the gross cochlear potentials provide some perspective on peripheral auditory dysfunction; however, the potentials are sometimes difficult to relate to psychophysical data because of biases inherent in the recordings, e.g., frequency specificity, absolute sensitivity, and onset response. The results of single-neuron studies on experimental animals partially deafened by either noise or ototoxic drugs can provide more detailed information on the changes that occur in the neural code, but unless the actual hearing performance of the animal can be measured or accurately estimated at the time of the experiment the generalizations one can make from the single neuron data are limited and not particularly revealing about the processes underlying the symptoms of SNHL.

The procedures and techniques from the fields of animal psychoacoustics, physiology, and anatomy can be integrated into an interdisciplinary approach that provides new insights into the processes responsible for the symptoms associated with SNHL. In the last 10 years, anatomists have made major improvements in histological techniques which have led to new understandings about cochlear innervation (Spoendlin, 1969, 1972; Warr, 1975). Auditory physiologists have refined single-neuron recording procedures so that it is now possible to sample the firing patterns of several hundred VIIIth nerve fibers from the same animal.

More subtle but equally important advances for developing an integrated approach to studying the dynamics of SNHL have come from psychophysics. The first advance was the development of a procedure to produce reliable hearing losses with small intersubject variability. Various laboratories have reported that when people and experimental animals are exposed to continuous noise, their hearing thresholds initially increase with exposure duraton, but eventually reach a stable, asymptotic threshold shift (ATS) after 8 to 24 hours (Mills *et al.*, 1970; Carder and Miller, 1972). The advantage of such procedures is that the actual hearing loss is quite predictable and uniform across animals. The second advance was the development of conditioning procedures that allowed animals to be evaluated on a variety of listening tasks. For example, with the chinchilla, it is possible to measure quiet thresholds, masked thresholds, tuning curves, amplitude-modulation thresholds, temporal integration, and gap thresholds (Henderson, 1969; Miller, 1970; Seaton, 1973; McGee *et al.*, 1976; Giraudi *et al.*, 1980; Salvi *et al.*, 1982). Thus, the effects of agents such as ototoxic drugs or excessive noise that produce SNHL can be investigated along a variety of auditory dimensions.

The purpose of this article is to review the current knowledge regarding the physiological basis of SNHL. Particular attention will be paid to a series of experiments in which SNHL is induced by noise exposure. Furthermore, an attempt will be made to relate the psychophysical changes associated with SNHL to the changes that occur in single-neuron firing patterns and the histopathologies in the cochlea.

Before examining the relationship between the symptoms of SNHL and the changes in the neural code it is important to review the discharge patterns of normal VIIIth nerve fibers to various stimuli.

II. RESPONSE PROPERTIES OF NORMAL VIIIth NERVE FIBERS

A. Afferent Innervation of the Cochlea

The auditory nerve is the only pathway for conveying acoustic information from the cochlea to the central auditory pathway. As illustrated in Fig. 1, most (90–95%) auditory nerve fibers project radially and innervate only one inner hair cell (IHC) (Spoendlin, 1969, 1972). Note that there is considerable redundancy since approximately 20 fibers synapse on each IHC. The dendrites of the few

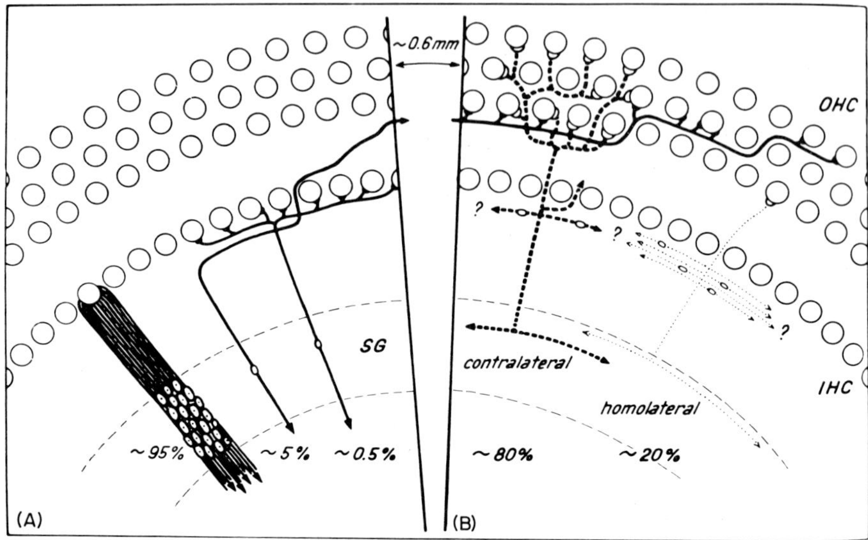

Figure 1   Innervation scheme of the organ of Corti with the different types of afferent neurons (A) and efferent neurons (B) along with their corresponding approximate percentages. SG, Spiral ganglion; OHC, outer hair cell; IHC, inner hair cell. (From Spoendlin, 1974.)

(5–10%) remaining afferents project outward from the habenular perforata and spiral basalward for varying distances, each neuron innervating approximately 10 outer hair cells (OHC). This pattern of afferent innervation should be contrasted with the predominant efferent innervation to the OHC shown in Fig. 1B. Since most afferent nerve fibers snapse on only one IHC, the response pattern of an individual fiber presumably provides information on the functional status of the IHCs in a limited region of the cochlea. By recording from many different fibers, it is possible to obtain an overall picture of the neural output of the cochlea flowing into the central auditory system.

B. Spontaneous Activity

When a microelectrode is advanced into the root of the auditory nerve as it exits from the internal auditory meatus, one can record the all-or-none action potentials (spike discharges) from individual nerve fibers as shown in Fig. 2. The spike waveform of these units is mainly monophasic and of positive polarity (Kiang *et al.*, 1965) with variable time intervals between successive spikes.

In the absence of controlled acoustic stimulation, most nerve fibers will discharge spontaneously. A typical distribution of spontaneous dischrage rates across a large sample of neurons is illustrated in Fig. 3. The rates generally fall within the range of 0–100 spikes/sec. The rate of spontaneous activity in VIIIth

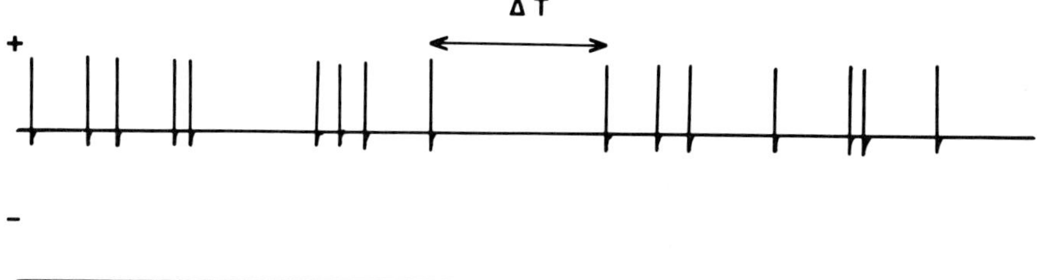

Figure 2   Upper trace represents the spontaneous neural discharges from an auditory nerve fiber in the absence of acoustic stimulation.

nerve fibers is particularly germane to a discussion of SNHL because it has been suggested that tinnitus may be the consequence of an irritative lesion in the cochlea which leads to a change in spontaneous activity (Loeb and Smith, 1967; Atherley *et al.*, 1968).

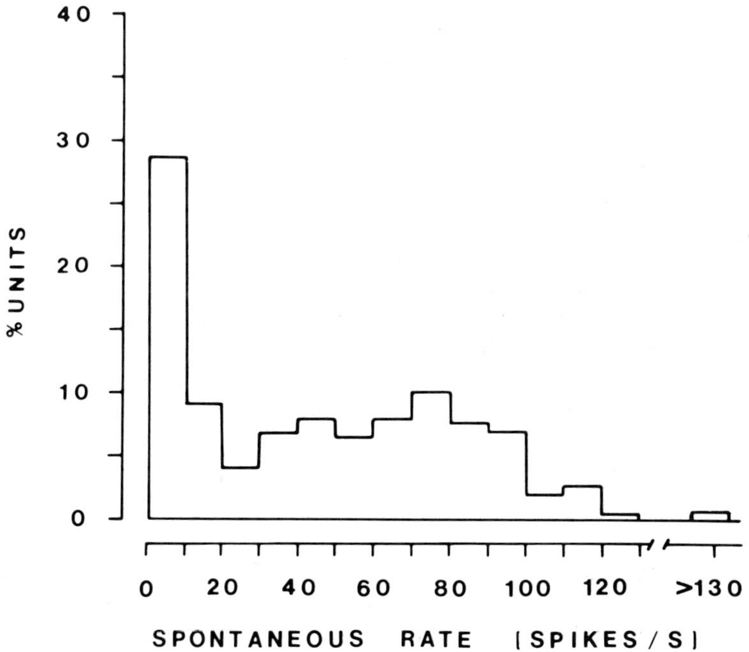

Figure 3   Distribution of spontaneous activity in a sample ($N=144$) of auditory nerve fibers from normal animals.

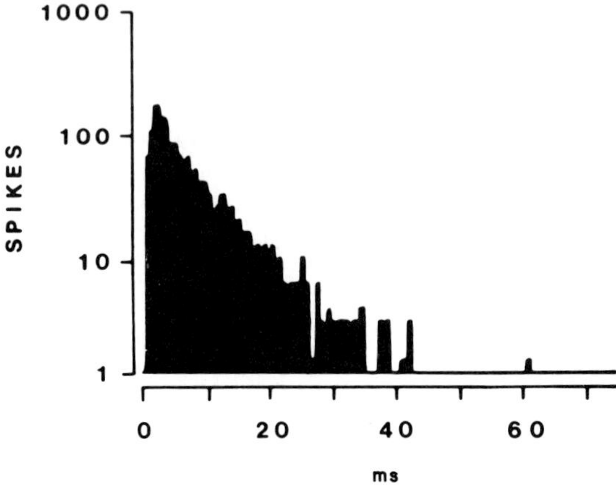

Figure 4   Interval histogram of spontaneous activity from a normal auditory nerve fiber.

The time pattern of spontaneous activity, as seen in Fig. 2, appears to be irregular. One way to characterize the temporal pattern of spontaneous activity is to compute a histogram which shows the distribution of time intervals (Δt) between adjacent spikes. The interval histograms from normal auditory nerve fibers show a modal value equal to or less than 10 msec and the decay from the mode is approximately exponential. When the number of spikes in each time interval is plotted on a logarithmic scale (ordinate), as in Fig. 4, the decay from the mode approximates a straight line (Kiang *et al.*, 1965).

C. Tuning Curves

If tone bursts are presented to the ear and the frequency and level of the signal are properly adjusted, one can observe an increase in the unit's dischrage rate during the time interval in which the tone is presented (Fig. 5). Furthermore, if low-frequency tones (<4 kHz) are presented, the spikes tend to occur within a particular half-cycle of the stimulus; this temporal synchronization or phase locking of neural activity can occur before there is an overall increase in firing rate above the spontaneous level (Rose *et al.*, 1971). At low intensities of sound stimulation, a unit will respond to a limited range of frequencies. The frequency to which the unit is most sensitive is called the characteristic frequency (CF). As the intensity of the stimulus is raised, a unit will respond to a wide range of frequencies above and below CF. The intensity at any stimulating frequency required to increase a unit's firing rate above the spontaneous rate is referred to as the unit's threshold at that frequency. The envelope of all such thresholds taken across frequency represents the tuning curve (TC) for that unit. A typical series of tuning curves for units with six different CFs spanning the range of

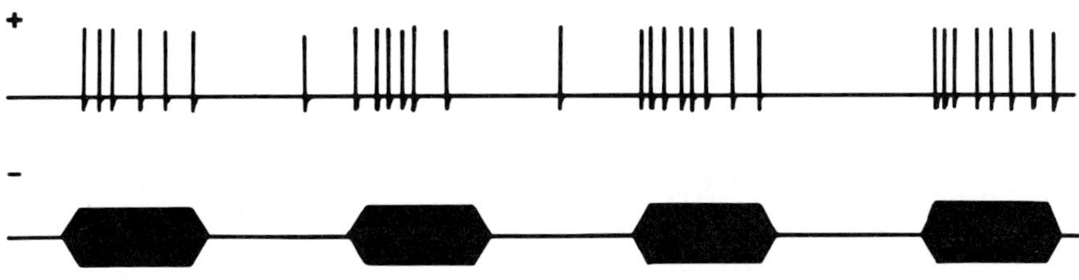

Figure 5 Discharge pattern of a normal auditory nerve fiber in response to tone burst stimulation.

audibility is shown in Fig. 6. The frequency–intensity combinations lying below the TC envelopes are not able to stimulate the unit, while those combinations lying within the envelope will increase the units firing rate. When frequency is plotted on a logarithmic scale, as in Fig. 6, the tuning curves of high-frequency

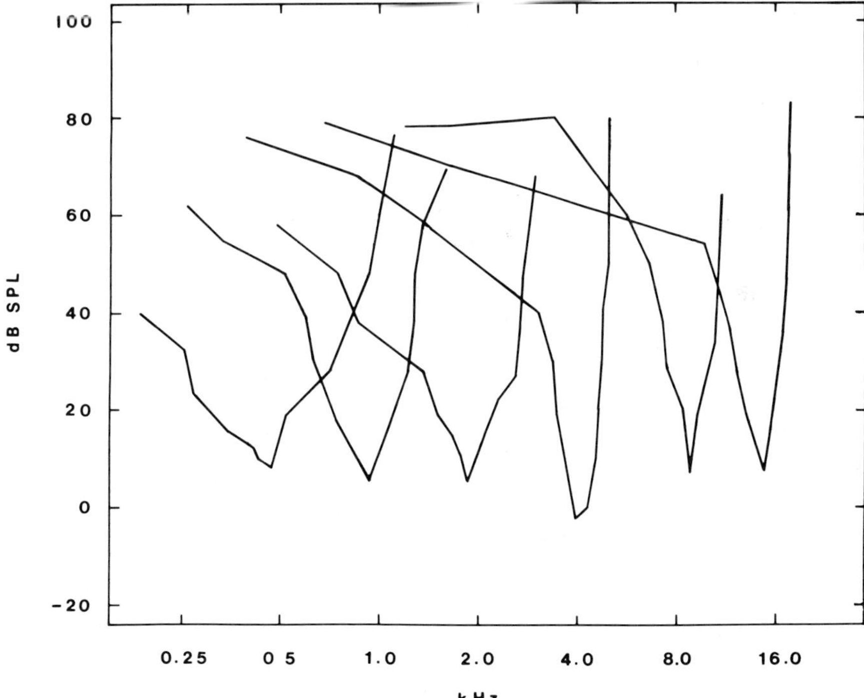

Figure 6 Auditory nerve fiber tuning curves from a normal chinchilla determined using audiovisual criteria.

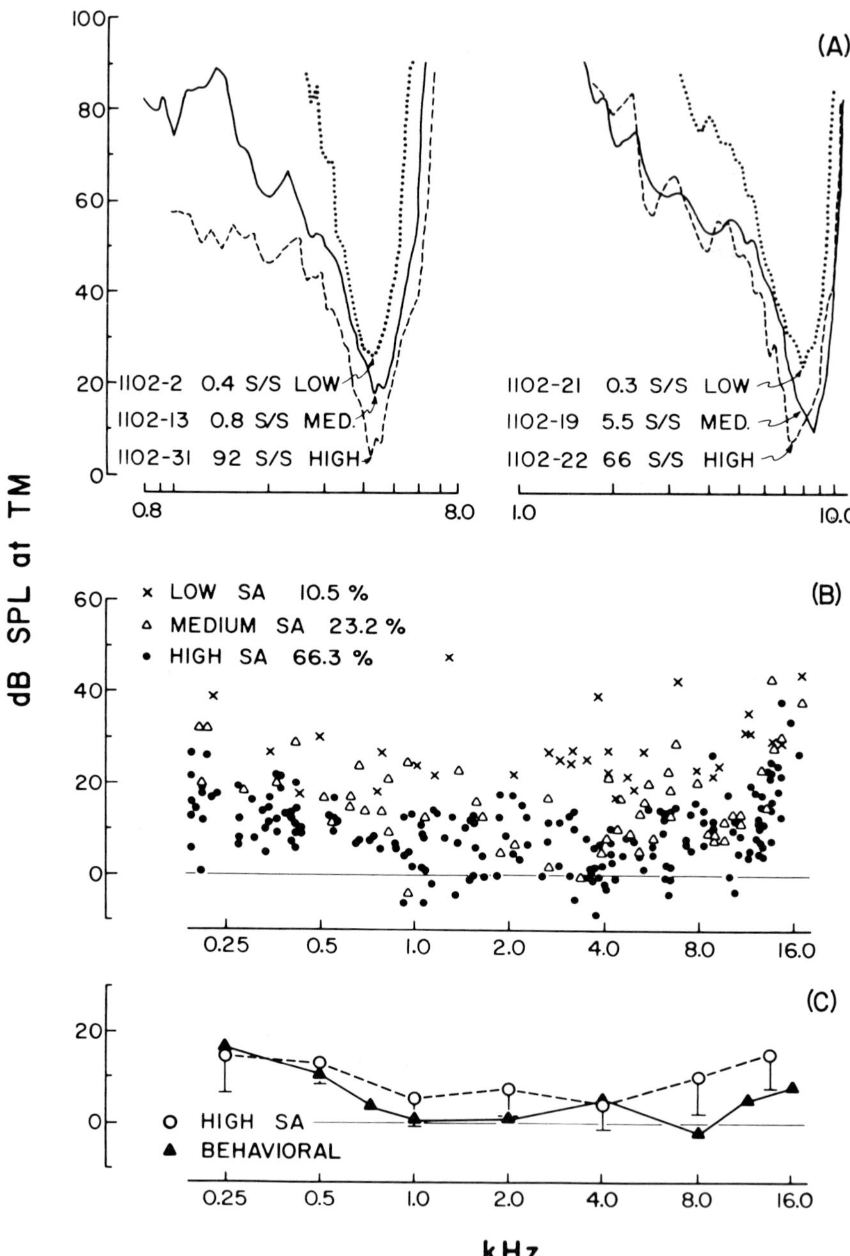

Figure 7 (A) Examples of computer-automated tuning curves from units having characteristic frequencies near 4 kHz (left) and 8 kHz (right) and having low (dotted line), medium (solid line), and high (dashed line) rates of spontaneous activity. Threshold is expressed in dB SPL at the tympanic membrane (TM). S/S, Spikes per second. (B) Distribution of unit thresholds plotted as a function of

units are asymmetrically shaped and appear to consist of two segments: a low-threshold, narrowly tuned tip near CF and a high-threshold, broadly tuned, low-frequency tail. By contrast, the tuning curves of low-CF units tend to be more symmetrically shaped (Kiang *et al.*, 1965). Although there are minor quantitative differences, it is important to recognize that the tuning curves from many different mammals have the same general shape (Kiang *et al.*, 1965; Moller, 1968; Evans, 1972; Geisler *et al.*, 1974; Salvi *et al.*, 1980). The tuning curves presumably reflect the pattern of mechanical vibration at a particular point along the basilar membrane.

If a computer is used to track a neuron's threshold it is possible to accurately trace out the tuning curves in great detail (Liberman, 1978). The threshold criterion for measuring the computer-automated tuning curves shown in Fig. 7A was based on a 1 spike difference between a 50-msec tone interval and 50-msec silent interval (Liberman, 1978; Salvi *et al.*, 1981). If a large sample of computer-automated tuning curves is obtained from a normal chinchilla, one finds a systematic relationship between the threshold at CF and the rate of spontaneous activity similar to that reported in the cat (Fig. 7B) (Liberman, 1978). Units with high spontaneous rates (18 spikes/sec) have the lowest thresholds and constitute approximately 66% of the sample. About 23% of the units have medium rates (0.5–18 spikes/sec) of spontaneous activity and thresholds which are roughly 7 dB higher than those in the high spontaneous rate group. The remaining 11% of the fibers have very low spontaneous rates (0.5 spikes/sec) and thresholds which are roughly 20 dB above those in the high rate group.

One popular idea related to the distribution of thresholds in Fig. 7B is the theory that the outer hair cells are much more sensitive than IHC. Thus, one might expect roughly 5% of the VIIIth nerve fibers, those innervating OHC, to have very low thresholds (Hallpike and Hood, 1960; Whitfield, 1967). Contrary to expectation, one finds that the majority of fibers, 66%, are very sensitive. Presumably a large proportion of these sensitive fibers innervate IHC.

A common hypothesis in auditory theory is that the most sensitive nerve fibers mediate the threshold of audibility. This assumption can be evaluated using audiometric and neural data from the chinchilla; however, to make a valid comparison it is necessary to express both classes of data in comparable units. By applying the outer ear transfer characteristic of the chinchilla to the behavioral audiogram (von Bismark, 1967), it is possible to express both the neural and

---

characteristic frequency. The percentage of units with low, medium, and high rates of spontaneous activity (SA) is shown (C) Mean behavioral thresholds of six normal hearing chinchillas compared with the mean threshold of units having high rates of spontaneous activity. The single unit data are averaged over octave intervals except for a half-octave interval at the highest frequency. (From Salvi *et al.*, 1981.)

behavioral results in terms of dB SPL at the tympanic membrane. As shown in Fig. 7C, there is extremely close agreement between the thresholds of the most sensitive auditory nerve fibers and the average behavioral threshold of the chinchilla. Whether such a relationship holds in animals with SNHL is a question that will be examined later.

D. Firing Pattern and Rate-Intensity Functions for Tones

When the intensity of a tone burst is increased above threshold a unit will respond at a high rate during the tone interval. However, the discharge pattern of the unit is probabilistic and varies from one burst to the next (Fig. 5). One approach to characterizing the average firing pattern of a unit is to generate a peri-stimulus (PST) histogram by presenting the same acoustic signal and repeatedly sampling the activity during the signal interval (Gerstein and Kiang, 1960). Figure 8 shows a series of PST histograms collected over a range of intensities using a 200-msec tone burst at the unit's CF (3740 Hz). Fortunately, auditory nerve fibers from several different species of normal animals respond in a pre-

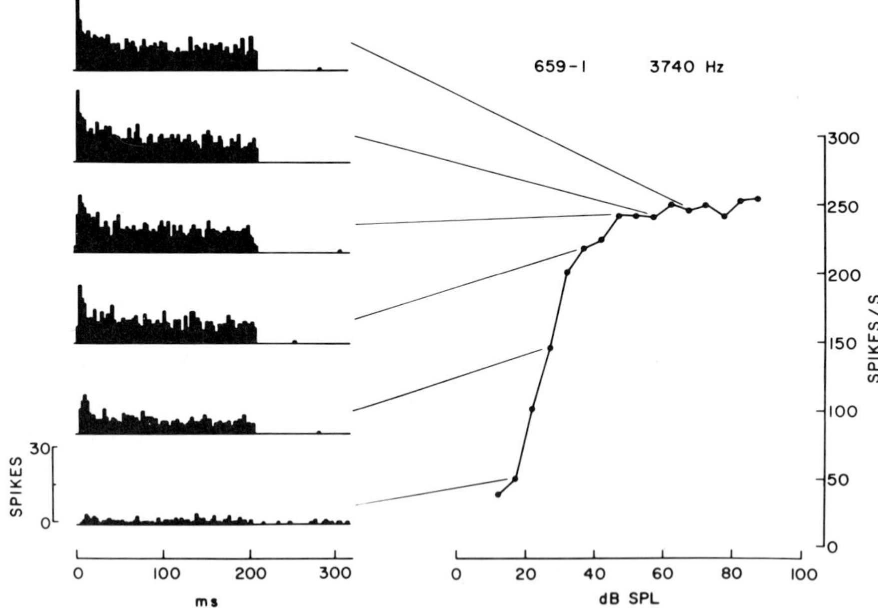

Figure 8 Peri-stimulus time (PST) histograms and an input/output function from a normal VIIIth nerve fiber. The left side of the figure shows a series of PST histograms obtained with 200-msec tone bursts at several intensities above threshold. The right side of the figure shows the unit's corresponding firing rate as a function of intensity.

dictable manner. At intensities near threshold, the firing rate is relatively low, and nearly constant over the duration of the tone burst. Consequently, the PST histograms have a nearly flat profile. As the intensity is raised, the overall firing rate increases. Now the discharge rate is highest near the beginning of the stimulus and then declines to a quasi-steady-state level for the duration of the tone. When the signal is terminated, the firing rate falls below the spontaneous rate, but then recovers.

Figure 8 also illustrates how the firing rate of a neuron varies with stimulus intensity. The spike rate increases monotonically over an intensity range of approximately 35 dB and then saturates. Nearly every unit in the auditory nerve reaches its maximum discharge rate within 20–50 dB of threshold. In general, units with the highest spontaneous rates have the highest saturation rates (Kiang *et al.*, 1965). Interestingly, the range of intensities over which a listener can make estimates of loudness is over 100 dB (Stevens, 1936; Viemeister, 1974). Clearly, using a neuron's firing rate as a criterion, there is no way to encode this range of loudness judgments. Phase locking also increases with intensity and the dynamic range is slightly greater than that for spike rate (Rose *et al.*, 1971); however, using phase locking as a code for loudness would be useful only at low frequencies. Presumably, the nervous system encompasses the range of such judgments by integrating the activity across a population of nerve fibers. Since loudness growth is altered with SNHL (i.e., recruitment), it will be interesting to see if the input/output function of individual nerve fibers or the aggregate response of the population of fibers is altered after noise exposure.

E. Response to Clicks

A useful stimulus for studying the response properties of VIIIth nerve fibers is an acoustic click. Since the energy spectrum of a click is relatively broad, clicks are capable of stimulating units with a wide range of CFs. Furthermore, a click is a relatively punctate acoustic event; thus the neural response to the click will be partially influenced by the initial forced vibration plus the damped response of the middle and inner ear. Auditory nerve fibers respond in a relatively consistent fashion when stimulated with clicks. The PST histograms from high-frequency fibers generally have a single large peak while those from low-frequency fibers (<4 kHz) have multiple peaks, some of which occur as late as 10–20 msec after the stimulus (Fig. 9).

The latency to the first peak (L) is related to the CF of the unit (Fig. 9). For high-frequency units, the latency is approximately 1–1.5 msec as shown in Fig. 10. As CF decreases, latency increases, presumably because of the time required for mechanical events to propagate from base to apex of the cochlea. Another important feature of the PST histograms is the time interval between peaks (ΔP) which is equal to 1/CF. In the histogram shown in Fig. 9, ΔP is approximately 1

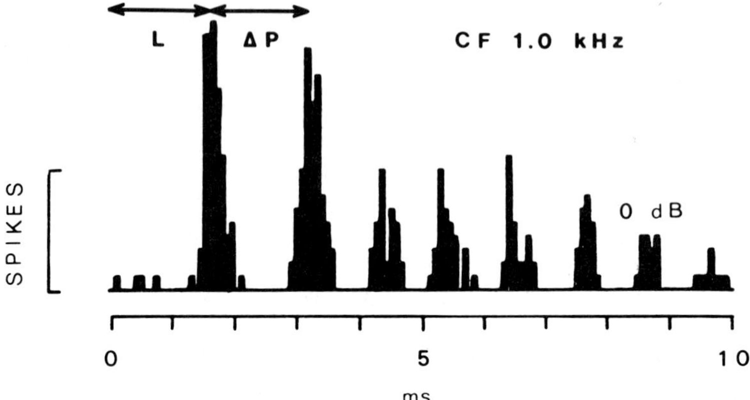

Figure 9   PST histogram obtained from a normal auditory nerve fiber using click stimuli. The latency (L), time interval between peaks (P), and CF are indicated.

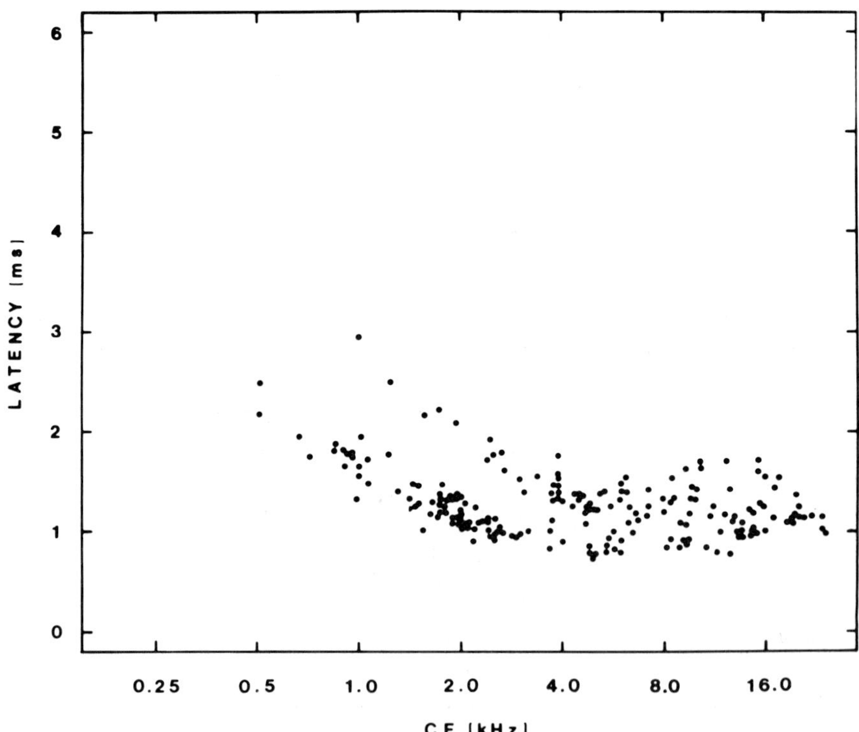

Figure 10   Distribution of latency as a function of CF in a population of normal auditory nerve fibers recorded from the chinchilla. Stimuli were clicks having a peak SPL of approximately 100 dB.

msec and the CF is roughly 1000 Hz; thus, it is possible to predict the CF of a low-frequency unit based on PST histograms obtained with clicks. Presumably, the multiple peaks in the PST histogram reflect the damped oscillatory motion of a particular point along the cochlear partition which is tuned to a specific frequency (Robles *et al.*, 1976).

F. Response to Multiple Tones

Much of the recent research on the physiology of the VIIIth nerve has focused on its response to multiple tones. If the auditory system processed these signals linearly, the response to a two-tone complex would be predictable, i.e., simply the sum of the responses to the individual signal components. However, the auditory system, like most biological systems, behaves nonlinearly; thus a primary aim of many physiological studies is to discern the source and degree of these nonlinearities.

1. Two-tone Inhibition (TTI)

Two tone inhibition (TTI)[1] is one of the prominent nonlinear responses that can be recorded in the auditory nerve (Kiang *et al.*, 1965; Arthur *et al.*, 1971). Two-tone inhibition can be readily demonstrated by stimulating a normal unit with a continuous tone at CF (f_1) and then presenting a tone burst (f_2) which is slightly above or below CF. As shown in Fig. 11, the discharge rate exceeds the spontaneous rate when either f_1 or f_2 is presented alone. However, when the two tones (f_1 and f_2) are presented simultaneously, the firing rate is less than that for either tone alone and temporarily less than the spontaneous rate. The time course of the response decrease is nearly the inverse of that of the PST histogram to an excitatory tone. Furthermore, the latency for TTI is very short; thus TTI most likely does not involve the efferent system.

2. Response to Distortion Products

Under certain acoustic conditions, an auditory nerve fiber will respond when two tones, f_1 and f_2, are presented together; however, it will not respond when either tone is presented alone (Goldstein and Kiang, 1968). The response to the two-tone complex is most significant when f_1 and f_2 are chosen such that the intermodulation distortion tone ($f_2 - f_1$) or ($2f_1 - f_2$) corresponds to the CF of the fiber. An interesting perspective on the cochlea's response to the two-tone complex can be found in Kim *et al.* (1980) where the neural firing patterns of several hundred neurons in one cat were examined using a two-tone complex. The neural

[1]TTI will be used here instead of TTS (two-tone suppression) to avoid confusion with the acronym for temporary threshold shift. The use of TTI in this context is meant to convey a neutrality on the part of the authors as to the origins of the phenomena.

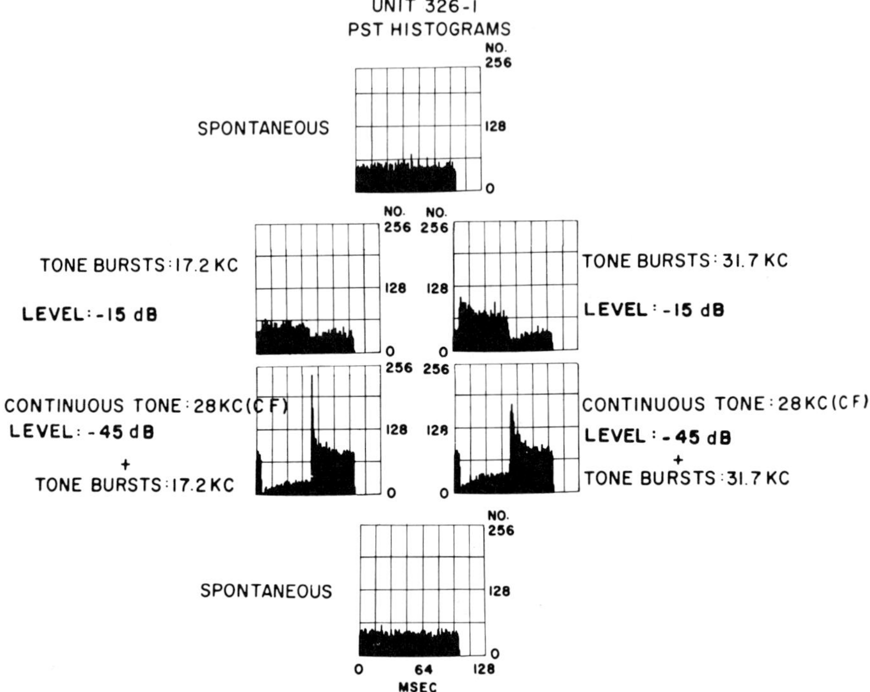

Figure 11   Response patterns of a unit with high CF to tone bursts at a frequency just within the tuning curve and to these same tone bursts in combination with a continuous tone at the CF. Rate of spontaneous discharges, 85.4 spikes/sec. Zero time of the histograms is 2.5 msec before the onset of the electric input to the earphone. Stimuli: tone bursts, 50-msec duration, 2.5-msec rise–fall time, 10 bursts/sec, −15 dB; continuous-tone level: −45 dB. Tone level reference is 200 V P-P. (From Kiang *et al.*, 1965.)

responses were repeatedly sampled over one period of the two-tone stimulus complex in order to obtain a period histogram. One period of the acoustic waveform generated by the combination of f_1 (2100 Hz = $7f_0$) and f_2 (2700 Hz = $9f_0$) is shown at the top of Fig. 12 and beside it is the acoustic spectrum. Below are shown the period histograms obtained from nerve fibers with different CFs. Although the acoustic waveform is the same in each case, the temporal pattern of the period histograms is significantly different for each unit. In order to determine which frequency components a unit was responding to, a discrete Fourier transform was performed on the period histogram. The amplitude spectrum derived from the Fourier analysis is shown to the right of the period histogram. The height of the peaks in the spectrum indicates the strength of the response to a particular frequency component (see Kim and Molnar, 1979, for a complete description of the analysis). As shown in Fig. 12, the response amplitude of

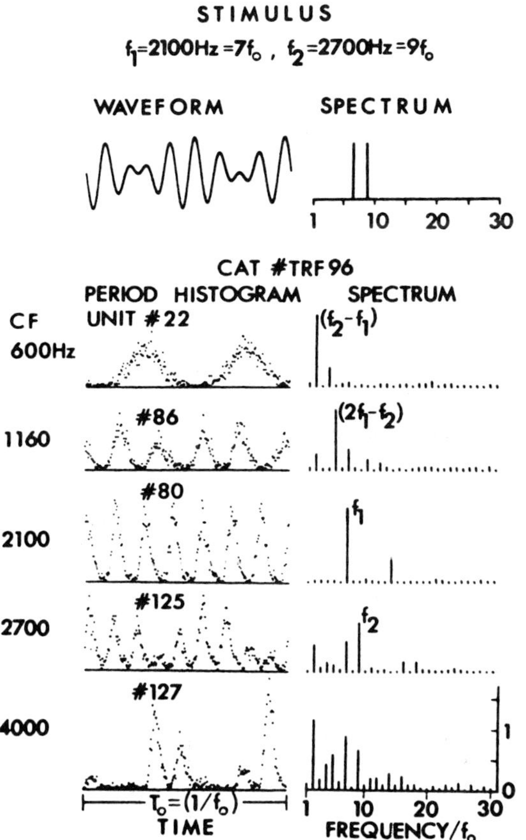

Figure 12   An example of a periodic two-tone stimulus waveform ($f_1=7f_0$, $f_2=9f_0$, $f_0=300$ Hz) and its spectrum in the top row, and five period histograms and their corresponding spectra for responses to this stimulus of five different cochlear nerve fibers in one cat. The sound pressure levels L_1 and L_2 at f_1 and f_2 frequencies, respectively, were both 64 dB. The spectrum of the period histogram shows the response–amplitude measure R(f)/R(0) for $f=f_0$, $2f_0$ . . . , $30f_0$, where R(f) is one of the Fourier components of the period histogram obtained with the complex signal, and R(0) is the average firing rate over one period of the signal. (From Kim *et al.*, 1980.)

some units is maximum at the primaries (f_1 or f_2), while in other units, the maximum response occurs to other frequencies that are not present in the acoustic waveform, e.g. (f_2-f_1) and ($2f_1-f_2$). When a large sample of fibers is studied with the same acoustic waveform, one can estimate the vibrational pattern in the cochlea by mapping the response amplitudes to the various components across a population of fibers with different CFs. The four lines in each of the panels of Fig. 13 represent the average response amplitude to the frequency components

$f_1, f_2, (f_2-f_1)$, and $(2f_1-f_2)$ across the distribution of neurons. When the intensity of the primaries is low (upper left panel) only neurons with CFs near f_1 or f_2 show a response and the response is limited to either f_1 or f_2. When the intensity is increased, units with CFs near the primaries continue to have large response amplitudes to f_1 and f_2. In addition, neurons tuned to (f_2-f_1) and $(2f_1-f_2)$ also respond vigorously. One interpretation of the results is that the distortion tone

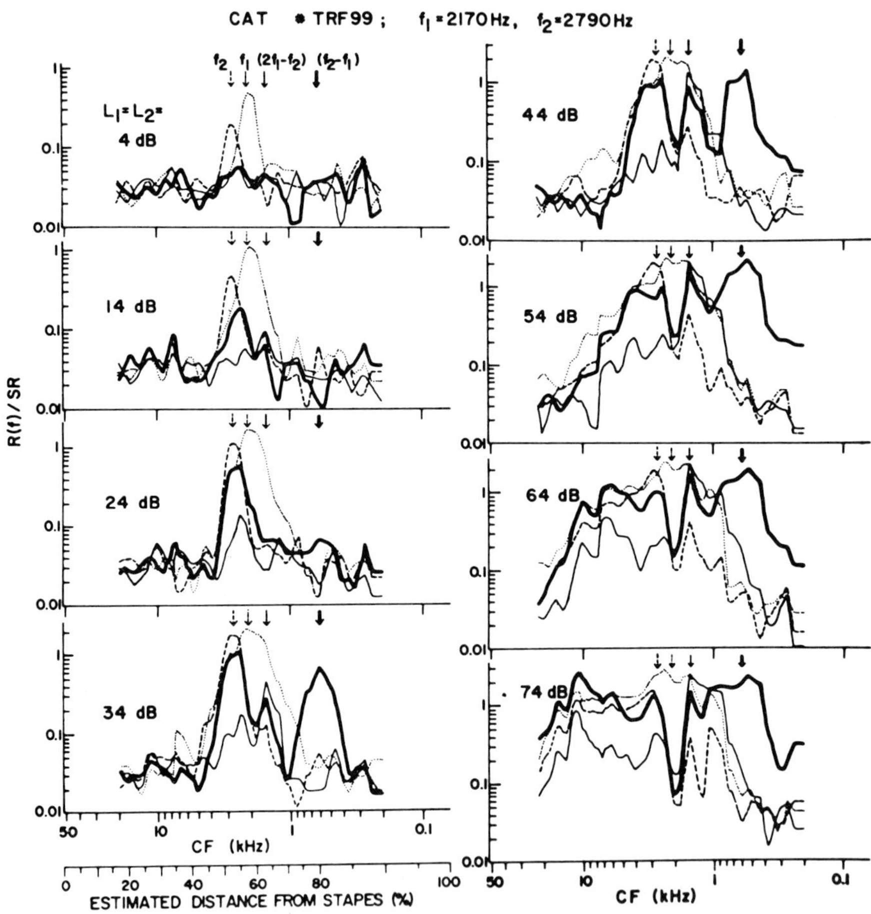

Figure 13 Spatial distributions of the response–amplitude measure R(f)/SR, for $f=f_1$ (dotted line), f_2 (dashed line), $(2f_1-f_2)$ (thin, solid line), and (f_2-f_1) (thick, solid line), plotted versus fiber CF and estimated distance from the stapes. The CF distance scale is derived from Schuknecht (1960). These continuous curves are moving-window averages calculated from responses of a total of 95 cochlear nerve fibers with SR=15 spikes/sec in one cat to two-tone stimuli at sound pressure level ranging from 4 to 74 dB. Each of the arrows represents the characteristic place of the labeled frequency. (From Kim *et al.*, 1980.)

responses $(2f_1-f_2)$ and (f_2-f_1) result from mechanical waves which are generated in the cochlea, perhaps in the region where f_1 and f_2 are transduced, and are then propagated through the cochlea to their characteristic places. Furthermore, the presence of the distortion products in the response of auditory nerve fibers of normal animals is an indication of the nonlinear processes that are part of the peripheral neuromechanical system. The presence of these distortion responses is intriguing since psychophysical studies have shown that normal listeners perceive the distortion tones $(2f_1-f_2)$ and (f_2-f_1) (Goldstein, 1967; Smoorenburg, 1972).

III. RESPONSES FROM NOISE-EXPOSED ANIMALS

The previous section outlined the response properties of VIIIth nerve fibers in animals with normal hearing. The following sections will review a series of studies on the peripheral neural code in animals with SNHL. Where it seems feasible, an attempt will be made to relate the changes in the neural code to the

TABLE I

TYPES OF ASYMPTOTIC THRESHOLD SHIFT EXPERIMENTS[a]

Noise Exposure	Type of Hearing Loss Studied	Dependent Measures
95-dB SPL octave band noise centered at 0.5 kHz; 5-day exposure	TTS	Hearing level VIIIth nerve responses Hair-cell loss
95-dB SPL octave band noise centered at 0.5 kHz; 5-day exposure	PTS	Hearing level Psychophysical tuning curve VIIIth nerve responses Hair-cell loss
86-dB SPL octave band noise centered at 4.0 kHz; 5-day exposure	TTS	Hearing level Cochlear nucleus responses Hair-cell loss
86-dB SPL octave band noise centered at 4.0 kHz; 5-day exposure	PTS	Hearing level VIIIth nerve responses Hair-cell loss

[a] Summary of the four types of asymptotic threshold shift experiments from which the data discussed in Section III were obtained. TTS indicates that the dependent measures were obtained within 2–15 hours following the noise exposure while PTS indicates that at least 4 months to 2 years hsa elapsed between the end of the noise exposure and the time at which the dependent variables were measured.

pattern of morphological damage in the cochlea and the psychophysical changes in auditory performance. As was mentioned in Section I, the intersubject variability in terms of audiometric symptoms and cochlear pathologies can be great, even for subjects with the same level of hearing loss. One way to minimize the amount of variability is to create the hearing loss using a noise that produces a state of asymptotic threshold shift (ATS). Since much of the data was obtained from experiments on ATS, Table I is included in order to summarize the conditions of the exposure, the type and extent of the hearing loss that was studied, and the dependent variables that were measured.

A. Threshold and Threshold Shifts

In normal animals, the thresholds at CF of the most sensitive VIIIth nerve fibers approximate the psychophysical quiet threshold. Thus, the first issue to resolve in animals with SNHL is the relationship between the shift in neural thresholds and the shift in behavioral thresholds during conditions of temporary threshold shift (TTS) and permanent threshold shift (PTS). Data relevant to TTS are shown in Figs. 14 and 15. Figure 14 shows the neural and behavioral threshold shifts obtained 3–15 hours after exposure to a low-frequency octave band of noise centered at 0.5 kHz (Table I). Figure 15 shows the neural and behavioral thresh-

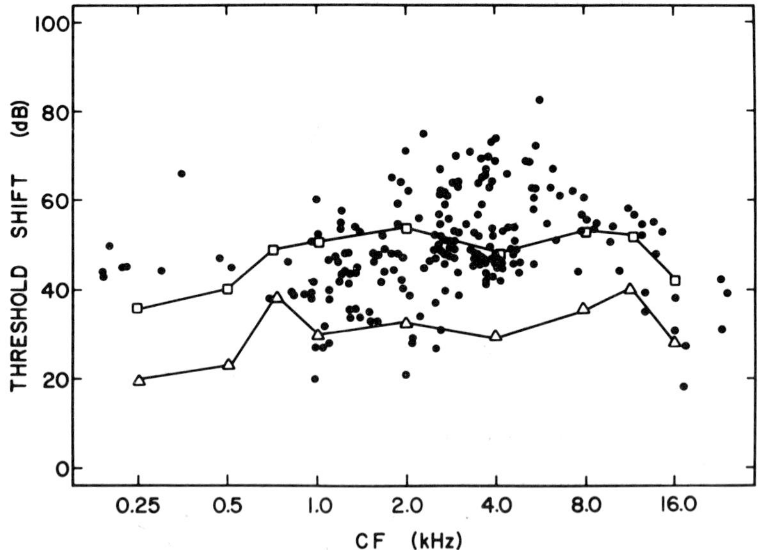

Figure 14 Average behavioral threshold shift during the noise exposure (□) and at 15 hours after the exposure (△). Threshold shifts (●) for 209 auditory nerve fiber obtained from noise-treated chinchillas between 2 and 15 hours postexposure.

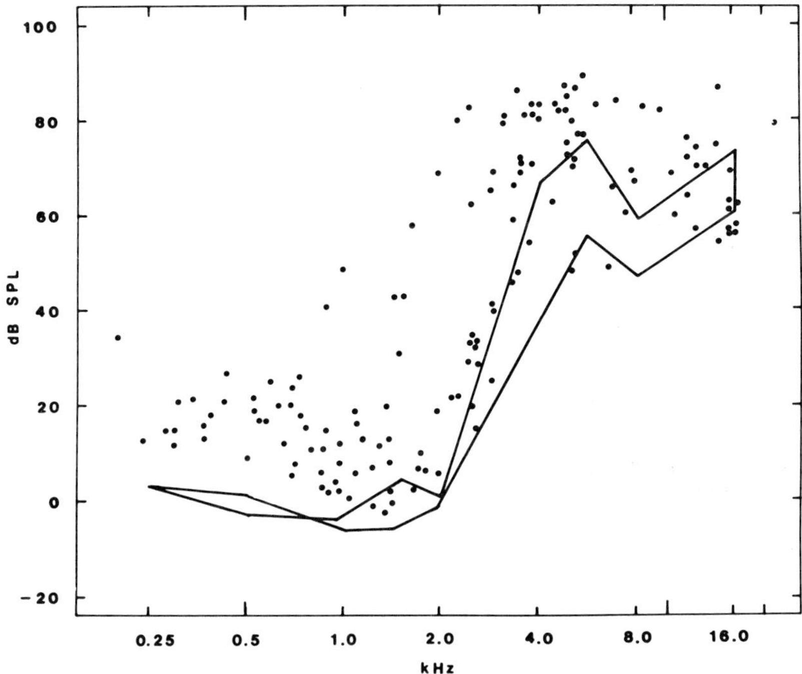

Figure 15 Solid lines represent mean behavioral thresholds and filled circles the single neuron thresholds 2–15 hours postexposure. (From Salvi *et al.*, 1978.)

olds obtained 2–12 hours after exposure to an octave band of noise centered at 4 kHz (Table I). The filled circles in each graph represent the neural data at CF for animals in the physiology experiment while the solid lines represent the psychophysical measures obtained from a separate group of animals exposed to the same noise. The low-frequency exposure (Fig. 14) produced a broad hearing loss in the behavioral group that recovered approximately 20 dB over the 3- to 15-hour period during which the single-neuron measurements were being made. The two sets of data can be compared directly because the measurements are expressed in terms of threshold shift. In order to compute the neural threshold shifts, a standard value for threshold was established for normal neurons having CFs within various octave bands. The ''normal threshold'' was then subtracted from the threshold of a neuron in the noise-treated animals. The threshold shifts of the individual VIIIth nerve fibers are in reasonably close agreement with the behavioral threshold shifts, except for a slightly greater threshold shift in the single neuron data in the 3- to 7-kHz region.

Similar data for the high-frequency exposure are shown in Fig. 15; however, the single-neuron data were obtained from four categories of units in the cochlear nucleus rather than from VIIIth nerve fibers (Salvi *et al.*, 1978). The neural and behavioral thresholds can be compared directly since both sets of data are expressed in terms of dB SPL at the tympanic membrane (von Bismark, 1967). The neural thresholds follow the contour of the behavioral audiogram across the full

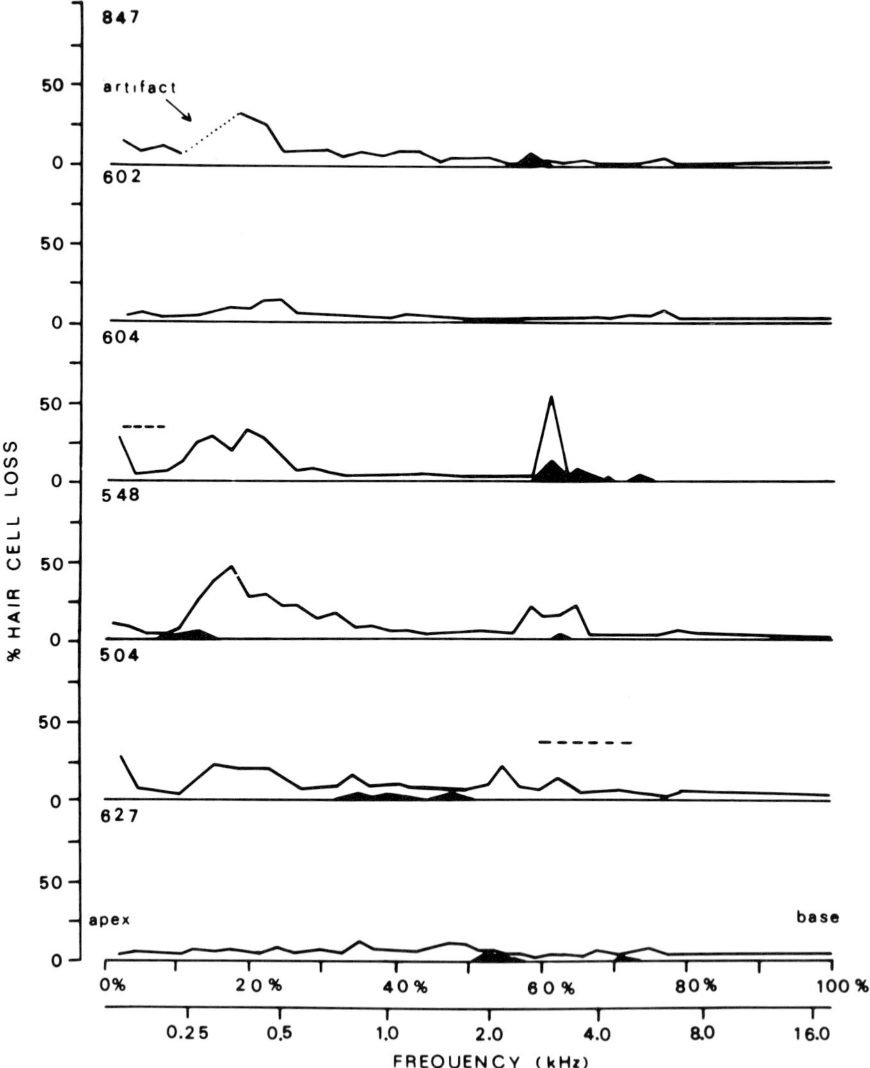

Figure 16 Percentage OHC (solid line) and IHC (black area) loss plotted as a function of percentage distance from the apex and as a function of frequency. Five-day exposure to an octave band of noise centered at 0.5 kHz and having an SPL of 95 dB.

range of frequencies. Thus, it appears from these two studies that the thresholds are primarily determined by the threshold at CF of the most sensitive neurons.

At the end of the physiology experiment, the chinchillas were killed and their cochleas were analyzed using standard surface preparation techniques (Salvi *et al.*, 1978). Figures 16 and 17 show the cochleograms from animals exposed to the low-frequency and high-frequency octave bands of noise, respectively. The actual size of the cochlear lesion is somewhat misleading because the animals were sacrificed 12–15 hours postexposure and the lesions had not yet fully developed. If the cochleograms had been measured at least 30 days postexposure they would have been somewhat larger. The most important point to be made, however, is the impressive consistency of the lesion pattern within each of the groups.

The animals in the behavioral experiments developed large temporary hearing losses; however, when they were allowed to recover (6 months to 2 years), only small amounts of PTS were measured. Physiological and anatomical measurements were then made from these animals. The behavioral, physiological, and

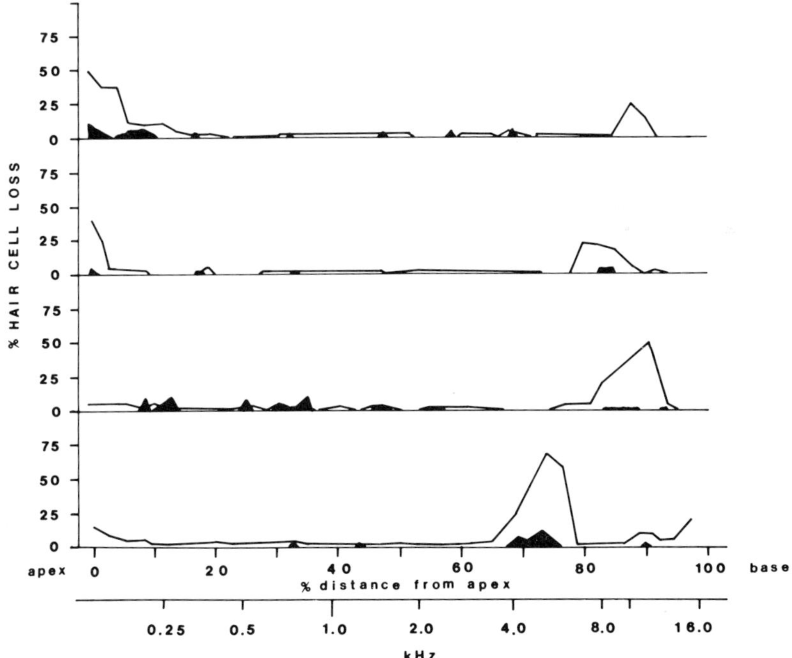

Figure 17 Percentage OHC (solid line) and IHC (black area) loss plotted as a function of percentage distance from the apex and as a function of frequency. Five-day exposure to an octave band of noise centered at 4.0 kHz and having an SPL of 86 dB. (From Salvi *et al.*, 1978.)

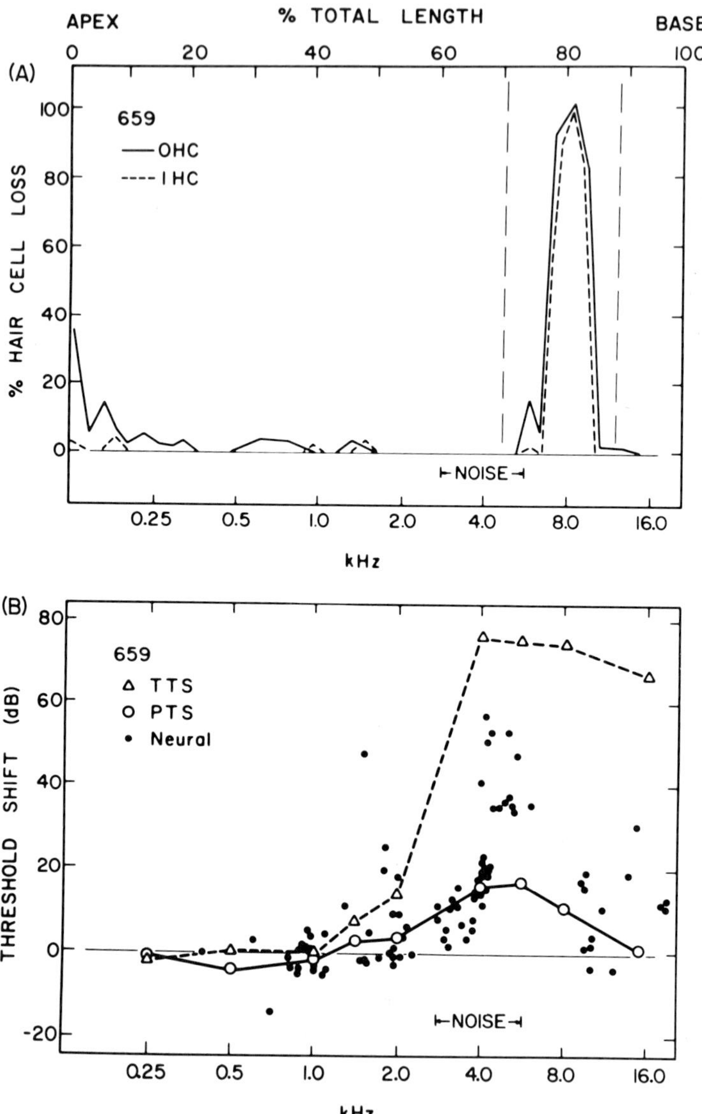

Figure 18 (A) Animal 659. Percentage outer (solid line) and inner (dashed line) hair cell loss plotted as a function of percentage total distance from the apex and as a function of frequency. Dashed vertical line indicates the region of the cochleas with anatomical defects. (B) Behavioral measures of the temporary threshold shift (TTS) (triangles) obtained during exposure and the permanent threshold shift (PTS) (open circles) obtained 6 months postexposure. Solid dots show the threshold shift of single units in the auditory nerve plotted as a function of CF. (From Salvi *et al.*, 1981.)

anatomical data taken from one of the chinchillas exposed to the octave band of noise centered at 4 kHz are shown in Fig. 18. Even though the ATS was substantial, the PTS for chinchilla 659 was only 15–20 dB between 4 and 8 kHz. The neural threshold shifts reached a maximum of 30–50 dB near 5 kHz and declined to 0 dB below 3 kHz; some units above 8 kHz also have normal thresholds. The threshold shifts are in reasonably good accord over much of the frequency range except between 5 and 9 kHz where the neural thresholds are much higher than one would expect from the behavioral data. This discrepancy, which was not uncommon, could result from an inadequate sample of units or it might indicate that the behavioral thresholds are mediated by units with CFs adjacent to the frequency of hearing loss.

The cochleogram from animal 659 is shown at the top of Fig. 18 and is plotted according to the frequency-place map developed by Eldredge *et al.* (1977). There is a total loss of IHC and OHC near the 8-kHz region which corresponds closely to the absence of units with CFs between 7.5 and 9 kHz. The correspondence between the gap in the hair cell and nerve fibers distribution is consistent with the innervation pattern of the cochlea (Spoendlin, 1969, 1972) and provides support for the frequency-place map of the chinchilla. Note that the maximum threshold shift and the location of the lesion are located one-half to one octave above the center frequency of the noise, a finding which is consistent with many human psychophysical studies (Hood, 1950; Davis *et al.*, 1950; Mills *et al.*, 1970). The neural and anatomical results strongly suggest that the half-octave shift has its origins in the cochlea.

There is a slight discrepancy between the neural and anatomical data in Fig. 18. The frequency range over which the neural thresholds are elevated tends to be wider than the region of hair cell loss, particularly near the low-frequency edge of the lesion. Better agreement can be obtained between the neural and anatomical data when the full range of anatomical defects is considered (e.g., distortion of the surface topography of the cochlea and loss of supporting cells); the dotted vertical lines in the top of Fig. 18 show the region of the cochlea surrounding the lesion which appeared structurally abnormal (Salvi *et al.*, 1979b).

Data from another animal exposed to the same noise are shown on Fig. 19. The temporary and permanent behavioral threshold shifts of animal 625 are nearly the same as those for animal 659. The behavioral PTS extends from 8 to 16 kHz and the neural threshold shifts are are in relatively close agreement over this frequency range. The hair cell lesion is centered about 1.5 octaves above the center frequency of the noise. Also note that the sensory cell loss is confined to OHCs and that the corresponding neural distribution is continuous through the region of damage, as one might expect based on the innervation pattern of the cochlea. Again, there is a discrepancy; the neural and behavioral thresholds are elevated over at least two octaves, whereas the OHC lesion occupies less than an octave. The area between the dotted vertical lines in the cochleogram of Fig. 19

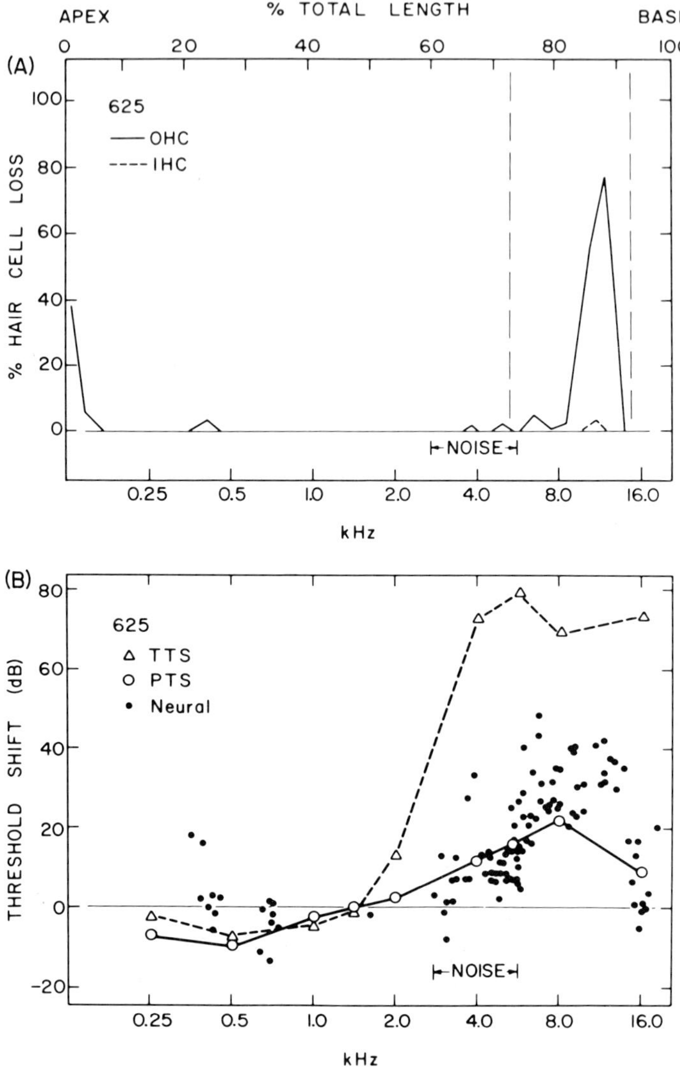

Figure 19 (A) Animal 625. Percentage outer (solid line) and inner (dashed line) hair cell loss plotted as a function of percentage total distance from the apex and as a function of frequency. Dashed vertical line indicates the region of the cochlea with anatomical defects. (B) Behavioral measures of the temporary threshold shift (TTS) (triangles) obtained during exposure and the permanent threshold shift (PTS) (open circles) obtained 6 months postexposure. Solid dots show the threshold shift of single units plotted as a function of CF. (From Salvi *et al.*, 1981.)

contains a variety of structural defects which effectively extend the width of the lesion. Some of the more serious histopathologies just apical of the focal lesion, where the OHC loss is less than 10%, are illustrated by the photomicrographs in Fig. 20. One prominent defect is the loss of pillar cells which affects the structural integrity of the organ of Corti and usually results in a partial collapse of the organ (Fig. 20A and B). Generally, the loss of outer pillar cells is accompanied by a loss of OHCs; sometimes only two to three OHCs are missing in the first row. When the OHC and pillar cell loss is more severe, the reticular lamina becomes distorted and, if enough pillar cells are missing, the reticular lamina distal to the tunnel of Corti is severely collapsed. Such defects could potentially alter the micromechanics of the cochlea, e.g., by changing the coupling between the stereocilia and tectorial membrane. Another defect is the loss of an inner pillar cell with the corresponding outer pillar cell left intact (Fig. 20C). This situation can also be found in areas of the cochlea where both inner and outer hair cells are present. In many cases of inner pillar cell loss, the adjacent IHCs are left intact (Fig. 20C–E); but the surrounding environment is grossly abnormal. Note the paucity of neural attachments at the base of the IHC in Fig. 20C and D; in this case, the IHC is directly exposed to the fluid of the tunnel of Corti. Localized defects such as these may influence the functioning of more widespread areas of the organ of Corti by reducing the number of spiral-running fibers in the vicinity of the IHC.

Liberman and Kiang (1978) have also examined the relationship between neural thresholds and cochlear pathologies in cats exposed to high-intensity noise. They noted that when there was a gap in the CF distribution, it was always associated with a total loss of OHC. Subtotal loss of OHC and normal IHC were correlated with a selected elevation of the tuning curve tip. In many cats, such as MCL 76 of Fig. 21, there was reasonably close agreement between the location of the hair-cell lesion and the units with elevated threshold at CF. However, the correlations were extremely poor in other animals such as MCL 64 (Fig. 21) where virtually all hair cells are present yet the thresholds are elevated by 40–50 in the mid-frequency region. Liberman and Kiang have reported that clumping of the cilia on IHC can sometimes be correlated with elevated neural thresholds; however, in the case of MCL 64 the clumping of IHC sterocilia is poorly correlated with the region in which the neural thresholds are elevated.

In summary, the thresholds of the most sensitive neurons in the VIIIth nerve or cochlear nucleus are similar to or slightly higher than the behavioral thresholds for both flat and high-frequency TTS or PTS. The relationship between either the neural or behavioral thresholds and the underlying cochlear pathologies is not nearly as direct. There are extremely limited data on the morphological basis of TTS; in fact, morphological changes that can be documented are probably more germane to permanent changes in hearing rather than to temporary ones. The permanent changes in thresholds can be accompanied by a host of morphological

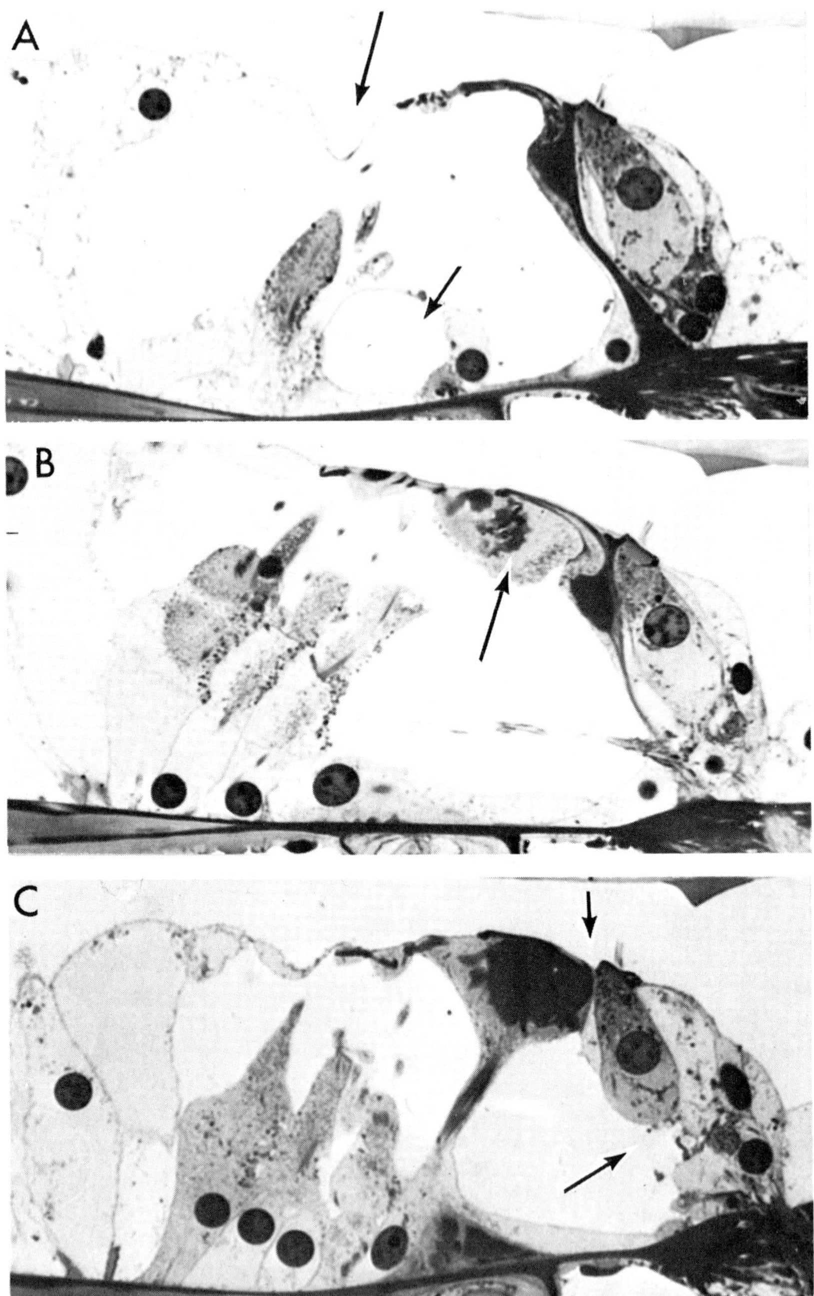

Figure 20 One micron radial section of the organ of Corti taken from a noise-damaged area in the cochlea of chinchilla 625. These sections were sampled from the 6- to 8-kHz region of the cochlea. (A) The OHCs are missing, the outer pillar cell is vacuolized, and the reticular lamina is distorted. (B) Partial loss of OHCs; the outer pillar cell head shows a nonuniform density distribution that is commonly seen in noise-exposed animals. (C) The OHCs are missing along with the inner

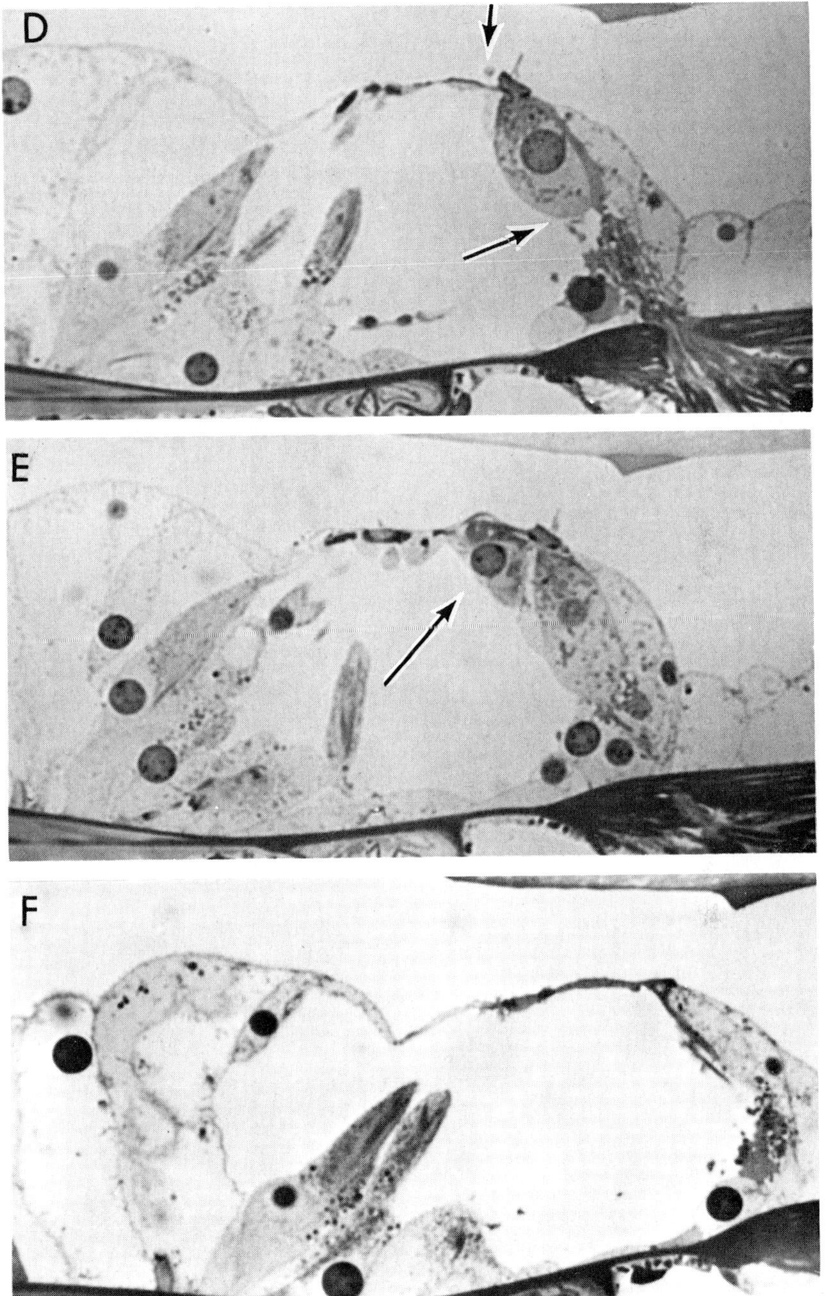

pillar cell. Note the paucity of neural elements at the base of the IHC. (D) OHCs are missing along with both inner and outer pillar cells. The structural and neural environments of the remaining inner hair cell are similar to the previous illustrations. (E) Similar to (D) except for the unusual displacement of a cell nucleus into the area of the pillar cell head. (F) Complete loss of OHCs, IHCs, pillar cells, and distortion of the reticular lamina. (From Salvi *et al.*, 1981.)

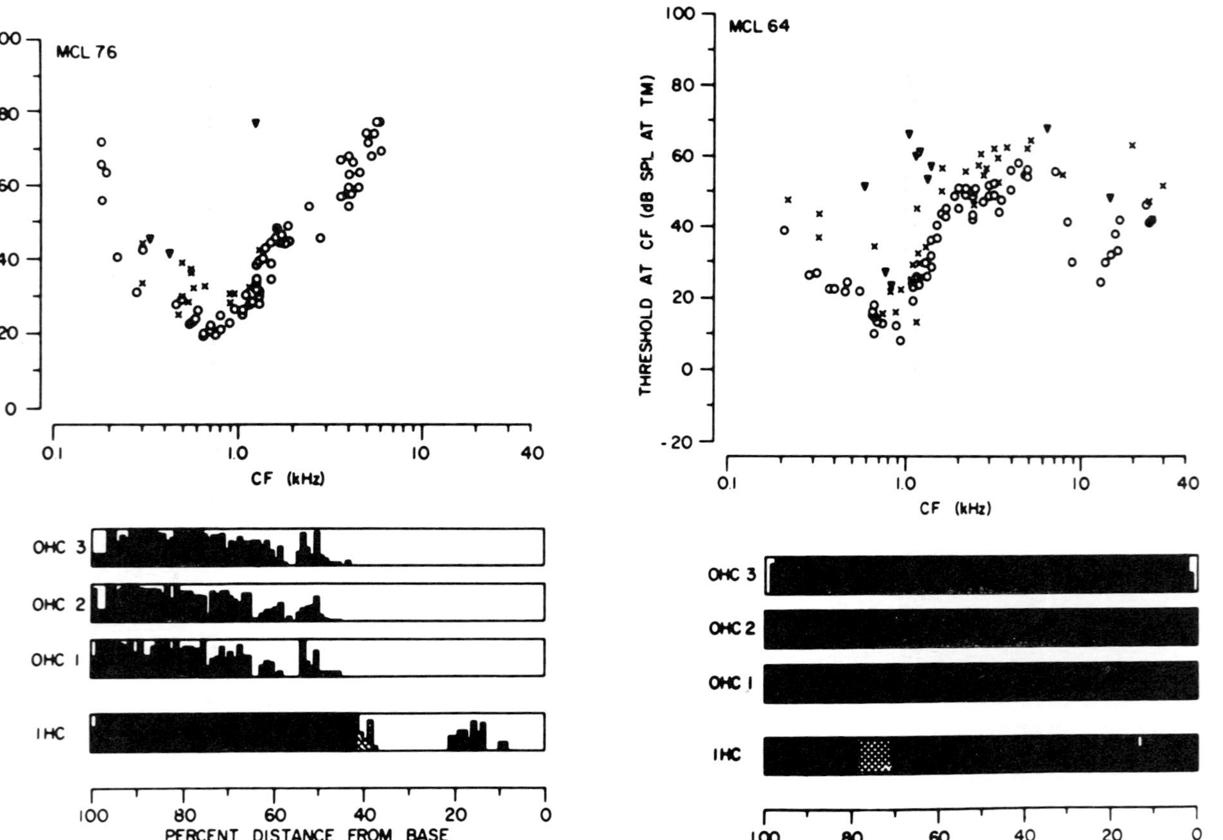

Figure 21 Comparison of cytocochleograms and CF-threshold plots from two cats exposed to intense acoustic stimuli. Cross-hatching in cochleograms indicates the area in which clumping of stereocilia was seen. White areas represent missing hair cells. (Adapted from Liberman and Kiang, 1978.)

changes (Fig. 20), but there is no set of rules to predict the types of morphological changes from either the behavioral or neural data.

B. Frequency Selectivity and Tuning Curves

Normal hearing listeners show a remarkable ability to detect and respond to selective frequency components in complex sounds. By contrast, the frequency selectivity of listeners with SNHL is often quite poor. The recent application of the psychophysical tuning curve (PTC) procedure to the clinical population has made it possible to isolate and dramatically document the deterioration of frequency selectivity in listeners with SNHL. The procedure for obtaining PTCs involves a simultaneous or forward masking paradigm using two tones. The listener's task is to detect a low-intensity probe of fixed frequency. Then a masking tone is introduced and adjusted in level until it just masks the probe. When the masking procedure is carried out across a range of frequencies, a masked threshold contour is obtained which is similar in shape to a neural tuning curve, i.e., there is a low-threshold, narrowly tuned tip and a high-threshold, broadly tuned tail. One interpretation of these results is that the detection of the low-level probe tone is based on the excitation of a few low-threshold units innervating a restricted region of the basilar membrane. The listener is prevented from detecting the probe when the masker invades the excitatory region and interferes with the response to the probe. Presumably, the PTC maps out the response areas of a few low-threshold units that respond to the probe.

Examples of PTCs from a patient with SNHL are shown in Fig. 22 (Wightman *et al.*, 1977). A consistent finding is that the tips of the PTCs become shallower and broader as the hearing loss increases; it has been suggested that this reduction in frequency selectivity is responsible for the poor performance of patients with SNHL in listening situations that require the discrimination of signals, such as speech, in a background of noise. The next section examines the changes in frequency selectivity in chinchillas with either noise-induced TTS or PTS; in one group of animals a direct comparison will be made between neural and psychophysical tuning curves.

Figure 23 shows the acute change in neural tuning 3–15 hours after exposure to an octave band of noise centered at 0.5 kHz (Table I). The exposure elevated the behavioral and neural thresholds approximately 20–60 dB across the full range of frequencies (Fig. 14). Three general types of tuning curves were observed during the recovery from ATS. Most (75%) of the tuning curves from the noise-exposed animals (Fig. 23A) are similar to those from normal animals except that the tip is shorter and wider than normal. The change in tuning occurs because there is a greater loss in sensitivity near the tip than in the tail of the tuning curve.

The frequency–threshold curves in Fig. 23B have been referred to as "W"-

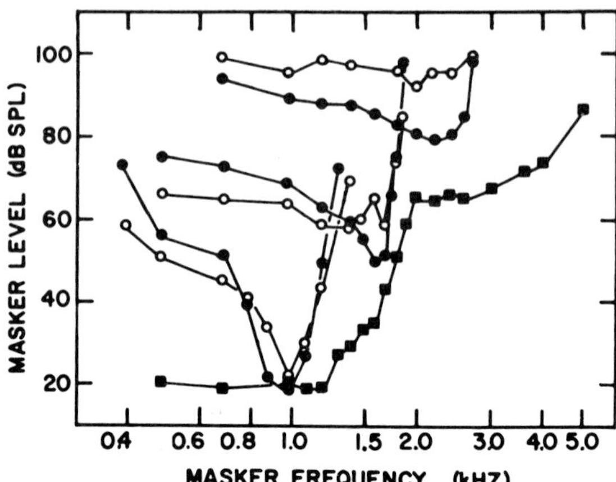

Figure 22 Psychophysical tuning curves obtained from hearing-impaired subject MM. The solid squares denote absolute threshold for the 20-msec probe (ordinate in this case gives probe level in dB SPL). A threshold of about 23 dB SPL is normal. The solid circles are data from forward-masking conditions; the open circles are data from simultaneous conditions. Probe frequencies used were 1.0 kHz (left curves), 1.7 kHz (middle curves), and 2.3 kHz (right curves). (From Wightman *et al.*, 1977.)

shaped tuning curves because there are two distinct tips (Liberman and Kiang, 1978). The presence of two threshold minima poses a problem in selecting CF. Our criterion was to assign CF to the tip nearest the high-frequency cutoff in keeping with the mechanical response of the basilar membrane (Bekesy, 1944; Rhode, 1971). The second tip with the lowest threshold was designated as the best frequency (BF). It is important to note that the unit with a CF near 8 kHz has a hypersensitive tail, i.e., the threshold at the BF is lower than the tail thresholds of normal units with CFs of 8 kHz. The "W"-shaped tuning curves comprised 17% of the sample, and only about a quarter of these had tail thresholds which could be considered hypersensitive.

The tuning curves shown in Fig. 23C were extremely broad and "U"-shaped. In some cases, the slope along the high-frequency side of the tuning curve was so shallow that there was considerable ambiguity in assigning CF using the high-frequency cutoff criterion mentioned earlier. It is conceivable that the "U"-shaped tuning curves actually represent the tails of the tuning curves of units with much higher CFs; the CFs could have been missed because the maximum stimulus intensity was below that necessary to excite the unit at CF. Thus, the actual CFs of the "U"-shaped tuning curves could be grossly underestimated; fortunately, only a small percentage (6%) of these units were encountered. Clearly, these results indicate that there can be a serious breakdown in neural frequency selectivity during TTS.

Several attempts have been made at relating the permanent changes in neural

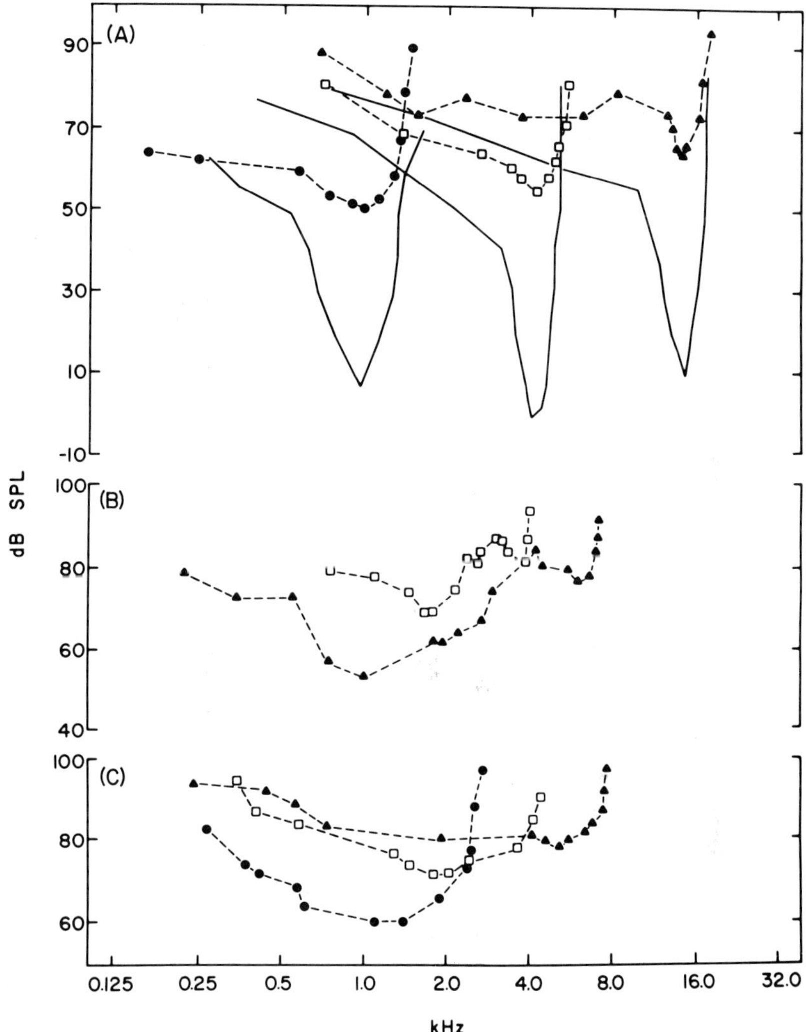

Figure 23 Normal tuning curves (solid line, A) and tuning curves from noise-treated chinchillas (symbols) having a blunt "V" shape (A), "W" shape (B), and broad "U" shape (C).

tuning to the underlying histopathologies. Liberman and Kiang (1968) have described two important classes of tuning curves. Tuning curves with a "W"-shape (Fig. 24B) have thresholds which are elevated in the region of the tip, and sometimes lower (hypersensitive) than normal in the tail region. The CFs of units with "W"-shaped tuning curves and hypersensitive tails are generally located just above the CFs of those units with the highest threshold (Fig. 24C). Units

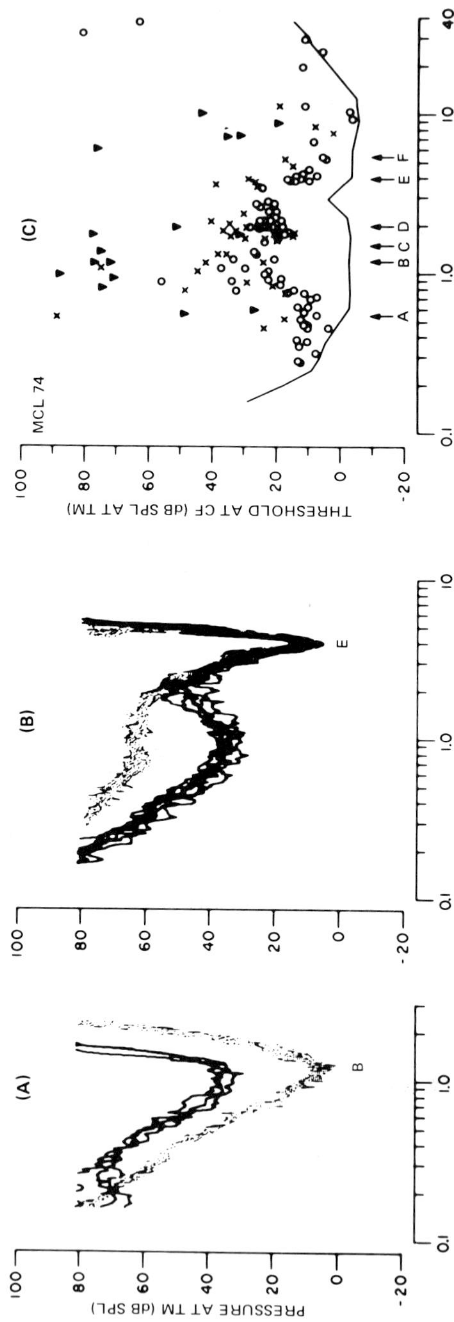

Figure 24 Abnormalities of the tuning-curve tail in several CF regions from one traumatized cat. A and B display the tuning curves (solid line) of several high spontaneous rate units from CF regions B and E of MCL 74. The stippling in each panel represents the tuning curve data from high spontaneous rate units obtained from an animal raised in a quiet chamber. C illustrates the distribution of CF thresholds for this cat; open circles represent units with SR>18/sec; filled triangles, SRL<0.5/sec; and crosses for units with intermediate rates. The solid curve represents the envelop of the best thresholds in a large sample of units from many cats. (Adapted from Liberman and Kiang, 1978.)

with "V"-shaped tuning curves have thresholds that are elevated in both the tail and the tip so that the units retain a substantial degree of tuning (Fig. 24A). Tuning curves with a "V"-shape were present only on the low-frequency side of the region where CF thresholds were elevated (Fig. 24C) and were strongly correlated with clumping of cilia on the IHC.

An interesting perspective on the interrelationship between cochlear pathology, auditory sensitivity, and frequency selectivity, measured both behaviorally and neurally, can be found in Fig. 25 and 26. The chinchilla was exposed to a low-frequency band of noise (Table I) and allowed to recover for 2 years. Although the noise exposure was centered at 0.5 kHz, the maximum PTS (30 dB) occurred at 2 kHz. The neural threshold shifts are in extremely close agreement with the behavioral data. The panels in Fig. 26 compare psychophysical and neural tuning curves having similar CFs. The psychophysical and neural tuning curves near 11.2, 8 and 4 kHz are in reasonably close accord. The curves at 11.2 and 8 kHz have low-threshold, sharply tuned tips and high-threshold, broadly tuned tails. Near 4 kHz, where there is a small hearing loss, the tuning curve tips are somewhat shorter and broader than at higher frequencies. The tuning curves near 4 kHz were located along the apical border of a discrete OHC lesion (Fig. 25A).

In the region of greatest hearing loss (2 kHz) the psychophysical tuning curves become grossly distorted and generally have a flattened "W" appearance. One tip is located near 2 kHz and a second more sensitive tip is found near 1 kHz. Furthermore, the high-frequency slope of the neural tuning curve is considerably steeper, and the tail of the neural tuning curve is flatter than that seen behaviorally. It is important to note that thse profound distortions in neural and behavioral tuning were correlated with a region of the cochlea in which virtually all hair cells were present and where there were no obvious anatomical defects. Near 1 kHz, the behavioral and neural thresholds approach normal values and the neural and behavioral tuning curves have tips which are narrower than those observed near 2 kHz; the curves are also less distorted.

The close agreement between neural and behavioral measures of tuning seen in Fig. 26 suggests that the peripheral auditory system plays a significant role in establishing the overall level of frequency selectivity of the ear. The general broadening of neural and behavioral tuning is important for understanding why hearing-impaired listeners have considerable difficulty understanding speech, particularly in noise (Olsen and Tillman, 1968). Rather than responding to selective frequency components in the speech signal, impaired neurons with broadened tuning curves respond to signals in the tail of the tuning curve as well as those near CF. This problem has the potential of becoming extrcmely severe when one recalls that the tail of the tuning curve may become hypersensitive after noise exposure. Consequently, a hearing aid may not be particularly helpful when the task is to discriminate a signal in a background of low-frequency noise.

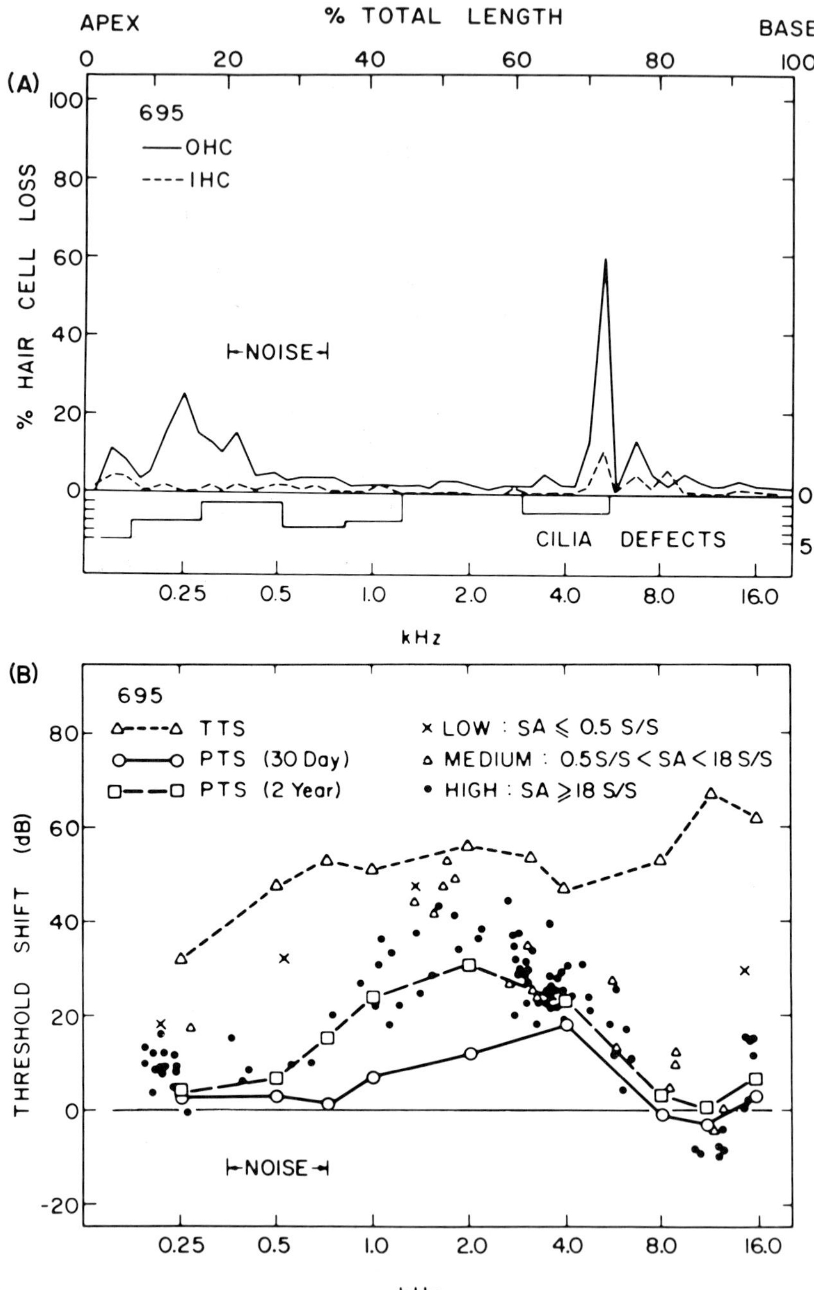

Figure 25 (A) Animal 695. Percentage outer (solid line) and inner (dashed line) hair cell loss plotted as a function of percentage total distance from the apex and as a function of frequency. The cilia defects were rated from 0 (normal) to 5 (grossly abnormal) and are indicated at the bottom of the cochleogram. (B) Behavioral measures of the temporary threshold shift (TTS) (triangles) obtained

As noted by Evans (1976), when the signal is amplified so that it can be detected, the impaired neurons will respond to both the signal and the noise, rather than to the signal alone.

C. Subjective Tinnitus and Spontaneous Activity

A common complaint expressed by listeners with noise-induced hearing loss is the perception of a ringing or buzzing sensation in the absence of any external sound. This phenomenon has been referred to as subjective tinnitus and there have been many clinical studies directed at its treatment (Atkinson, 1947; Passe, 1953; Flottorp and Wille, 1954). Effective treatment of a disorder, however, often requires knowledge of the underlying mechanisms of the disorder. One popular, but unsupported explanation for tinnitus involves the concept of an irritative lesion in the cochlea which presumably gives rise to high rates of spontaneous activity in auditory nerve fibers (Loeb and Smith, 1967; Atherley *et al.*, 1968; Feldman, 1971). Presumably, the pitch of the tinnitus is correlated with the CFs of units with high spontaneous rates while loudness relates to the rate of spontaneous activity.

While there is no effective means of having an animal report on the subjective experience of tinnitus, it is possible to examine the preceding hypothesis by sampling spontaneous activity in animals that are likely to have tinnitus, i.e., animals with noise-induced TTS or PTS. Figure 27 compares the spontaneous discharge rates of normal units with those obtained during TTS (see Fig. 14). Although the neural thresholds of the noise-exposed animals were elevated 20–60 dB above normal, the spontaneous rates of the two groups were not statistically different. Note, however, that there was a slight tendency for units in the noise-exposed groups to have rates greater than 100 spikes/sec. Similar results were obtained from chinchillas with PTS at the high frequencies (Fig. 28). The animals were exposed to an octave band of noise centered at 4 kHz and developed little or no hearing loss below 2 kHz (Figs. 18 and 19). Thus, the spontaneous rates of low CF units serve as a control for evaluating the rates of high CF units whose thresholds were elevated 20 dB or more. The distribution of spontaneous activity is not grossly different between low and high CF units; however, there is a slightly greater tendency for the high CF units to have spontaneous rates greater than 100 spikes/sec. Note also that there is a greater percentage of units with rates between 20 and 40 spikes/sec.

Liberman and Kiang (1978) have also measured spontaneous activity in noise-exposed cats (Fig. 29). The spontaneous rates of units in the low-threshold

during exposure and the permanent threshold shift (PTS) measured 1 month (open circles) and 2 years (open squares) postexposure. Small dots, triangles, and squares show the threshold shift of single units plotted as a function of CF. (From Salvi *et al.*, 1981.)

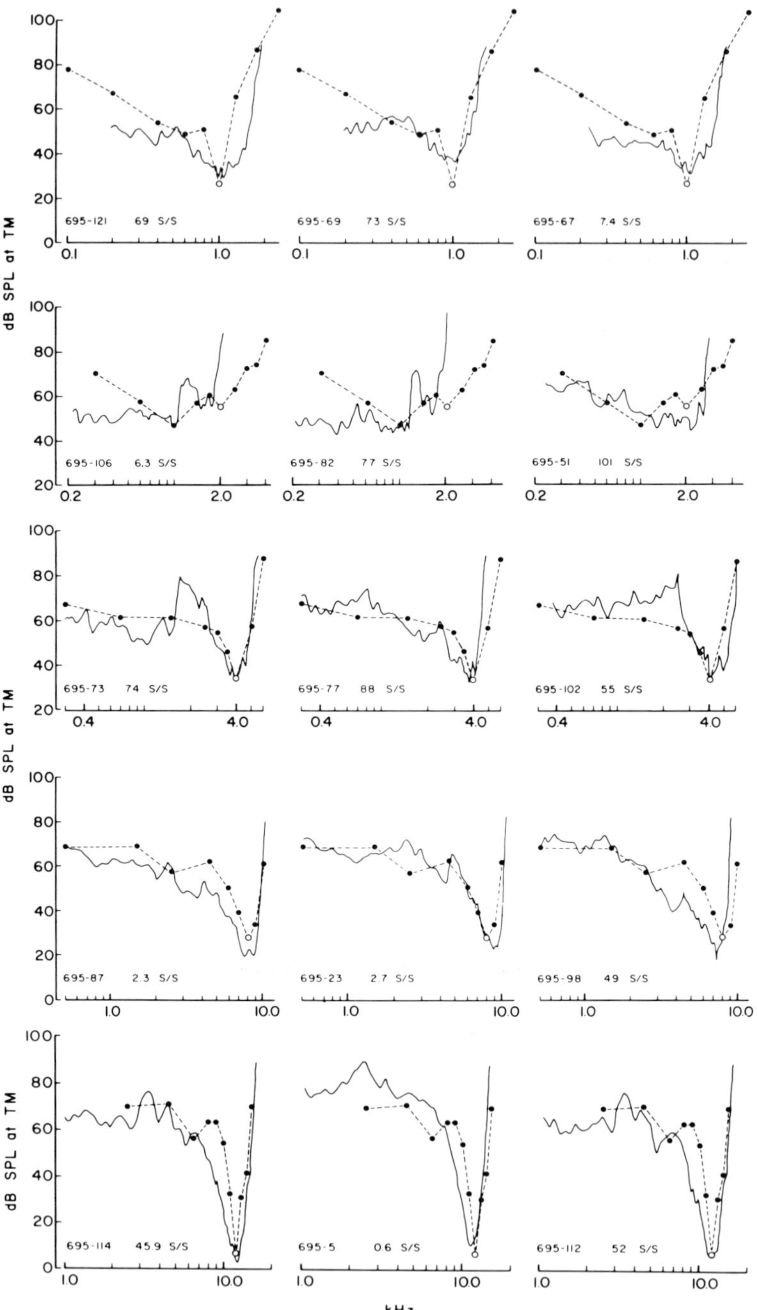

Figure 26 Psychophysical tuning curves obtained with a 11.2, 8, 4, 2, and 1 kHz probe. Masker level is expressed in dB SPL at the tympanic membrane for probe (open circle) and off-probe (solid circle) frequencies. The neural tuning curves (solid line) from units having different spontaneous rates are compared with the psychophysical tuning curves (dashed line). (Adapted from Salvi *et al.*, 1981.)

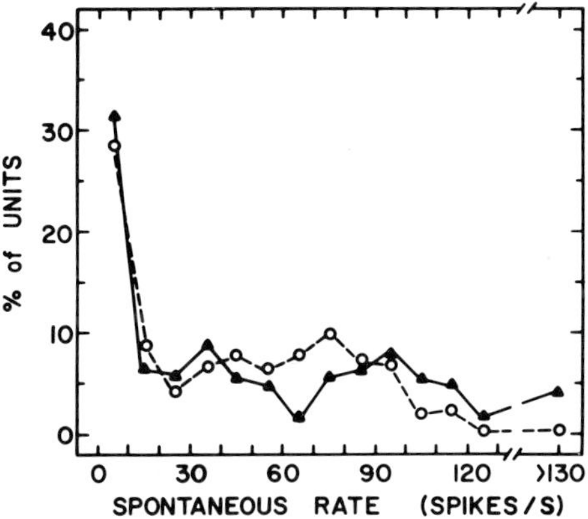

Figure 27 Percentage of units in the normal (▲) and noise-treated group (○) with the indicated rates of spontaneous activity.

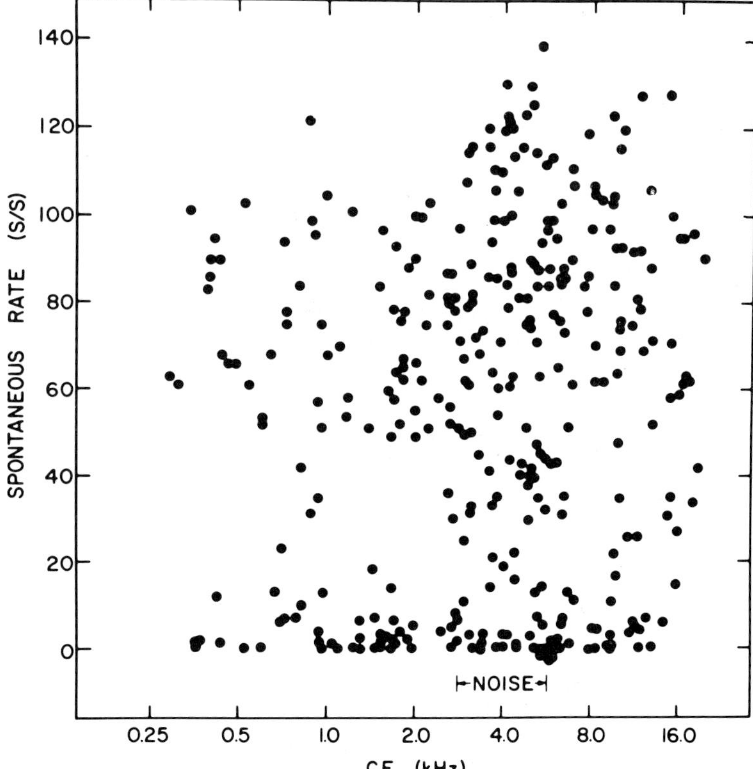

Figure 28 Distribution of spontaneous rates as a function of CF. Data pooled from four animals exposed to an octave band of noise centered at 4.0 kHz.

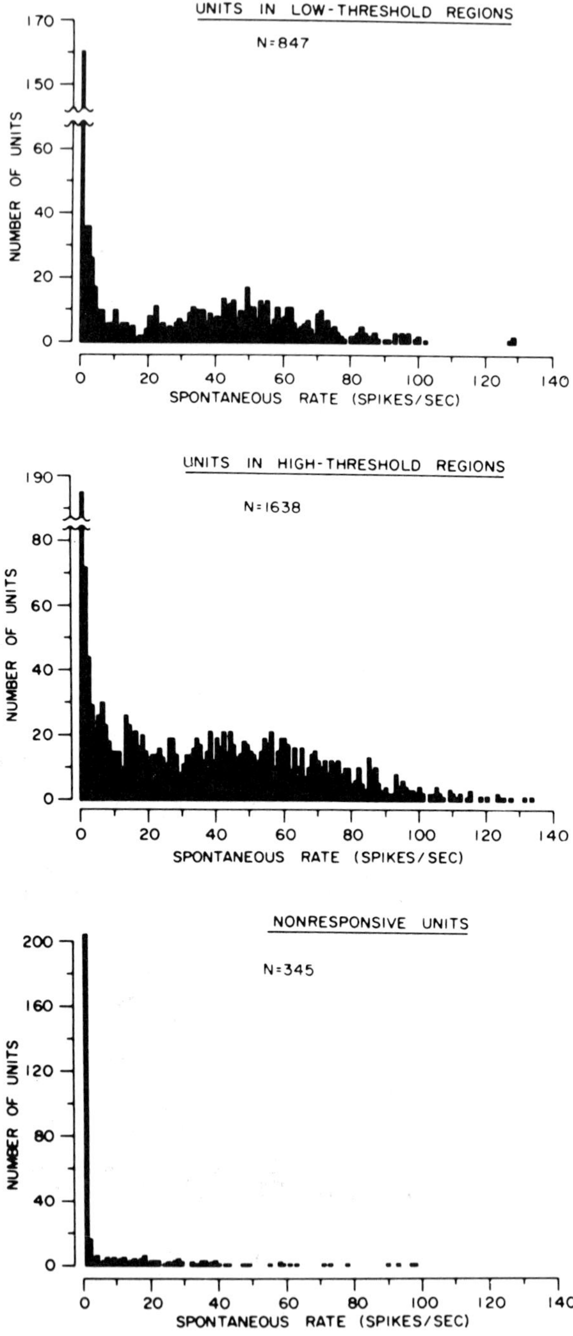

Figure 29 Comparison of the distribution of spontaneous rates for units with low and high thresholds and those unresponsive to sound. (Adapted from Liberman and Kiang, 1978.)

regions are clustered below 10 spikes/sec and between 40 and 60 spikes/sec. However, among the high-threshold units there is an increased proportion of units with rates between 10 and 30 spikes/sec. An abnormally high percentage of units with V-shaped tuning curves have rates between 10 and 30 spikes/sec. Finally, most units that were not responsive to sound had no spontaneous activity or rates below 40 spikes/sec.

The temporal pattern of spontaneous activity of most units in noise-exposed ears remains normal as illustrated by the interval histogram in Fig. 30A. However, a few units with significant threshold shifts have interval histograms with an abnormally large peak at short interspike intervals and a decay from the mode which is faster than normal (Fig. 30B).

Earlier, it was suggested that tinnitus was signaled by a substantial increase in spontaneous activity; however, the previous data provide little or no support for this hypothesis. One alternative mechanism for tinnitus, suggested by Kiang *et al.* (1970), is that the pitch of the tinnitus is related to an ''edge effect,'' that is, a sudden change in the average spontaneous rate across the population of fibers with different CFs. Presumably, the pitch of the tinnitus is matched to units with CFs at the transition region.

Although pitch studies of tinnitus have not been done with animals, such data are available from humans. When humans are exposed to a high-frequency band of noise, the tinnitus induced by the noise has a pitch which is matched to a frequency just below the frequency of maximum TTS (Loeb and Smith, 1967; Atherley *et al.*,– 1968). Such a transition has been observed in the distribution of spontaneous activity in units from the cochlear nuclus. As shown in Fig. 31, exposure to an octave band of noise centered at 4 kHz results in a significant high-frequency hearing loss with a peak at 5.6 kHz. The spontaneous rates are extremely low among units with CFs between 4 and 8 kHz and higher on either side. Thus, there is a boundary between spontaneously active and inactive units.

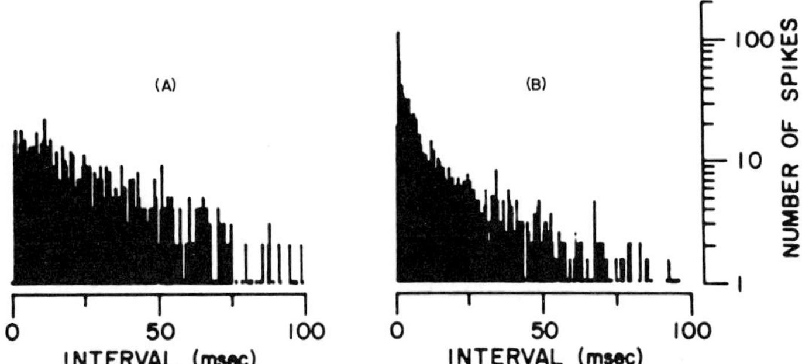

Figure 30 Interval histograms of spontaneous activity from two high threshold units with high spontaneous rates. (Adapted from Liberman and Kiang, 1978.)

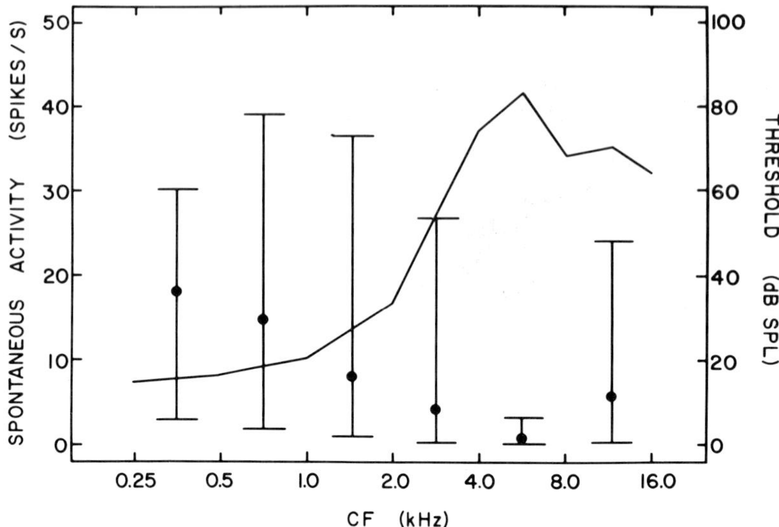

Figure 31 Comparison of the octave band distribution of spontaneous activity (median, ●; interquartile range, I) of units in the cochlear nucleus (left axis) and the average behavioral audiogram (right axis) of chinchillas exposed to an octave band of noise centered at 4 kHz. (From Salvi *et al.*, 1978.)

The low-frequency boundary corresponds to the pitch of the tinnitus reported in human psychophysical studies.

D. Temporal Summation and Response to Tone Bursts

It is well known that acoustic trauma modifies the normal process of auditory temporal summation. This is illustrated in Fig. 32A using the relationship between the threshold of a tone and its duration. In normal listeners, the threshold for a long-duration tone is approximately 12 dB lower than that to a short-duration tone. However, the threshold difference for a hearing-impaired listener is reduced to as little as 2 to 3 dB (Jerger, 1955; Wright, 1968; Henderson, 1969; Mills *et al.*, 1970). Explanations for the reduction in temporal summation have assumed that acoustic trauma causes an abnormally rapid decay over time in the output of the cochlea at intensities near threshold (Wright, 1968). Figure 32B is a schematic which shows the normal discharge pattern of a unit to a tone and the abnormally rapid decay pattern ''predicted'' for a neuron from hearing-impaired listeners. Presumably, long-duration signals are less effective in signaling threshold in the impaired ear because of abnormally rapid adaptation which leads to fewer neural dischrages for a centrally located physiological summator to integrate over time.

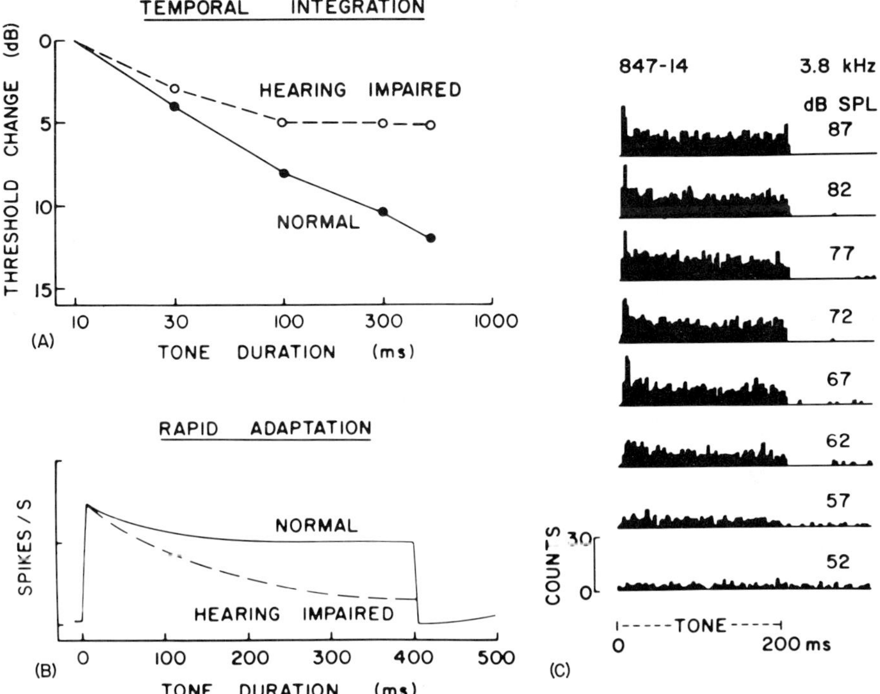

Figure 32   A Shows typical psychophysical data which illustrate the improvement in threshold with increasing signal duration for normal and hearing-impaired listeners. B illustrates the firing rate over time near threshold in normal auditory nerve fibers and the firing rate which is "presumed" to occur in hearing-impaired ears. C shows a series of PST histograms from a unit in a noise-treated animal with a threshold shift of approximately 40 dB.

Unfortunately, the response patterns of units from noise-exposed chinchillas do not give any evidence of abnormally rapid adaptation. Noise-exposed chinchillas were tested at several intensities using 200-msec tones at the unit's CF. The PST histograms shown in Fig. 32C were typical of those obtained from noise-treated animals. The unit's threshold was elevated approximately 40 dB. Just above threshold, the unit fires at nearly a constant rate over the duration of the stimulus, consequently the PST histogram is nearly flat. At higher levels of stimulation there is a peak near the beginning of the PST histogram followed by a plateau. These features of the tone-burst PST histograms are essentially the same as those obtained from units with normal sensitivity (Fig. 8). Such findings are paradoxical because acoustic trauma damages the cochlea and reduces temporal summation, yet it does not seem to alter significantly the temporal firing pattern of peripheral auditory neurons during TTS or PTS (Salvi, 1976; Henderson, 1976). Perhaps the reduction in temporal summation is the result of some other change in the neural code, such as an increase in the bandwidth over which neural information is integrated at higher auditory centers.

E. Loudness Recruitment and Rate-Intensity Functions

Loudness recruitment, or the abnormally rapid growth of loudness, is a common disorder associated with SNHL (Davis *et al.*, 1950; Hickling, 1967). Intuitively, one might expect that there would be a relationship between loudness, intensity, and neural firing rate. Thus, one potential mechanism for explaining the abnormally rapid growth of loudness involves a steepening of the slope of a neuron's dischrage rate-intensity function. The predicted neurophysiological change is shown by the solid line in Fig. 33A. Presumably, a small increment in stimulus intensity would produce an abnormally large increment in firing rate.

To test this hypothesis, the neural rate-intensity functions were measured in

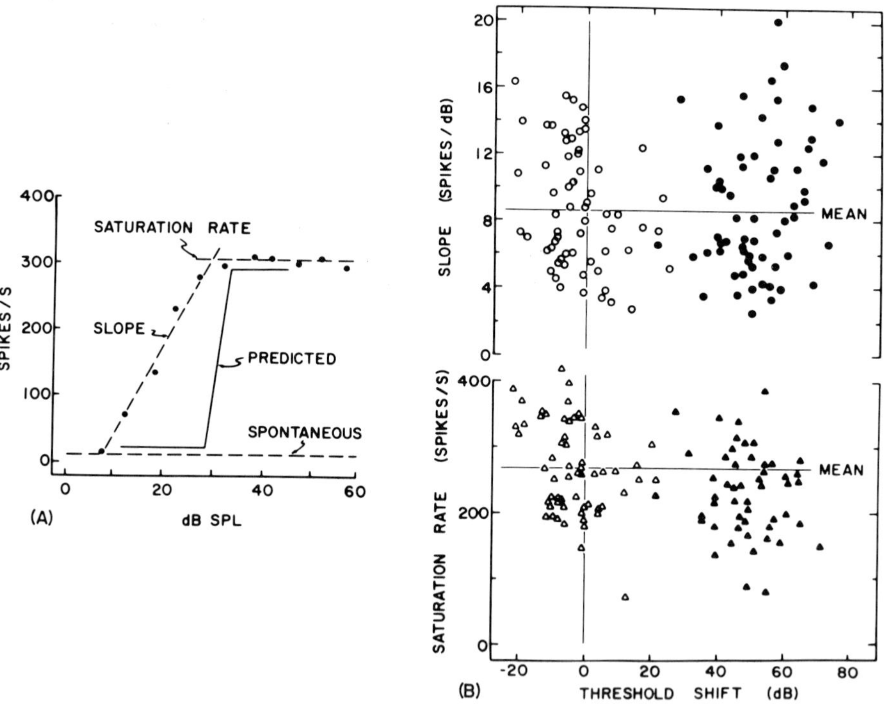

Figure 33   A shows the slope and saturation rate of the input/output function of a normal unit (- - -) and the "predicted" input/output for a neuron in a hearing-impaired ear (———). The predicted increase in the slope of the input/output function would presumably account for loudness recruitment. B shows the slopes and saturation rates obtained from units in normal (open symbols) and noise-treated (filled symbols) animals plotted as a function of the unit's threshold shift.

animals following exposure to a low-frequency band of noise (Fig. 14). Rate-intensity functions were measured with 20-msec tone bursts at the unit's CF. The two measures used to describe quantitatively the rate-intensity functions were the saturation discharge rate and the slope along the rising segment of the function. Figure 33 shows the slopes and saturation rates of units from normal and noise-treated animals plotted as a function of the threshold shift of the unit. The thresholds in the noise-treated animals are elevated approximately 50 dB above normal; however, the slopes and saturation rates of units in the noise-treated group were not significantly different from those of normal units. The noise exposure appears to have simply shifted the origin of the rate-intensity function without creating a recruitment-like change in the slope.

An alternative explanation of loudness recruitment suggested by Kiang *et al.* (1970) and Evans (1976) is based on the proportion of active units in the population of nerve fibers. In normal animals, neural tuning curves have a low-threshold, sharply tuned tip near CF and a high-threshold, broadly tuned tail below CF. Thus, at low intensities, only a few neurons will respond to a tone which is located near the low-threshold tip of the tuning curves. At higher intensities, the tone is capable of exciting other units, particularly those with CFs above the tone. These high-CF units are excited by tones located in the tail of the tuning curve. The threshold difference between the tip and tail of the tuning curve influences the rate at which new units are activated as intensity is increased; presumably this affects the rate of loudness growth. Figure 34A illustrates the theoretical model proposed by Kiang *et al.* (1970) and Evans (1976). The dashed line in Fig. 34A indicates the frequency of the stimulus. An individual unit begins to contribute to the population of active neurons when the intensity of the tone exceeds the threshold at that point on the tuning curve. As the stimulus level is increased more neurons respond; however, for a given increment in intensity, a larger percentage of units will become activated in the pathological group than in the normal population. Figure 34B shows the result of applying such a model to normal units and units from animals exposed to a low-frequency band of noise (Fig. 14). The solid line represents the percentage of normal units ($N = 144$) in our sample that responded to a 2-kHz tone as intensity was increased; the dashed line shows similar results for units ($N = 96$) in the noise-treated group. A comparison of the two curves shows that units in the noise-treated group begin to respond at a level which is roughly 40 dB higher than that for the normal sample. Within the first 20 dB of "threshold," the slope of the noise-treated group is shallower than normal; however, at higher intensities the slope becomes steeper than normal so that the function catches up with that of the normal group. Thus, the population response of the noise-treated units appears to parallel the psychophysical findings of loudness recruitment.

Although the preceding model and data appear reasonable, certain loudness measurements obtained by Viemeister (1974) from normal listeners pose a prob-

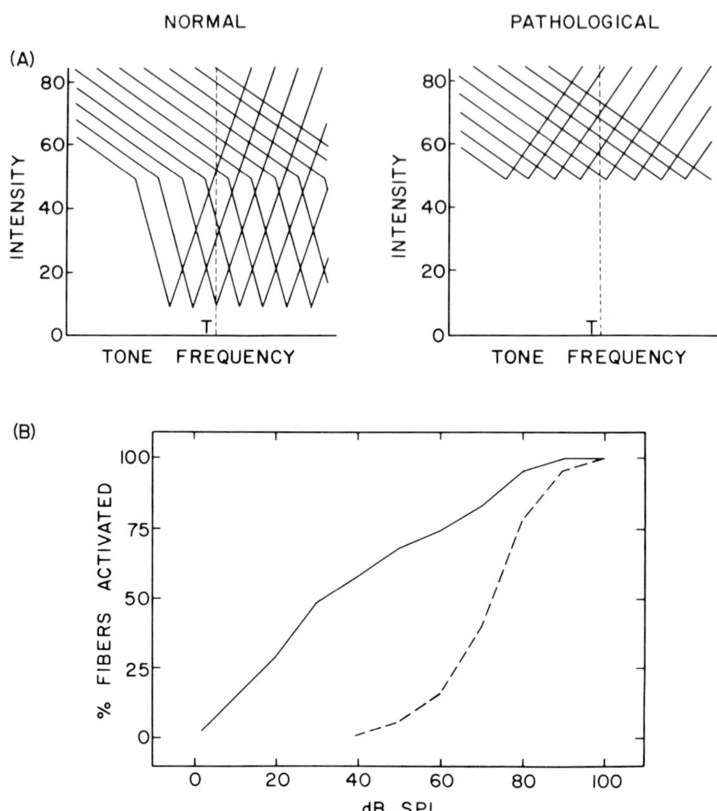

Figure 34 Idealized tuning curves in normal and pathological (A) animals according to Evans (1976). Units begin to respond to the tone (dashed line) at the intensity where the dashed line cuts across the tuning curve. B shows the percentage of the units in the normal (solid line) and noise-treated (dashed line) chinchillas that were activated as the intensity at 2 kHz was increased.

lem for loudness growth based on the recruitment of fibers having CFs adjacent to the stimulating tone. Viemeister placed a band-reject noise masker around the test signal used for the loudness judgments. The band-reject noise presumably forced the listener into making loudness judgments using the information supplied by units having CFs near the narrow-band test signal. It is assumed that units with CFs above or below the test signal would be saturated all of the time and thus unable to signal a change in loudness upon the introduction of the test signal. Under such conditions, listeners were still able to make loudness judgments over an 80-dB range. Thus, it appears that units with CFs above or below a narrow-band signal contribute little to the loudness percept of that signal. Clearly, this creates a problem for the preceding model of loudness recruitment.

F. Temporal Resolution and Neural Timing

Another important aspect of auditory temporal processing is temporal resolution, i.e., the ability to resolve rapid fluctuations in stimulus intensity such as those found in speech. Since it is well known that speech discrimination deteriorates with SNHL, one might expect to find some deterioration in the temporal resolving power of the auditory system. There are a number of psychophysical tasks which provide quantitative estimates of the systems temporal resolving power (Plomp, 1964; Jesteadt *et al.*, 1976; Viemeister, 1977); however the procedure which has seen the most widespread use among the hearing-impaired population involves the detection of gaps or silent intervals in an otherwise continuous noise.

The minimum gap that can be detected by normal listeners is approximately 3 msec; however, when the sensation level of the noise falls below about 30 dB the gap thresholds begin to increase (Plomp, 1964). Boothroyd (1978) and Fitzgibbons (1979) have reported that certain human listeners with SNHL exhibit poor temporal resolution; generally listeners with severe to moderate hearing losses had gap thresholds that were larger than normal. A closer examination of individual data, however, reveals substantial intersubject variability, with some hearing-impaired subjects having gap thresholds within normal limits. More recently, a comprehensive picture on the relationship between temporal resolution (gap threshold) and degree of hearing loss was provided by Giraudi *et al.* (1982). They exposed chinchillas to an octave band of noise centered at 0.5 kHz which caused a relatively flat hearing loss (e.g., Fig. 14). The level of the noise was systematically varied in order to produce different levels of ATS and at each level of ATS, the gap thresholds were measured. No change in gap thresholds was noted for mild hearing loss (15 dB). With moderate levels of ATS (30 dB) temporal resolution began to deteriorate, but normal resolution could be reinstated by compensating for the change in sensation level of the test signal. When ATS exceeded 40–50 dB temporal resolution was degraded beyond the point where it could be corrected by compensating for the effect of sensation level.

Since abnormal gap detection has been documented in hearing-impaired chinchillas, it would be interesting to see if the nerve fibers in such animals were capable of following these rapid amplitude fluctuations; unfortunatley such studies of temporal resolution have not yet been conducted. There are indications, however, that the temporal characteristics of VIIIth nerve firing patterns are remarkably resistent to changes in auditory sensitivity.

Harrison and Evans (1979) measured the phase-locking characteristics of VIIIth nerve fibers in guinea pigs with hearing losses caused by kanamycin poisoning. Although the neural thresholds were significantly higher than normal, the temporal coding properties (coefficient of synchronization, interspike interval histograms) of the units to speech stimuli were essentially normal when the stimuli were presented at suprathreshold levels.

Because speech signals are relatively complicated, it is difficult to analyze and interpret any changes in neural response from hearing-impaired animals. A more direct measure of temporal processing changes in VIIIth nerve fibers can be obtained with click stimuli; such data have been obtained from chinchillas with approximately 40–60 dB of TTS following exposure to an octave band of noise centered at 0.5 kHz (Fig. 14). Figure 35 shows a typical series of PST histograms obtained with clicks in normal and noise-exposed animals. Near threshold, the normal unit has a relatively long latency; as intensity is raised the latency systematically decreases. In the noise-exposed animal, the latency shift is absent. As illustrated in Fig. 36B, the latencies measured near threshold tend to be shorter than normal in noise-exposed animals; however, if latencies are measured at a fixed SPL, the latencies for the normal and noise-exposed group are similar (Fig. 36A). Thus, latency appears to be more closely related to absolute intensity than to the intensity relative to the neuron's threshold.

Another important feature of the histograms obtained with clicks is the time interval between peaks. In both normal and noise-exposed ears, ΔP is approximately equal to 1/CF. One difference between the PST histogram from normal

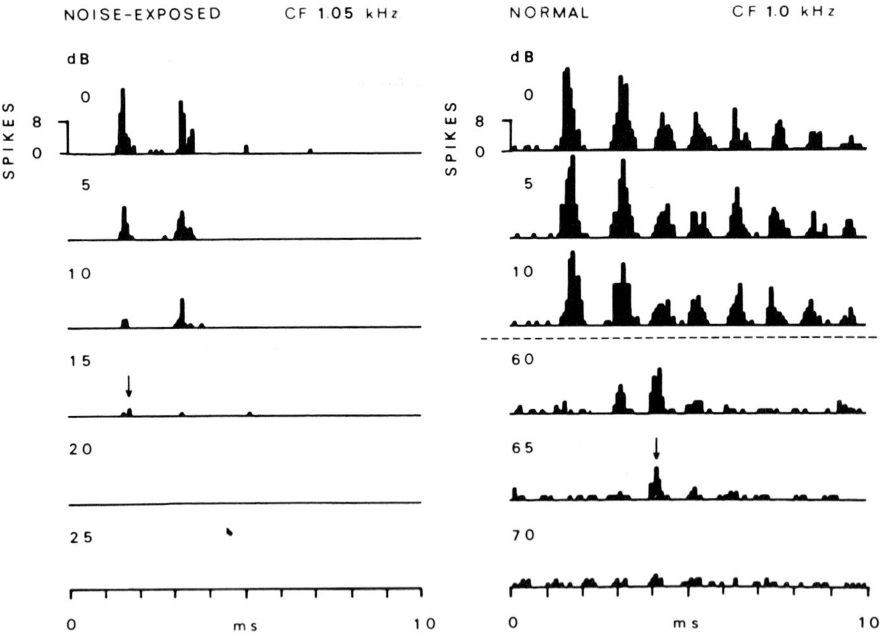

Figure 35   Histograms obtained with clicks from normal and noise-treated auditory nerve fibers. Histograms can be compared at the threshold (arrow), 15 and 65 dB attenuation for the noise-treated and normal fiber, respectively, or at the same intensity, 0–10 dB attenuation. (From Salvi *et al.*, 1980.)

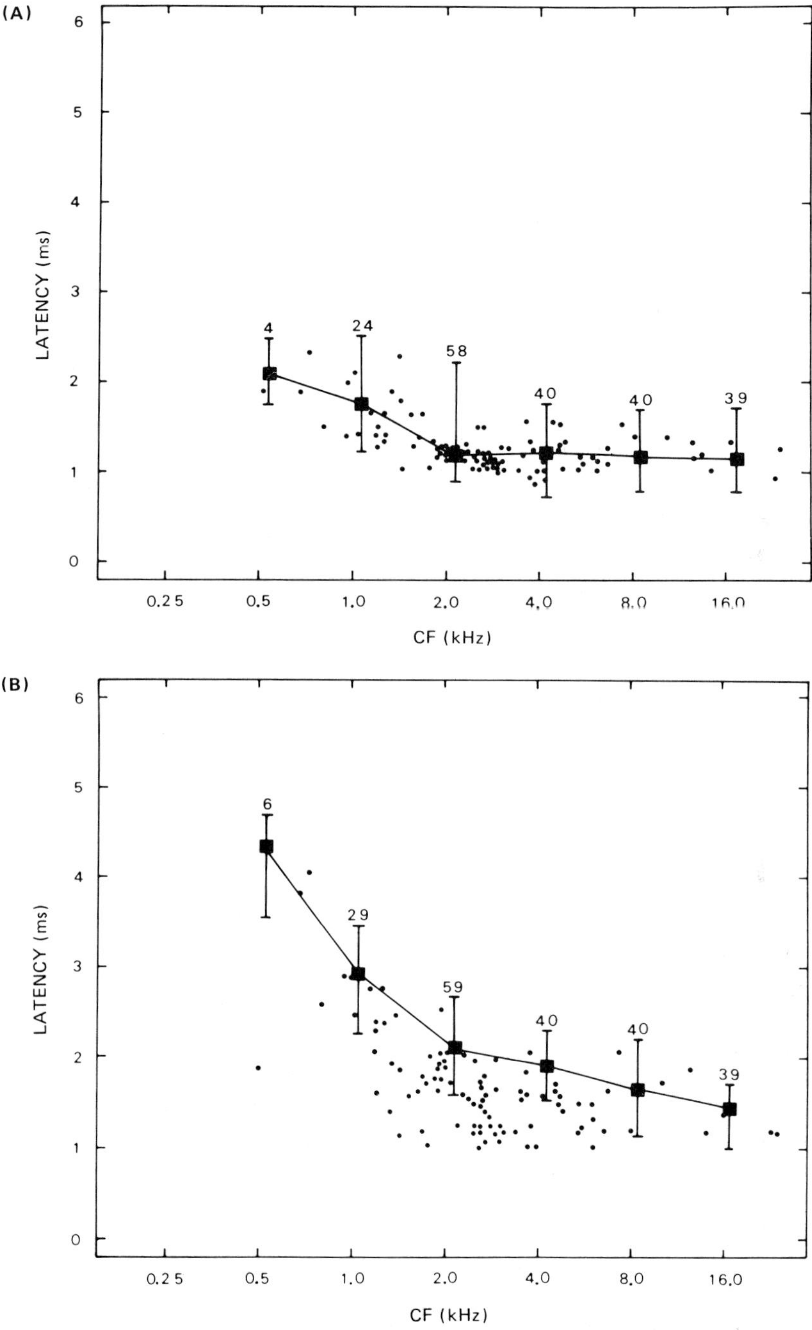

Figure 36 Single fiber latencies as a function of CF at 0 dB attenuation of the click (A) and at the click threshold (B). The click thresholds varied as a function of the CF of the unit. The range (vertical bars), median (■), and number of units in each octave band for normal chinchillas are compared with those from noise-treated animals (●). (From Salvi *et al.*, 1980.)

and noise-exposed animals, however, is the number of peaks measured at a fixed intensity above threshold; the units in the noise-exposed animals tend to have fewer peaks (Fig. 35), i.e., they lack the lightly damped, ringing characteristics seen in normal units.

The changes in the click response of units in noise-exposed animals have interesting parallels in the transient mechanical response of the basilar membrane observed by Robles *et al.* (1976). First, in impaired animals, there was a loss of the lightly damped nonlinear tail of the basilar membrane velocity response; this correlates with the reduced number of peaks in the PST histogram. Second, the largest peak in the PST histogram occurred earlier in time as intensity was increased. If the neural latency is determined by the largest peak in the mechanical response, then the high-threshold unit should have shorter latencies at threshold than low-threshold units as seen in Fig. 36 (Salvi *et al.*, 1979a).

The greater damping seen in the PST histogram measured with clicks is difficult to reconcile with the psychophysical gap detection data. One would expect the rapid decay of firing seen in the PST histogram to lead to even better gap detection; however, as reported above, the gap detection threshold systematically increased with SNHL. Perhaps the change in gap detection is the result of an alternation in the temporal code across the population of VIIIth nerve fibers rather than a change in firing patterns of individual fibers.

The neural latencies measured in noise-exposed animals (Fig. 36) have interesting implications for understanding the processes involved with sound localization. The timing of neural events plays an important role in models of sound lateralization. Sounds are normally lateralized to the midline if the sound arrives at the same time (latency) and if the intensity is the same at both ears. On the other hand, a sound will be lateralized to one side of the head if the sound arrives earlier (shorter latency) and/or is more intense at that side. Given that timing is an important cue, what predictions can be made about lateralization in listeners with a unilateral, noise-induced hearing loss? Recall that neural latencies in noise-exposed ears are a function of absolute intensity, and not intensity relative to threshold. If a suprathreshold sound is presented simultaneously to both ears at the same intensity, the neural latency in the impaired ear should be the same as that in the normal, contralateral ear. Thus, a patient with a pure cochlear lesion should localize the sound at the midline; this is exactly what has been reported clinically (Wang and Dallos, 1972). On the other hand, listeners with conductive losses should show a much different lateralization pattern.

G. Suppression and Two-Tone Inhibition

Simple stimuli, such as tone bursts, are seldom encountered in natural environments; however, they are used extensively in laboratory and clinical settings in order to isolate fundamental auditory processes. When these simple, but well-controlled, stimuli are combined it is possible to extract additional information about more complex auditory processes. One of the nonlinear properties of the auditory system that can be assessed with a combination of simple stimuli is known as suppression. The behavioral measure of suppression is especially interesting since it is similar to TTI observed in VIIIth nerve fibers. If suppression and TTI are in fact governed by the same cochlear mechanisms, then SNHL should affect these two nonlinear processes in the same general way.

The psychophysical paradigm for demonstrating suppression involves the use of two-tone bursts (f_m and f_v) of fixed intensity which precede and ultimately mask a third tone burst (f_p) of variable intensity (f_m—forward masker of fixed frequency; f_v—forward masker of variable frequency; f_p—frequency of probe tone). The intensity of f_v is generally 20 dB greater than that of f_m. Tones f_m and f_p are at the same frequency. Initially, only f_m and f_p are presented and the subject adjusts the intensity of f_p so it is just detectable. This establishes the baseline condition for the suppression experiment. Next, the tone of variable frequency (f_v) is presented simultaneously with f_m. At each frequency of f_v, the subject adjusts the intensity of f_p so that it is, again, just detectable. If the threshold of f_p rises above the baseline threshold for f_p, then the assumption is that f_v assists f_m in masking f_p. However, if the threshold of f_p falls below the baseline, then this is taken as evidence that f_v improves the detectability of f_p by suppressing the masking effect of f_m.

Wightman *et al.* (1977) have measured suppression areas in human subjects with normal and impaired hearing (Fig. 37). The normal listener (MK) shows suppression areas (i.e., a reduction in probe intensity re baseline intensity) when the frequency of f_v is slightly above f_p; this occurs at all three probe frequencies. Subject JA has a high-frequency hearing loss which rises steeply beginning at 1.6 kHz. The suppression areas are present at the low frequencies where hearing is normal; however, at the highest probe frequency, suppression is totally absent. Apparently when tone f_v falls within the region of hearing loss, it is unable to suppress the masking effect of f_m.

Similar measures of suppression are unavailable for hearing-impaired animals; however, neurophysiological measures of TTI have been obtained which appear to mirror the suppression data obtained from humans with SNHL. Following acoustic trauma, the normal pattern of TTI (Fig. 11) observed in auditory nerve fibers can be altered to varying degrees. The exact effect, however, may depend on the type and location of the cochlear lesion.

Schmeidt *et al.* (1980) exposed gerbils to impulse noise and found changes in TTI that seemed to be related to the location of the OHC lesion. Units that were associated with an OHC lesion in the basal turn had broad tuning curves, elevated thresholds at CF, and generally showed a reduction or total loss of TTI on the high-frequency side of CF. On the other hand, units that were associated with mid-cochlear lesions generally exhibited TTI above CF, although sometimes the amplitude of TTI was reduced. TTI did not appear to be strongly correlated with the degree of threshold shift at CF; thus, some units with threshold shifts as great

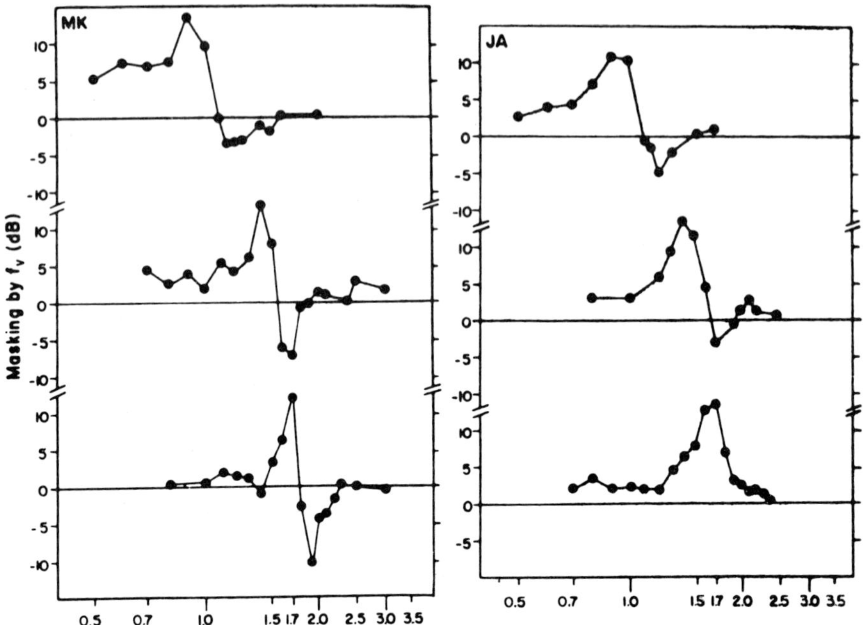

Figure 37   Suppression measurements from a normal subject (MK) and a hearing-impaired subjects (JA). Probe frequencies were 1.0 kHz (top), 1.5 kHz (middle), and 2.0 kHz (bottom). In all cases the fixed masker ($f_m=f_p$) was at 40 dB SPL and the variable masker (f_v) was at 60 dB SPL. (From Wightman *et al.*, 1977.)

as 40–60 dB showed normal TTI. Finally, units with hypersensitive thresholds in the tail of the tuning curve failed to demonstrate TTI for inhibitory tones (f_2) placed below CF; in fact, the firing rate sometimes increased when f_1 and f_2 were presented together. The variability in this study may be attributed to the diverse set of pathologies associated with exposure to impulse noise. What the study by Schmiedt *et al.* shows, however, is that TTI is altered with cochlear lesions.

A somewhat more orderly set of TTI results were obtained from a chinchilla exposed to an octave band of noise centered at 4 dHz. Figure 38 shows how the magnitude of TTI varies across the population of auditory nerve fibers, the neural

---

Figure 38   (A) Animal 679. Percentage outer (solid line) and inner (dashed line) hair cell loss plotted as a function of percentage total distance from the apex and as a function of frequency. Dashed vertical line indicates the region of the cochlea with anatomical defects. (B) Behavioral measures of temporary threshold shift (triangles) and permanent threshold shift (open circles). Solid dots indicate permanent neural threshold shifts at CF. (C) Maximum amount of two-tone inhibition (TTI) expressed as a percentage of the driven discharge rate and plotted as a function of the characteristic frequency of the unit (solid dot). The degree of inhibition increases in the negative direction. R_{TT}—two tone response rate; R_{SA}—spontaneous rate; R_E—excitatory response rate. (Adapted from Salvi *et al.*, 1981.)

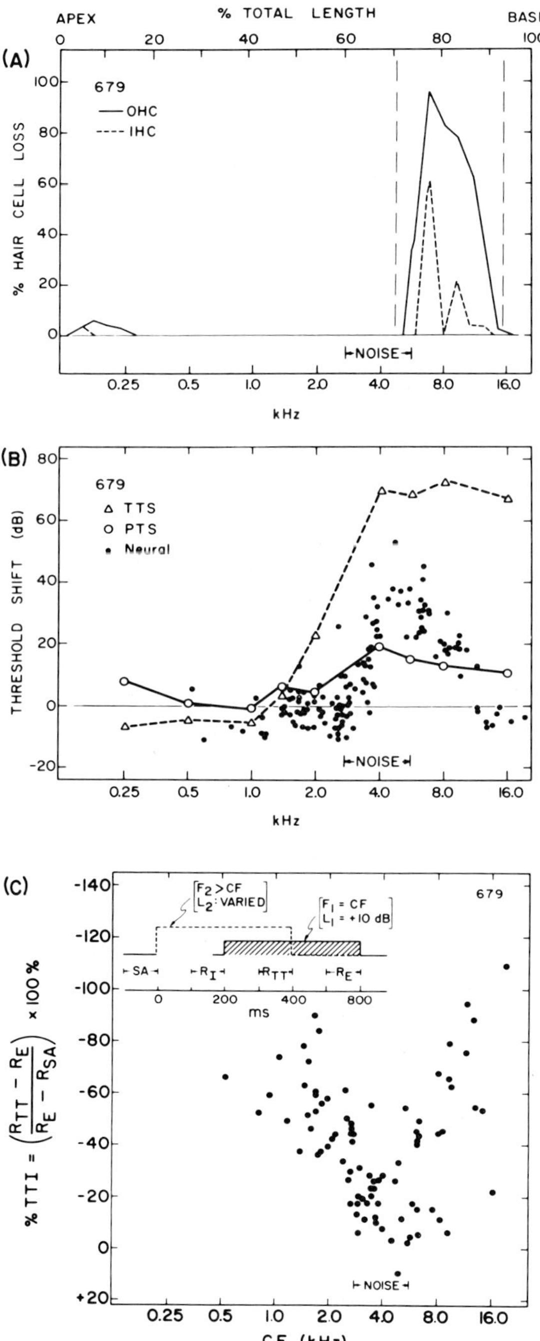
APEX
% TOTAL LENGTH
BASE
0
20
40
60
80
100
(A)
100
% HAIR CELL LOSS
80
60
40
20
0
679
OHC
IHC
NOISE
0.25
0.5
1.0
2.0
4.0
8.0
16.0
kHz

(B)
80
679
TTS
PTS
Neural
THRESHOLD SHIFT (dB)
60
40
20
0
-20
NOISE
0.25
0.5
1.0
2.0
4.0
8.0
16.0
kHz

(C)
-140
-120
-100
-80
-60
-40
-20
0
+20
679
F2 > CF
L2 : VARIED
F1 = CF
L1 = +10 dB
SA
RI
RTT
RE
0
200
400
800
ms
% TTI = ((RTT - RE) / (RE - RSA)) × 100 %
NOISE
0.25
0.5
1.0
2.0
4.0
8.0
16.0
CF (kHz)

and behavioral thresholds, and the cochlear lesion. Note that the PTS is rather mild, less than 20 dB, yet substantial changes occur in TTI. Each dot represents the greatest reduction (negative values) in TTI that could be found at any frequency–intensity combination of f_1 ($f_2 > f_1$) with f_2 at CF. TTI is weak and nearly absent among units with the greatest threshold shift; this corresponds to the frequency where the behavioral PTS is greatest and parallels the human data in Fig. 37. These results strengthen the relationship between TTI and suppression and suggest that suppression may be an expression of nonlinear processes in the cochlea.

H. Perceptual and Neural Responses to Combination Tones

When normal human listeners are presented with two tones (f_1 and f_2) having the appropriate frequency separation and level, they not only can detect the primary tones, but also combination tones, the most prominent of which are $(2f_1 - f_2)$ and $(f_2 - f_1)$ (Goldstein, 1967; Smoorenburg, 1972). There is still a debate as to the loudness level of the combination tones relative to the loudness of the primaries; however, psychophysical measurements of combination tones in hearing-impaired listeners have provided insights on the approximate site of generation. Smoorenburg (1972) reported that a listener with SNHL was unable to detect the combination tones when one of the primaries was located in the region of loss. Later, Dallos (1977) showed similar data from a chinchilla with an OHC lesion induced by kanamycin intoxication. When f_1 and f_2 were located within the region of hearing loss, the combination tones $2f_1 - f_2$, which falls within the region of normal sensitivity, could not be detected by the chinchilla. These results strongly suggests that combination tones are generated by some neuromechanical process at the level of the cochlea. If so, parallel changes should be observed in VIIIth nerve fibers from animals with SNHL.

As shown earlier (Fig. 12), auditory nerve fibers will normally respond to the intermodulation-distortion frequencies $(f_2 - f_1)$ and $(2f_1 - f_2)$ even though only the primaries are present in the acoustic signal. Figure 39, from Siegel and Kim (1981), shows the magnitude of the distortion tone response $(f_2 - f_1)$ and the response to a single tone (f_2) across the population of neurons in a normal animal (Fig. 39A) and in a noise-exposed animal (Fig. 39B). The frequency of f_s (320 Hz) is equal to the frequency of the distortion tone $(f_2 - f_1)$ where $f_1 = 3680$ Hz and $f_2 = 4000$ Hz. In normal chinchillas, the two primaries (f_1 and f_2) generate a significant response among units having CFs corresponding to the distortion frequency ($f_2 - f_1 = 320$ Hz). In the region of the distortion frequency, the magnitude and distribution of neural activity across CF approximate the pattern of neural activity when f_s is presented alone. The data in Fig. 39B were obtained from a noise-exposed chinchilla with a sizable hair-cell lesion in the basal turn; the location of the lesion corresponds to the frequencies of the primaries. In this

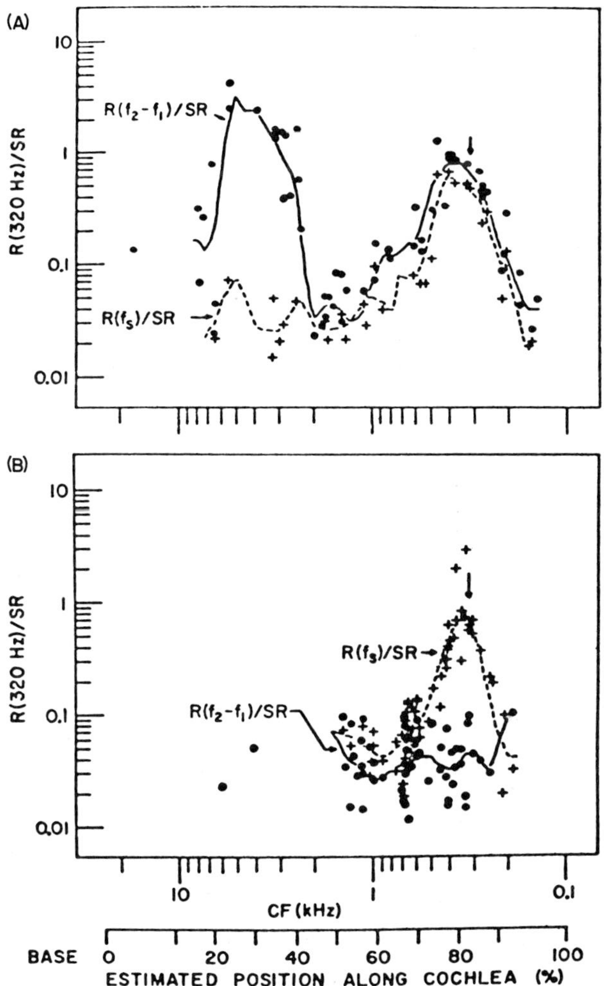

Figure 39 Comparison of (f_2-f_1) and single-tone responses of cochlear nerve fibers in an unexposed chinchilla (9) (A) and chinchilla (14) with basal turn damaged by noise exposure (B). The CF-distance scale is from Eldredge *et al.* (1977). In both cases $f_1 = 3680$ Hz, $f_2 = 4000$ Hz, $L_1 = L_2 = 50$ dB for the two-tone stimulus, while $f_s = 320$ Hz, $L_s = 5$ dB for the single tone. (solid line, two-tone data; + dashed line, single tone data). (A) the unexposed animal shows a large propagating distortion produce (f_2-f_1) near the 320-Hz characteristic place (arrow), corresponding to a peak in the single-tone response. In the exposed animal, no propagating distortion product is seen even through the sensitivity to 320 Hz is normal. Lines through the data points are moving-window averages. (From Siegel and Kim, 1981.)

animal, the two tones (f_1 and f_2) fail to generate a response among units with CFs corresponding to the distortion frequency; however, a single tone ($f_2 = 320$ Hz) matching the distortion tone frequency is capable of exciting units in this CF region in a normal manner. Thus, when the primary tones are placed in a region where the neural thresholds are elevated, the tones fail to generate a neural response in normal units with CFs corresponding to the distortion tone frequency ($f_2 - f_1$). These results are consistent with the failure of listeners to detect the combination tone when the primaries are placed in the region of the hearing loss. Based on recent evidence (Siegel et $al.$, 1981), one could interpret these results as follows. In normal listeners, the neuromechanical events surrounding the transduction of f_1 and f_2 presumably give rise to secondary vibrations corresponding to the distortion tones; these mechanical waves propagate to their characteristic places within the cochlea and result in a pattern of neural activity similar to that produced by a single tone corresponding to the distortion tone frequency. When the region of the cochlea corresponding to the primaries is damaged by noise or drugs, the secondary vibrations are no longer generated.

IV. SUMMARY AND DISCUSSION

The hearing loss caused by exposure to high levels of noise is considered to be primarily of cochlear origin. It follows that the symptoms of noise-induced hearing loss should be reflected in the neural output of the cochlea. In fact, some of the symptoms are clearly expressed in the output of the VIIIth nerve, while others are not. The audiogram and pattern of hearing loss are most easily understood in terms of the distribution of VIIIth nerve fiber thresholds. In four experiments involving noise-induced TTS and PTS, the distribution of thresholds at CF followed the general contour of the behavioral audiogram. However, in a few instances there were discrepancies between the behavioral and neural thresholds. For example, in Fig. 18, no units with CF of 8 kHz were found, yet the animal responded to moderate intensity tones at this frequency. Presumably the animal was able to hear the 8-kHz tone by using information conveyed through air cells adjacent to the lesion. Unfortunately, the relation between the changes in sensitivity observed physiologically and behaviorally do not always map neatly on to the regions of sensory cell damage. Frequently, thresholds are elevated with little or no cell loss. Presumably there are very subtle anatomical changes which can lead to a deterioration in auditory performance.

The exceptional frequency selectivity of normal listeners has been shown to deteriorate after noise exposure. The breakdown in frequency resolution with SNHL appears to have a clear physiological bases in the auditory periphery. It has been known for some time that hearing loss of cochlear origin usually results in a detuning in VIIIth nerve fibers; however, the results are complicated. For example, units with the same CF may have tuning curves with a V-, W-, or U-shaped profile. The broadening of the tuning curve, especially with hypersensitivity of the tail, is particularly intriguing with respect to dyplacusis, i.e., distorted pitch. In psychophysical studies of TTS, human subjects generally report an upward shift in pitch of a half octave or more after noise exposure. The pitch shifts are pronounced when tones are placed in the region of greatest TTS (Ruedi and Furner, 1946; Piazza, 1966). Presumably the pitch shift occurs because a greater proportion of units with CFs above the tone frequency are activated relative to units with CFs corresponding to the tone. Obviously such large pitch shifts will adversely affect the perceptual characteristics of more complex sounds such as speech or noise.

The broadening of both the psychophysical and physiological tuning curves may be useful in understanding the problems of fitting hearing aids. Patients with essentially the same hearing loss often derive much different benefits from the same aid. Thus, the hearing loss per se may not adequately describe the patient's hearing problem. Psychophysical tuning curves are difficult to measure, but they may help in discriminating successful from unsuccessful hearing aid users. Patients with predominantly "V"-shaped tuning curves might be expected to perform differently than patients with especially broad or "W"-shaped tuning curves. Presumably, the patients with poorer tuning will have much more difficulty in discriminating signals from background noise.

Even if the patient showed good frequency resolution, a conventional hearing aid would not correct for other auditory deficits such as recruitment, tinnitus, temporal resolution, temporal integration, suppression, and distortion tones. Our understanding of the neural underpinnings of each of these symptoms varies. The breakdown in temporal resolution and temporal integration does not appear to have an obvious correlate in the timing of discharges of a single VIIIth nerve fiber. Presumably, the change in temporal processing depends on the relative timing of neural activity across the distribution of units.

One of the audiometric symptoms which has some neurophysiological support is loudness recruitment. The model and data indicate that in hearing-impaired subjects the nerve fibers are added to the active population at a faster rate than normal rate as intensity is increased. This model relies on the abnormally rapid spread of excitation toward units with CFs above the tone frequency. While the model is intriguing, it clearly would not account for the normal pattern of loudness growth observed when a test signal is sandwiched within band-reject noise (Viemeister, 1974).

Another symptom, subjective tinnitus, was originally thought to arise from elevated rates of spontaneous activity. Experimental results, however, indicate that the rates remain unchanged or in some instances decline. In cases in which the rate of spontaneous activity changes abruptly across CF, it is possible to account for tinnitus using an "edge" effect model. Unfortunately, animal psychophysical data necessary to test the model rigorously are unavailable.

The two psychophysical nonlinearities, suppression and the perception of combination tones, appear to have the appropriate neural analogs in two-tone inhibition and in the neural responses to combination tones. The data from listeners with SNHL have helped to strengthen the linkage between the psychophysical and neurophysiological nonlinearities since the neural and behavioral measures appear to deteriorate in the same general fashion. Exactly how important the loss of these two nonlinearities is to the hearing-impaired listener is not well understood.

In summary, it has been possible to gain a better understanding of the symptoms associated with SNHL by combining the techniques from psychophysics, anatomy, and neurophysiology. In addition to the techniques, each discipline formulates or conceptualizes the problem from a slightly different point of view; this scientific cross-fertilization often leads to a reformation or refinement of the problem and issues.

Acknowledgments

The research was supported in part by grants from the National Institutes of Health (1-R01-NS1676), National Institute of Occupational Safety and Health (1-R01-OH-00364), and the U.S. Army Medical Research and Development Command (DAMD-17-80-C-0133). The authors wish to thank Patricia Robinson and George Turrentine for their technical assistance.

References

Ades, H. W., Trahiotis, C., Kokko-Cunningham, A., and Averback, B. V. (1974). Comparison of hearing thresholds and morphological changes in the chinchilla after exposure to 4 kHz tones. *Acta Oto–Laryngol.* **78,** 192–206.

Arthur, R. M., Pfeiffer, R. R., and Suga, N. (1971). Properties of two-tone inhibition in primary auditory neurons. *J. Physiol.* **212,** 593–609.

Atherley, G. R. C., Hempstock, T. I., and Noble, W. G. (1968). Study of tinnitus induced temporarily by noise. *J. Acoust. Soc. Am.* **44,** 1503–1506.

Atkinson, M. (1947). Tinnitus aurium: Some consideration concerning its origin and treatment. *Arch. Otolaryngol.* **45,** 68–76.

Bekesy, G., von (1944). Uber die mechanische Frequenz Analyse in der Schnecke vershiedener Tiere. *Akust. Z.* **9,** 3–11.

Bismark, G., von. (1967). "The Sound Pressure Transformation from Free-Field to the Eardrum of the Chinchilla." Master's Thesis, Massachusetts Institute of Technology.

Boothroyd, A. (1978). "Detection of Temporal Gaps by Deaf and Hearing Subjects." SARP #12, Clark School for the Deaf, Northampton, Massachusetts.

Cardner, H. M., and Miller, J. D. (1972). Temporary threshold shift from prolonged exposure to noise. *J. Speech Hear. Res.* **15,** 603–623.

Dallos, P. (1977). Comment following W. S. Rhode. *In* "Psychophysical and Physiology of Hearing" (E. F. Evans and J. P. Wilson, eds.). Academic Press, New York.

Davis, H., Morgan, C. T., Hawkins, J. E., Galambos, R., and Smith, F. W. (1950). Temporary deafness following exposure to loud tones and noise. *Acta Oto–Laryngol. Suppl.* **88.**

Dolan, T. R., Ades, H. W., Bredberg, G., and Neff, W. D. (1975). Inner ear damage and hearing loss after exposure to tones of high intensity. *Acta Oto–Laryngol.* **80,** 343.

Eldredge, D. H., Miller, J. D., Bohne, B. A., and Clark, W. W. (1977). Frequency-position maps for the chinchilla cochlea. *J. Accoust. Soc. Am.* **62,** S-35.

Evans, E. F. (1972). The frequency response and other properties of single fibers in the guinea pig cochlea nerve. *J. Physiol.* **226,** 263–287.

Evans, E. F. (1976). Temporary sensorineural hearing loss and VIIIth nerve changes. *In* "Effects of Noise on Hearing" (D. Henderson, R. P. Hamernik, D. S. Dosanjh, and J. Mills, eds.). Raven, New York.

Feldmann, H. (1971). Homolateral and contralateral masking of tinnitus by noise-bands and by pure-tones. *Audiology* **10,** 138–144.

Fitzgibbons, P. J. (1979). "Temporal Resolution in Normal and Hearing-impaired Listeners." Doctoral Dissertation, Northwestern University, Evanston, Illinois.

Flottorp, G., and Wille, C. (1954). Nicotinic acid treatment of tinnitus: A clinical–audiological examination. *Acta Oto–Laryngol.* **118,** 85–97.

Geisler, C. D., Rhode, W. S., and Kennedy, D. T. (1974). Response to tonal stimuli of single auditory nerve fibers and their relationship to basilar membrane motion in the squirrel monkey. *J. Neurophysiol.* **37,** 1156–1172.

Gerstein, G. L., and Kiang, N. Y. S. (1960). An approach to the quantitative analysis of electrophysiological data from single neurons. *Biophys. J.* **1,** 15–24.

Giraudi, D., Salvi, R., Henderson, D., and Hamernik, R. P. (1980). Gap detection by the chinchilla. *J. Acoust. Soc. Am.* **68,** 802–806.

Giraudi, D., Salvi, R., and Henderson, D. (1982). Gap detection in hearing-impaired chinchillas. *Meet. Assoc. Res. Otolaryngol., Jan. 18–21, St. Petersburg, Florida.*

Goldstein, J. L. (1967). Auditory nonlinearity. *J. Acoust. Soc. Am.* **41,** 676–689.

Goldstein, J. L., and Kiang, N. Y. S. (1968). Neural correlates of the aural combination tone $2f_1 - f_2$. *Proc. IEEE* **56,** 981–992.

Hallpike, C. S., and Hood, J. D. (1960). Observations on the neurological mechanism of the loudness recruitment phenomenon. *Acta Oto–Laryngol.* **50,** 472–486.

Harrison, R. V., and Evans, E. F. (1979). Some aspects of temporal coding by single cochlear fibers from regions of cochlear hair cell degeneration in the guinea pig. *Arch. Oto–Rhino–Laryngol.* **224,** 71–78.

Henderson, D. (1969). Temporal summation of acoustic signals by the chinchilla. *J. Acoust. Soc. Am.* **46,** 474–475.

Henderson, D. (1976). Cochlear nucleus firing patterns during asymptotic threshold shift. *In* "Hearing and Davis" (S. K. Hirsch, D. H. Eldredge, I. J. Hirsh, and S. R. Silverman, eds.). Washington University Press, St. Louis, Missouri.

Henderson, D., Hamernik, R. P., and Sitler, R. W. (1974). Audiometric and histological correlates of exposure to 1-msec noise impulses in the chinchilla. *J. Acoust. Soc. Am.* **55,** 795.

Hickling, S. (1967). Hearing test patterns in noise induced temporary hearing loss. *J. Audit. Res.* **7,** 63–76.

Hood, J. D. (1950). Studies in auditory fatigue and adaptation. *Acta Oto–Laryngol.* **92,** 1–57.

Hunter-Duvar, I. M., and Bredberg, G. (1974). Effects of intense auditory stimulation: Hearing losses and inner ear changes in the chinchilla. *J. Acoust. Soc. Am.* **55,** 795–801.

Hunter-Duvar, I. M., and Elliot, D. N. (1972). Effects of intense auditory stimulation: Hearing losses and inner ear changes in squirrel monkey. *J. Acoust. Soc. Am.* **52,** 1181–1192.

Jerger, J. F. (1955). Influence of stimulus duration on the pure-tone threshold during recovery from auditory fatigue. *J. Acoust. Soc. Am.* **27,** 121–124.

Jesteadt, W., Bilger, R. C., Green, D., and Patterson, J. H. (1976). Temporal acuity in listeners with sensorineural hearing loss. *J. Speech Hear. Res.* **19**, 357–370.

Kiang, N. Y. S., Watanabe, T., Thomas, E. C., and Clark, L. F. (1965). "Discharge Patterns of Single Fibers in the Cat's Auditory Nerve." Research Monograph No. 35. MIT Press, Cambridge, Massachusetts.

Kim, D. O., and Molnar, C. E. (1979). A population study of cochlear nerve fibers: Comparison of spatial distribution of average-rate and phase-locking measures of responses to single tones. *J. Neurophysiol.* **42**, 16–30.

Kim, D. O., Molnar, C. E., and Matthews, J. W. (1980). Cochlear mechanics: Nonlinear behavior in two-tone responses as reflected in cochlear nerve fiber responses and in ear canal sound pressure. *J. Acoust. Soc. Am.* **67**, 1704–1721.

Liberman, M. C. (1978). Auditory-nerve response from cats raised in a low-noise chamber. *J. Acoust. Soc. Am.* **63**, 442–445.

Liberman, M. C., and Kiang, N. Y. S. (1978). Acoustic trauma in cats. Cochlear pathology and auditory-nerve activity. *Acta Oto–Laryngol. Suppl.* **358**, 1–64.

Lindquist, S. E., Neff, W. D., and Schuknecht, H. F. (1954). Stimulation deafness: A study of hearing losses resulting from exposure to noise of blast impulses. *J. Comp. Physiol. Psychol.* **47**, 406.

Loeb, M., and Smith, R. (1967). Relation of induced tinnitus to physical characteristics of the inducing stimuli. *J. Acoust. Soc. Am.* **42**, 453–455.

McGee, T., Ryan, A., and Dallos, P. (1976). Psychophysical tuning curves of chinchillas. *J. Acoust. Soc. Am.* **60**, 1146–1150.

Miller, J. D. (1970). Audibility curve of the chinchilla. *J. Acoust. Soc. Am.* **48**, 513–523.

Mills, J. H., Gengel, R. W., Watson, C. S., and Miller, J. D. (1970). Temporary changes of the auditory system due to exposure to noise for one or two days. *J. Acoust. Soc. Am.* **48**, 524–530.

Moller, A. (1968). Unit responses in the cochlear nucleus of the rat to pure tones. *Acta Physiol. Scand.* **75**, 530–541.

Olsen, W. O., and Tillma, T. W. (1968). Hearing aids and sensorineural hearing loss. *Ann. Oto–Rhinol–Laryngol.* **77**, 717–726.

Passe, E. R. G. (1953). Surgery of the sympathetic for Meniere's disease, tinnitus and nerve deafness. A.M.A. *Arch. Oto–Laryngol.* **57**, 257–266.

Piazza, R. S. (1966). The effect of the auditory fatigue upon the loudness and the pitch. *Acoustica* **17**, 179–183.

Plomp, R. (1964). Rate of decay of auditory sensation. *J. Acoust. Soc. Am.* **36**, 277–282.

Rhode, W. S. (1971). Observations of the vibration of the basilar membrane in squirrel monkeys using the Mossbauer technique. *J. Acoust. Soc. Am.* **49**, 1218–1231.

Robles, L., Rhode, W. S., and Geisler, C. D. (1976). Transient response of the basilar membrane measured in squirrel monkeys using the Mossbauer Effect. *J. Acoust. Soc. Am.* **59**, 926–939.

Rose, J. E., Hind, J. E., Anderson, D. J., and Brugge, J. F. (1971). Some effects of stimulus intensity on response of auditory nerve fibers in the squirrel monkey. *J. Neurophysiol.* **34**, 685–699.

Ruedi, L., and Furrer, W. (1946). Das akustische Trauma. *Pract. Oto–Rhino–Laryngol.* **8**, 177–372.

Salvi, R. (1976). Central components of the temporary threshold shift. *In* "The Effects of Noise on Hearing: Critical Issues" (D. Henderson, R. P. Hamernik, D. Dosanjh, and J. Mills, eds.). Raven, New York.

Salvi, R., Hamernik, R. P., and Henderson, D. (1978). Discharge patterns in the cochlear nucleus of the chinchilla following noise induced asymptotic threshold shift. *Exp. Brain Res.* **32**, 301–320.

Salvi, R. J., Henderson, D., and Hamerik, R. P. (1979a). Single auditory nerve fiber and action potential latencies in normal and noise-treated chinchillas. *Hear. Res.* **1**, 237–251.

Salvi, R. J., Hamernik, R. P., and Henderson, D. (1979b). Auditory nerve activity, and cochlear morphology after noise exposure. *Arch. Oto–Rhino–Laryngol.* **224**, 111–116.

Salvi, R., Henderson, D., Hamernik, R. P., and Parkins, C. (1980). VIIIth nerve response to click stimuli in normal and pathological cochleas. *Hear. Res.* **2**, 335–342.

Salvi, R., Perry, J., Hamernik, R. P., and Henderson, D. (1981). Relationship between cochlear pathologies and auditory nerve and behavioral responses following acoustic trauma. *In* "New Perspectives on Noise-Induced Hearing Loss" (R. P. Hamernik, D. Henderson, and R. Salvi, eds.). Raven, New York.

Salvi, R., Giraudi, D., Henderson, D., and Hamernik, R. P. (1982). Detection of sinusoidally amplitude modulated noise by the chinchilla. *J. Acoust. Soc. Am.*, **71**, 424–429.

Schmeidt, R. A., Zwislocki, J. J., and Hamernik, R. P. (1980). Effects of hair cell lesions on responses of cochlear-nerve-fibers. I. Lesions, tuning curves, two-tone inhibition, and responses to trapezoidal-wave patterns. *J. Neurophysiol.* **43**, 1367–1389.

Schuknecht, H. F. (1960). Neuroanatomical correlates of auditory sensitivity and pitch discrimination in the cat. *In* "Neural Mechanism of the Auditory and Vestibular Systems" (G. L. Rasmussen and W. Windle, eds.). C. C. Thomas, Springfield, IL.

Seaton, W. (1973). A comparison of critical ratios and critical bands in the monaural chinchilla. *J. Acoust. Soc. Am.* **53**, 376(A).

Siegel, J. H., and Kim, D. O. (1981). Cochlear bio-mechanics: Vulnerability to acoustic trauma, and other alterations as seen in neural responses and ear canal sound pressure. *In* "New Perspectives on Noise-Induced Hearing Loss" (R. P. Hamernik, D. Henderson, and R. Salvi, eds.). Raven, New York.

Smoorenburg, G. F. (1972). Combination tones and their origin. *J. Acoust. Soc. Am.* **52**, 615–632.

Spoendlin, H. (1969). Innervation patterns in the organ of Corti of the cat. *Acta Oto–Laryngol.* **67**, 239–254.

Spoendlin, H. (1972). Innervation densities of the cochlea. *Acta Oto–Laryngol.* **73**, 250–263.

Spoendlin, H. (1974). Neuroanatomy of the cochlea. *In* "Facts and Models of Hearing" (E. Zwicker and E. Terhardt, eds.). Springer-Verlag, Berlin and New York.

Stevens, S. S. (1936). A scale for the measurement of a psychological magnitude: Loudness. *Psychol. Rev.* **43**, 405–416.

Viemeister, V. F. (1974). Intensity discrimination of noise in the presence of band-reject noise, *J. Acoust. Soc. Am.* **56**, 1594–1600.

Viemeister, V. F. (1977). Temporal factors in audition: A system analysis approach. *In* "Psychophysics and Physiology of Hearing" (E. F. Evans and J. P. Wilson, eds.). Academic Press, New York.

Wang, C. Y., and Dallos, P. (1972). Latency of whole-nerve action potentials: Influence of hair-cell normalcy. *J. Acoust. Soc. Am.* **52**, 1678–1686.

Warr, W. B. (1975). Olivocochlear and vestibular efferent neurons of feline brainstem: Their location, morphology and number determined by retrograde axonal transport and acetylcholinesterose histochemistry. *J. Comp. Neurol.* **161**, 159–182.

Whitfield, I. C. (1967). "The Auditory Pathway." Arnold, London.

Wightman, F. L. (1981). Psychoacoustic correlates of hearing loss. *In* "New Perspectives on Noise-Induced Hearing Loss" (R. Hamernik, D. Henderson, and R. Salvi, eds.), Raven, New York.

Wightman, F., McGee, T., and Kramer, M. (1977). Factors influencing frequency selectivity in normal and hearing-impaired listeners. *In* "Psychophysics and Physiology of Hearing" (E. F. Evans and J. P. Wilson, eds.). Academic Press, New York.

Wright, H. N. (1968). The effect of sensorineural hearing loss on threshold-duration functions. *J. Speech Hear. Res.* **11**, 842–852.

Frequency Selectivity: Physiological and Psychophysical Tuning Curves and Suppression

John H. Mills and Richard A. Schmiedt

Department of Otolaryngology
Medical University of South Carolina
Charleston, South Carolina

I. INTRODUCTION

The data reported here are applicable to theoretical and applied issues in hearing. In regard to theory an issue of historical and current interest is the mechanism that determines the frequency selective properties of the auditory system. One of the more commonly used measures of frequency selectivity is the tuning curve. Tuning curves are measured physiologically from single nerve fibers within the peripheral and central auditory nervous systems, or from gross neural responses arising within those systems. Tuning curves can also be measured psychophysically by employing variations of the paradigm used to measure the masking of a pure tone by a pure tone and by using both simultaneous masking and temporal (forward and backward) masking paradigms. Scientific questions regarding tuning curves sometimes apply only to single-unit data or sometimes to gross neural data, sometimes to specific cases of psychophysical tuning curves, and sometimes to tuning curves in general. In the last case, for example, a commonly raised question involves the mechanical and micro-mechanical properties of the cochlea: namely, is "tuning" achieved principally by the mechanical properties of the ear? What is the influence of suppression on tuning? Is suppression of neural or mechanical origin or both? What are the effects of sensorineural hearing loss on tuning and suppression? Is frequency selectivity determined mostly by the peripheral or central systems? Answers to these general questions and to a nearly endless list of more specific questions are incomplete or unavailable.

In regard to applied issues, there is a need to explore and validate psycho-physical and physiological measures of hearing which are appropriate for use with human subjects and patients and which are more sensitive to injury of the auditory system than traditional procedures, particularly the audiogram. The need for more sensitive measures of injury to the peripheral auditory system is based on studies that demonstrate normal or nearly normal auditory sensitivity in the presence of injury to the cochlea and auditory nerve (Eldredge *et al.*, 1973; Schuknecht and Woellner, 1955, for example), and studies that show large differences in performance among individuals on auditory tasks differences that are not predictable given traditional audiometric data (for example, see Martin and Pickett, 1970). Lastly, with the low cost and easy access of averaging computers and their wide-ranging applications to clinical audiology and otoneurology, there is a need for basic information on physiological acoustics in human subjects, and the establishment of correlations between human phys-iological data and sensory–perceptual skills.

Our experimental approach involves physiological and psychophysical experi-ments with human subjects in combination with experiments on animals. The strategy is to obtain as much information as is possible on human subjects and to complement the human research project with experimental data from animals. The story is far from complete, but our efforts continue. The data reported here reflect some of our recent research. An explanation of our efforts may be achieved best by first considering the concept of frequency selectivity in physical systems and some of the rich history of frequency selectivity in physiological and psychological acoustics.

II. FREQUENCY SELECTIVITY IN PHYSICAL SYSTEMS

A. Relations between Time and Frequency

1. Fourier Transforms

In its usual connotation, the term "tuning curve" refers to a measure of the frequency response of the auditory system. In this section we shall briefly define some of the more pertinent terms and general concepts dealing with how physical systems behave in the frequency and time domains. The following discussion is necessarily elementary in scope, and the more knowledgeable reader may want to skip this section entirely. Our purpose here is to acquaint the beginning student with the background necessary to understand the results presented in later sections. The following is brief. We include this section to give the reader a feel for some of the tradeoffs in examining a system by means of its time or its frequency response. Many engineering texts are available that cover Fourier analysis, filters, and system theory in general; these include Papoulis (1966), Lathi (1965, 1968), and Carlson (1968). A more mathematical approach to resonance and system theory can be found in Kreyszig (1962), whereas good introductory material can be found in Smith (1966) or Leshowitz (1978).

All acoustic and electric signals that can be physically generated in the laboratory can be described mathematically either as a function of time, $x(t)$, or as a function of frequency, $X(f)$. Further, given a signal fully represented in the time domain, we can uniquely map it into the frequency domain and vice versa. Some 150 years ago Jean Baptiste Fourier first developed the mathematical transforms by which time and frequency functions could be related. (Note that the transform variables need not be time and frequency; any pair of independent variables can be substituted. In this article we are interested only in transforms relating time and frequency.) Let us now review the transforms and some of their properties for two classes of signals: periodic and nonperiodic.

a. Periodic Signals. A signal is defined as being periodic if

$$x(t) = x(t+T) \qquad (-\infty < t < \infty) \tag{1}$$

In other words, the signal repeats itself after a period of time, T. If the function $x(t)$ is continuous in time it follows that

$$x(t) = x(t+nT) \tag{2}$$

where n is any integer. The transform that applies under these circumstances is the Fourier series expansion, which in trigonometric terms is

$$x(t) = a_0 + \sum_{n=1}^{\infty} [a_n \cos(n\omega t) + b_n \sin(n\omega t)] \tag{3}$$

where

$$\omega = 2\pi f = \frac{2\pi}{T} \tag{4}$$

and

$$a_0 = \frac{1}{T}\int_0^T x(t)dt \tag{5}$$

$$a_n = \frac{2}{T}\int_0^T x(t)\cos(n\omega t)dt \tag{6}$$

$$b_n = \frac{2}{T}\int_0^T x(t)\sin(n\omega t)dt \tag{7}$$

While seemingly complex, the above relations are often fairly simple to solve. In essence, a periodic time function can be expressed alternatively as an infinite number of positive frequency components represented by the sinusoidal functions in Eqs. (6) and (7). There is also an average-value term, a_0, which represents the DC ($f=0$) level of the time waveform over a single period.

In other words a continuous, periodic signal will have associated with it a line spectrum in the frequency domain, i.e., the frequency function will be a series of lines, weighted by the coefficients a_n and b_n, placed at integer multiples of the fundamental frequency, f. A vector analogy is appropriate here. The time waveform, $x(t)$, can be considered an n-dimensional vector, where the sinusoidal components are the n axes needed to define the position of the time vector. A rather trivial example is obtained when the time signal is a simple sum of two sinusoids that are integrally related:

$$x(t) = A \cos 2\pi f_1 t + B \cos 2\pi f_2 t \tag{8}$$

By inspection we see that the frequency spectrum will consist of two lines at f_1 and f_2 each weighted by A and B, respectively.

b. Nonperiodic Signals. Signals in the time domain which are not periodic can be transformed to the frequency domain using the Fourier integral transform:

$$X(f) = \int_{-\infty}^{\infty} x(t)e^{-j\omega t}dt \tag{9}$$

In Eq. (9), the time variable is integrated out with the result that $X(f)$ is a continuous function of frequency and is not a line spectrum as in the case of periodic signals. Conversely, given a signal in the frequency domain, the time signal may be obtained by

$$x(t) = \int_{-\infty}^{\infty} X(f)e^{j\omega t}df \tag{10}$$

Returning to our vector analogy, a very convenient way to represent a vector is in terms of its magnitude and its phase relative to a given reference. Likewise, a complete spectral analysis requires both the magnitude and phase of the transform to be specified in order to describe a time signal uniquely. This is true for both the line spectra of periodic signals as well as the continuous spectra of time limited, nonperiodic signals. In auditory work, phase is often not as important as how energy is distributed over frequency within the signal spectrum. We define the energy spectral density, $S(f)$, as

$$S(f) = |X(f)|^2 \tag{11}$$

where the vertical lines denote absolute values. Thus, $S(f)$ is always positive and real; however, the original time signal cannot be uniquely obtained from just $S(f)$ because the phase information has been lost.

Note that the Fourier transform is double sided and includes positive as well as negative time and frequency. In the real world, negative frequencies are often ignored; however, negative frequencies can make their presence known in practical circumstances. For instance, under conditions of frequency translation whereby a time signal is multiplied by a high-frequency sinusoid or carrier, f_c, the resulting spectrum is shifted from being symmetric about $f=0$ to being symmetric about $f=f_c$, and the negative frequencies appear as real (positive) frequencies which can be measured with a wave analyzer.

2. Time–Bandwidth Reciprocity

An extremely important feature inherent in the Fourier transform is that the shape and extent of the signal spectrum, i.e., its bandwidth characteristics, are determined by the characteristics of the signal in the time domain and vice versa. As it turns out, signals sharply delineated in time have spectra that involve a large range of frequencies (large bandwidths). Conversely, signals that are characterized by small bandwidths cover a large extent of the time domain. This reciprocity relationship between time and bandwidth is illustrated in Fig. 1 for signals commonly used in auditory research. Both the duration of a tone burst and its rise–fall time will have an effect on its bandwidth. Thus, a short tone pip with a fast rise–fall time will have the largest bandwidth, and a long tone burst with a slow rise–fall time will have the smallest.

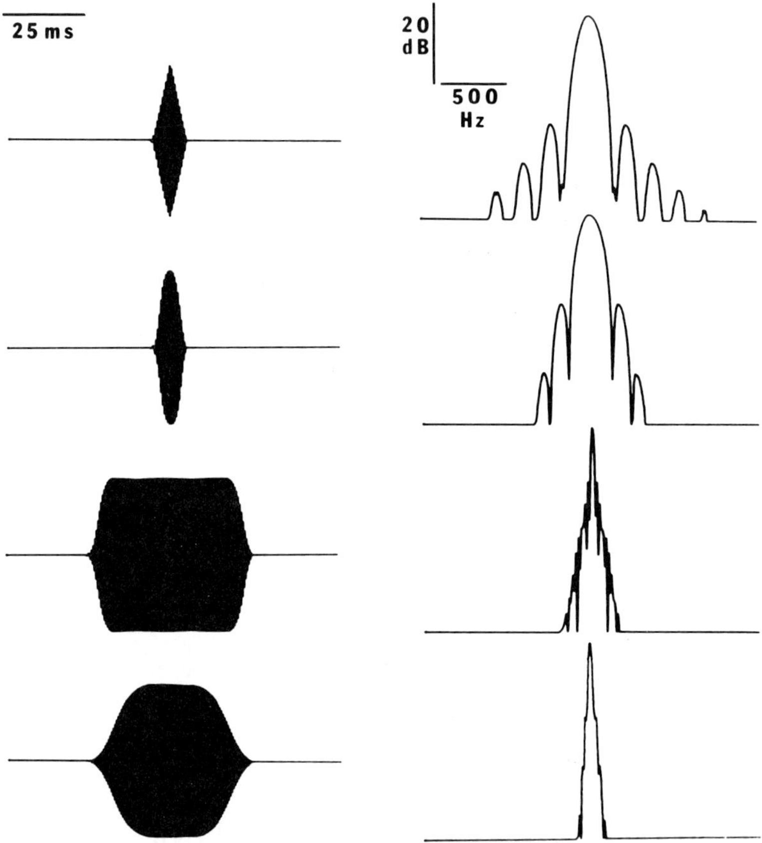

Figure 1   Four time signals commonly used in auditory research (left) and their respective power spectral densities (right). All tone bursts are at 2 kHz which corresponds to the central frequency peaks of the spectra. The two upper time signals both have a total duration of 10 msec with 5 msec rise–fall times. The two lower signals have 50 msec durations with 5 and 12 msec rise–fall times, respectively. The rise–fall envelope is a linear ramp (top) or a nonlinear function of time (bottom three signals). Compare the difference in the spectra of the tone pips with linear and nonlinear rise–fall envelopes, and note the inverse relation between time extent and bandwidth. The probe stimulus used to obtain the psychophysical tuning curves presented by the authors in this article corresponds to the 10-msec burst with a nonlinear rise–fall envelope. Likewise, physiological tuning curves were obtained with the 50-msec burst with a 5 msec nonlinear rise–fall envelope.

B. General Filter Terminology

1. Bandwidth

Filters are devices that selectively emphasize or deemphasize a band of frequencies within a spectrum. Filters operate on both the magnitude and phase components of a signal. The types of filters used in auditory research can be broken down into five overall categories termed, appropriately, allpass, lowpass, highpass, bandpass, and bandreject. Allpass filters do not alter the magnitude spectrum of a signal, but operate only on its phase spectrum. Lowpass, highpass, and bandpass filters, respectively, emphasize low, high, or a particular band of frequencies. Bandreject filters, sometimes called notch filters, strongly deemphasize a given region in the frequency domain.

Within the bandpass of a filter, the magnitudes of the frequency components of a signal are relatively unaltered. Outside the bandpass, the components are attenuated, often at some constant rate of rejection with respect to a given interval in frequency. In order to define bandwidth in a more quantitative fashion, we often refer to a boundary frequency at which the energy at the output of the filter is one-half that at the center of the bandpass. The magnitude of the filter response (or gain) at the output is often plotted in terms of decibels (dB) relative to the input energy as a function of frequency (Fig. 2), or

$$\text{Filter gain in dB} = 10 \log\left[\frac{E_{\text{out}}}{E_{\text{in}}}\right] = 20 \log\left[\frac{V_{\text{out}}}{V_{\text{in}}}\right] \qquad (12)$$

We see that the one-half power frequencies correspond to the frequencies at which the filter response is

$$10 \log(\tfrac{1}{2}) = -3.01 \text{ dB} \qquad (13)$$

or 3 dB down from the maximal response.

Figure 2 is a plot of the magnitude and phase response of a simple lowpass filter made up of a single resistor and shunt capacitor (RC). The upper thick line is simply the magnitude of the output energy of the filter as measured with a constant input across frequency. At low frequencies ($f \ll f_{3\ \text{dB}}$), the filter gain is 1, or in terms of dB, 0 dB. At high frequencies ($f \gg f_{3\ \text{dB}}$) the filter attenuates the input magnitude at a rate of 20 dB for each factor of 10 increment in frequency (20 dB/decade). A more common description of this rejection rate is in terms frequency doubling or octaves. In these terms the filter rejection rate is

$$20\log(2) = 6.02 \text{ dB} \qquad (14)$$

or approximately 6 dB/octave. The thin line in Fig. 2 is an asymptotic measure of the frequency response of the filter developed by H. W. Bode (1930). Note that the breakpoint of the line, where it goes from a slope of 0 to -6 dB/octave, is at $f_{3\ \text{dB}}$ and is often referred to as the corner frequency. It is here that the largest

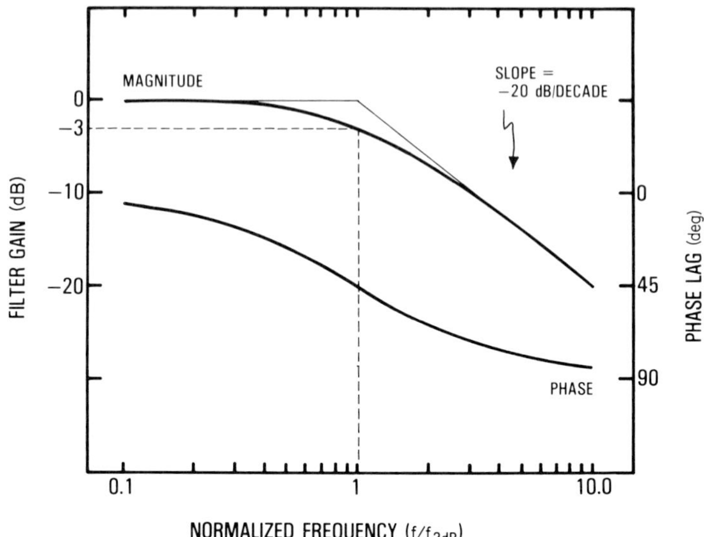

Figure 2   Magnitude and phase characteristics of the output of a simple RC lowpass filter normalized to the input. The frequency scale has been normalized to the cutoff frequency ($f_{3\ dB}$) at which the output power is one-half that at the center frequency of the bandpass (in this case $f=0$ or DC). Thick lines are the actual magnitude and phase curves; thin lines are the asymptotic values according to Bode. The phase at the cutoff frequency is 45° lag referred to the input. Such curves are often termed the *transfer functions* of the filter.

error is incurred (3 dB) with the use of the Bode asymptotic plot. A useful result of cascading two identical lowpass filters is that the rejection rate will simply double; for *n* filters in series, the rate will be 6*n* dB/octave.

Also in Fig. 2 is plotted the phase response of the lowpass filter. The phase response of a filter is needed to characterize fully how a particular filter will respond to transient signals in the time domain. For a simple RC filter, the phase of the output as referenced to the input is essentially 0 within the bandpass and asymptotes to 90° lag outside the bandpass. At $f_{3\ dB}$, the phase shift is 45°.

Figure 2 also represents the response of a simple highpass RC filter, except that the 6 dB/octave rejection rate would appear for $f \ll f_{3\ dB}$ and the phase would asymptotically lead by 90° at $f \ll f_{3\ dB}$. If a lowpass and high pass with identical corner frequencies are properly cascaded, the resulting filter would be a bandpass with a center frequency at $f_{3\ dB}$ and center frequency gain of −6 dB.

2. Resonance

The simple RC filters described above will not oscillate or "ring" when the input is a sharp transient in the time domain. These filters can be simply described by a first-order differential equation and are not resonant systems. Many systems, manmade or in nature, can emphasize certain frequencies to the exclusion of others. Take for example the familiar mass–spring–damper system. By adjusting the parameters of the spring and the size of the mass, we can get the system to oscillate at different frequencies. The frequency at which the system oscillates is called the resonant frequency. By adding an inductor (L) to the RC filters described above, the new RLC filter will exhibit a resonant frequency. Depending on how the RLC components are configured, a lowpass, bandpass, or highpass filter can result.

Figure 3 illustrates some important aspects of resonant systems. In the left panel are normalized filter responses in the frequency domain for two RLC filters. The frequency and amplitude axes are both linear. The one-half power bandwidth is marked at 0.707 on the amplitude scale (energy is proportional to amplitude squared, thus 0.707 in normalized amplitude is equivalent to -3 dB). The obvious difference between the upper and lower curves lies in their sharpness of tuning. The tuning difference stems from the amount of damping (resistance) in the system: the upper curve represents a system with high damping, the lower curve, little damping. A measure of the amount of damping, and therefore the bandwidth, of a simple resonant system is the quality factor, Q, where

$$Q \propto \frac{\text{maximum energy stored}}{\text{energy dissipated/cycle}} \tag{15}$$

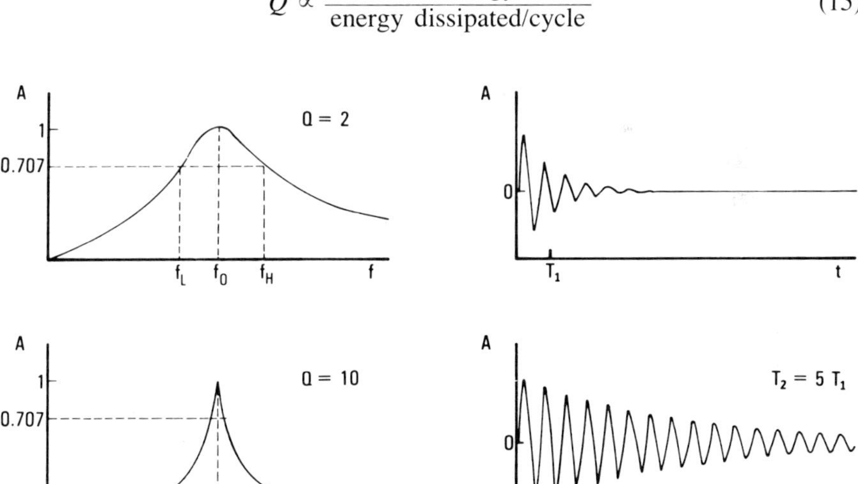

Figure 3 Normalized frequency–response (left) and time–response (right) curves of resonant systems described by a second-order differential equation. Top curves correspond to a system with high damping (large energy loss per cycle); bottom curves correspond to a system with five times less damping. Note reciprocity between sharpness of tuning in the frequency domain and the extent of the ringing in the time domain.

Because energy is dissipated only in the damping (resistance) term, highly damped systems have low Q values. Energy storage is accomplished by the mass and spring (inductance and capacitance) components. The Q value is related to the one-half power bandwidth in this second-order system by

$$Q = \frac{f_0}{f_H - f_L} \tag{16}$$

Thus the larger the bandwidth, the lower the Q.

We can relate the frequency response of the system with its time domain characteristics as shown in the right panels of Fig. 3. If the highly damped system is excited by an impulse in the time domain, its transient response amplitude (A) is shown in the upper right panel: a ringing that exponentially decays with a time constant, t_1; mathematically

$$A = e^{-t/t_i} \sin(\omega_0 t) \tag{17}$$

The less-damped system under the same circumstances rings with a much longer time constant, t_2. If $Q_1 = 2$ and $Q_2 = 10$, then $t_2 = 5t_1$. (Note that the time constant, t_c, is defined as that point in time when the ringing is about 37%, or $1/e$, times its initial value.) A relationship between Q and t_c can be formulated for a simple resonant system where

$$t_c = \frac{Q}{\pi f_0} \tag{18}$$

It is instructive to realize that time–bandwidth reciprocity is present once again. Sharply tuned bandwidths are associated with long response times and vice versa. Thus, a filter that is sharply tuned to a narrow band of frequencies will have time-domain characteristics with long duration rise and decay envelopes, i.e., the filter will need a long time for the output to build up to a steady-state value when a steady input signal is applied. On the other hand, when the input is switched off, the filter output will only slowly decay to a zero value.

3. Types of Filters

There are many types of filters that have applications to auditory research. Each type has its own advantages and disadvantages. The following is a brief description of three types, beginning with the previously discussed RC filter.

RC filters are easily understood theoretically and can be built with minimal circuit elements. Other advantages lie in the fact that they can be configured in a variety of ways to yield highpass, lowpass, and bandpass filters with easily adjustable rejection rates. Filter slopes will always be some integer multiple of ±6 dB/octave. Therefore, a lowpass RC filter with a −24 dB/octave cutoff rate necessarily will be made up of four RC filters in series. A final advantage is that an RC filter is not a resonant system; thus, it performs well with transient inputs with no ringing in its output.

Disadvantages of the RC filter are due mainly to the rather gradual rolloff of the filter response around the cutoff frequency. In the example above, if four RC filters are cascaded each with an identical cutoff frequency, f_c, then the response of the overall filter will be 12 dB down at f_c (because each filter section will have contributed -3dB at f_c). Thus signals are attenuated relatively severely within the passband of a multistage RC filter.

A type of filter that overcomes this disadvantage is the so-called maximally flat, or Butterworth, filter first described by Butterworth (1930). Unlike the RC filter, the Butterworth has a relatively flat bandpass characteristic right up to the cutoff frequency. At frequencies outside the bandpass, the rejection rate very quickly approaches an asymptotic value of an integer multiple of -12 dB/octave. As a point of comparison, a Butterworth filter configured to yield a 24 dB/octave rejection rate will have an attenuation at the cutoff frequency of only 3 dB, whereas the attenuation of the RC filter at the same cutoff will be 12 dB. The disadvantage to the Butterworth filter lies in its transient response. The output of the Butterworth will ring considerably with transient signal inputs.

Perhaps the best of both worlds, with regard to time and frequency response, is embodied in the Bessel filter, so named because it can be described mathematically by Bessel polynomials. In short, it is a compromise between the RC and Butterworth filters in terms of its frequency domain characteristics. With a 24 dB/octave rejection rate, a Bessel filter will yield an attenuation of 7.5 dB at the cutoff frequency as compared to 12 and 3 dB, respectively, of the RC and Butterworth. However, where the Butterworth filter has a disadvantage in the time domain to transient inputs, the Bessel filter is well behaved and has minimal ringing in its output. Therefore, the Bessel design is ideally suited for filtering impulsive signals like nerve-fiber activity.

III. FREQUENCY SELECTIVITY IN THE COCHLEA

A. Historical Perspective

1. Resonance Theories

The middle of the nineteenth century was an active period in hearing theory. The new mathematics of Fourier in 1829 brought a clearer light to bear on the concepts relating tonal frequency and resonance. Georg Ohm (1843) hypothesized that the auditory periphery worked on the principles of Fourier analysis, i.e., the ear somehow was able to resolve the individual frequency components of a tonal complex. In 1863 Helmholtz proposed that Ohm's frequency analysis was carried out by a series of independent resonators within the cochlea. Helmholtz at first proposed that the tuned elements involved were the rods of Corti (pillar cells). These rods are shorter in the base of the cochlea than in the apex, so Helmholtz correctly assigned high-frequency analysis to the base, and low-frequency analysis to the apex. Thus was born the "place" theory of hearing, whereby auditory frequency analysis is accomplished by the fact that tuning in the cochlea varies as a function of place along the organ of Corti. On the basis of Johannes Muller's doctrine of specific nerve energies, Volkmann (1844) proposed that single fibers in the auditory nerve would be tuned to a single frequency. Helmholtz was able to put a physiological basis behind Volkmann's theory by suggesting that each nerve fiber was excited by just one resonator. Additional anatomical evidence gathered by Hensen (1863) convinced Helmholtz that the rods could not be the resonating elements—their length varied only by a factor of two, and the nerve fibers ended at the hair cells, not the rods. Thus, the fibers of the basilar membrane became the favored tuned structures. As time went on, however, better and more detailed anatomical data led to more and more theories of cochlear analysis.

It was left to Georg von Békésy, a physicist and communications engineer, to make the observations which form the basis of modern auditory theory. First in models comprised of a rubber membrane of varying compliance, and later in cochleas obtained from cadavers, Békésy (1928, 1947, 1960) observed that the vibration along the cochlear duct took the form of a traveling wave. The traveling wave always started at the base and proceeded toward the apex. Further, the vibration envelope had a place of maximum displacement for any given frequency: a low-frequency tone was associated with a maximum nearest the apex, a high-frequency tone, nearest the base. For his work empirically describing the traveling wave, Békésy was awarded the Nobel Prize in Physiology and Medicine in 1961.

A mathematical description of Békésy's traveling wave was first successfully developed by J. J. Zwislocki (1946, 1948). A comparison of Békésy's observations and Zwislocki's original theory is shown in Fig. 4. Zwislocki demonstrated that a vibration maximum could occur solely due to an interaction between the compliance gradient and damping along the basilar membrane. Indeed, according to Zwislocki (1948, 1953, 1965) the point of resonance for the traveling wave is just beyond the apical cutoff of the wave. The basic equations that Zwislocki (1953) derived are still valid today. Thus, in modern theories of basilar membrane mechanics, the traveling wave is not at all a phenomenon of resonance.

A confirmation in a living cochlea of Békésy's traveling wave was obtained by Tasaki *et al.* (1952) using the cochlear microphonic (CM). The CM magnitude and phase was recorded differentially across each of the four turns in the guinea

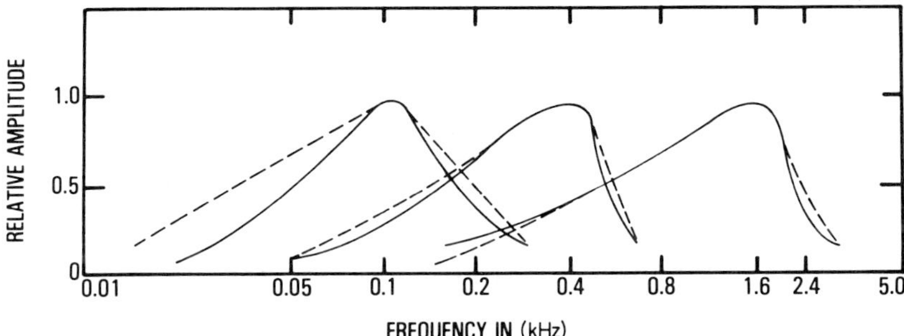

Figure 4 Empirically measured curves of Bekesy (solid lines) and theoretical curves of Zwislocki (dashed lines) describing the envelopes of the vibration pattern of the basilar membrane for three frequencies. The curves have been normalized at their maxima. (Adapted from Zwislocki, 1950.)

pig cochlea. By assuming that the CM waveform is proportional to basilar membrane displacement, the results of Tasaki *et al.* closely followed the observations of Békésy.

2. Neural Tuning

The era of analysis of single-cell and single-fiber responses in the auditory periphery began with the report of Galambos and Davis (1943). In this study they probed the auditory nerve of the cat with glass microelectrodes and described the first neural response areas to pure tones. Galambos and Davis defined the response areas as those coordinates of the tone in the frequency–intensity domain which produced excitation over the spontaneous rate of discharge of the fiber (see Fig. 5). Spontaneous rate, defined as neural firing in the absence of external stimuli, was found to be a characteristic of the individual neuron under study. The boundary of the response area corresponding to a criterion change in rate is now commonly termed the ''tuning curve.''

Some important conclusions reached by Galambos and Davis were that response areas are most sensitive at a best or characteristic frequency (CF) and extend asymmetrically more toward lower frequencies (below CF) than toward frequencies greater than CF. Moreover, toward high frequencies the response area is sharply cut off. These results seemed to confirm Békésy's model observations, except that the neural response was much more sharply tuned than the traveling wave envelope—a controversy that has managed to survive to this day.

Galambos and Davis (1948) later concluded that their recordings were from second-order cell bodies in the anteroventral cochlear nucleus rather than from primary fibers in the auditory nerve. Tasaki (1954) was finally able to record from single fibers in the auditory nerve of the guinea pig. This breakthrough was probably in large part due to better glass micropipets. Whereas Galambos and

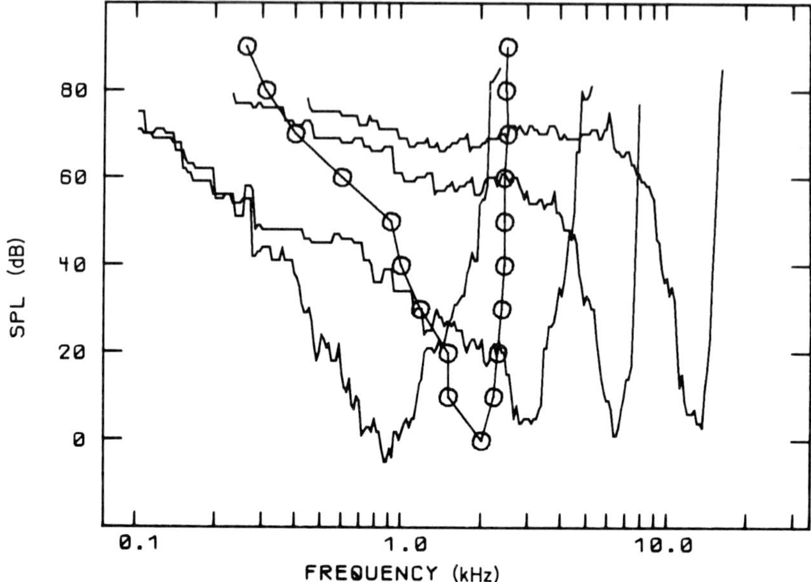

Figure 5   Tuning curves from single auditory nerve fibers in gerbils as compared to one of the first physiological tuning curves ever obtained in the auditory system by Galambos and Davis (1943) in cat (circles). The latter curve was most probably obtained from a cell body in the cochlear nucleus (see text). The four gerbil curves were obtained by the automated tracking procedures described by Kiang and Moxon (1974) and Liberman (1978). More details on the methods can be found in Schmiedt (1982b). Note the curves of the low-CF fibers are V shaped, whereas those of the high-CF fibers have a sharply tuned and sensitive tip around their CF and a broadly tuned, high-threshold tail at lower frequencies below CF. All the gerbil fibers had spontaneous activities in excess of 18 spikes/sec. Gerbil fiber identification in order of increasing CF is CG9-9, CG9-41, CG9-27, and CG9-1.

Davis used tip diameters of about 5 μm, Tasaki was able to obtain electrodes with tip sizes as small as 0.25 μm. (Note there were no mechanical electrode pullers as such in the early 1950s. Tasaki's electrodes were pulled by hand by his wife!) Tasaki's results obtained from primary fibers essentially replicated those of Galambos and Davis: single fibers were sharply tuned about a CF and most had spontaneous activities; however, unlike the earlier results, spontaneous activity was not usually suppressed with single tones.

In the early and mid 1960s, Kiang and his colleagues completed the first systematic study of the responses of auditory nerve fibers in cat to a variety of stimuli (Kiang *et al.*, 1965). In this monograph, Kiang presents the first clear picture of physiological tuning in the neural output of the cochlea. An important outcome was that low-CF fibers (around 1 kHz) are approximately V shaped, whereas higher CF fibers have a sensitive ''tip'' region around CF and a broadly tuned ''tail'' extending to low frequencies (see Fig. 5).

3. Neural Suppression

In 1944 Galambos and Davis published the first account of inhibitory phenomena in the auditory system. As in their 1943 paper, they assumed they were recording from primary fibers but actually were recording from cell bodies in the anteroventral cochlear nucleus. Their findings, for the most part, paralleled the results of later work in primary fibers with regard to two-tone stimuli. In the paradigm of Galambos and Davis, the response rate to an excitor tone placed at CF within the response area could be inhibited by the simultaneous addition of a second (inhibitor) tone. The frequency–intensity combinations of the second tone producing inhibition fell into regions they termed "inhibitory areas." For most neurons, there were two of these areas: one at frequencies above CF and another below CF. The inhibitory effect of one tone on the response of another was called "two-tone inhibition." As we shall see, the term now has evolved to "two-tone rate suppression."

Nomoto *et al.*, in 1964, demonstrated that primary fibers in squirrel monkey

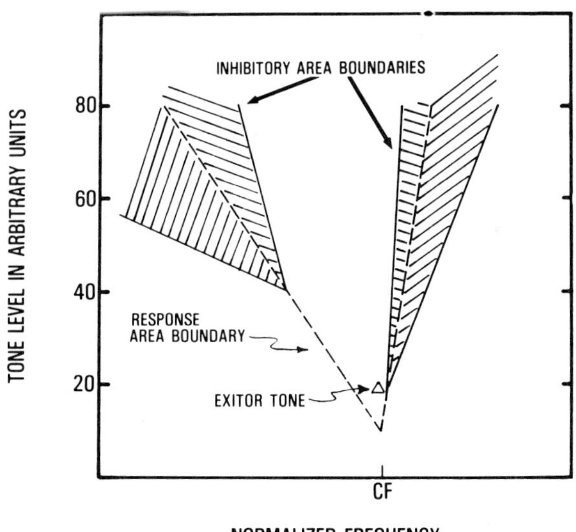

Figure 6 Schematic diagram of the excitatory and two-tone inhibitory areas of primary auditory nerve fibers. The excitatory area is also referred to as the response area, and its boundary is defined as the tuning curve. The inhibitory areas are defined as those frequency and intensity coordinates of a second tone that will inhibit the response of the fiber to a simultaneously presented excitor tone. The excitor (triangle) is usually placed at the fiber characteristic frequency (CF) at a level of about 10–20 dB above threshold. Note that there are two inhibitory areas flanking the tuning curve: one above CF, the other below CF. Because there is no time lag associated with two-tone inhibition in primary fibers, nor any evidence that it is neurally mediated, the inhibitory areas are now termed suppression areas. (Adapted from Sachs and Kiang, 1968.)

have two-tone inhibitory areas similar to those described by Galambos and Davis in the cochlear nucleus. The first thorough and quantitative study on primary-fiber inhibition was done by Sachs (1969) and Sachs and Kiang (1968). A diagrammatic interpretation of the relationship between the response and inhibitory areas of a single auditory nerve fiber is shown in Fig. 6.

More on the history of the study of the ear can be found in Wever's (1949) excellent book as well as in Békésy (1960) and Zwislocki (1981). Readings in Stevens and Davis (1938), Stevens (1951), and Schubert (1978) are all of historical interest.

B. Current Views

Auditory physiology with regard to neural tuning has advanced considerably in the last four decades since Galambos and Davis. What follows is a review of some of the highlights that have occurred since that time as well as some new data that reflect the authors' current views on tuning and suppression within the auditory system. By necessity we are leaving out most of the auditory literature written over the last 40 years. Specifically, there is little discussed of the cochlear analyses of sounds in the time domain. For example, we do not cover the phenomenon of the synchronization of fiber activity to the cycles of low-frequency stimuli, and the related phenomena of synchrony tuning and synchrony suppression (Hind *et al.*, 1967; Rose *et al.*, 1967; Brugge *et al.*, 1969; Anderson *et al.*, 1971; Johnson, 1980; Javel, 1981). From our earlier discussion of the relations between time and bandwidth, it is apparent that the tuning and suppression results presented here in the frequency domain with respect to firing rate have similar counterparts in the time domain with respect to synchrony. This duality should be kept in mind throughout this article.

1. Cochlear Mechanics

The discrepancy between the broad tuning of Békésy's traveling wave and the sharp tuning of primary and secondary neurons has intrigued auditory physiologists over the last four decades. Békésy (1960) linearly extrapolated, from his mechanical observations at 140 dB SPL, that at 0 dB SPL the vibration of the basilar membrane would be on the order of 0.1 Å (one tenth of the diameter of a hydrogen atom). The extrapolation carried with it the feeling that something was not quite right. Is it really valid to assume any biomechanical system could be linear over seven orders of magnitude with regard to vibration amplitude? Is it possible that a second filter is interposed somewhere between basilar membrane motion and single-fiber response to sharpen the neural tuning? Answering both of these questions has proven to be the basis of a large segment of the current research effort directed toward understanding the auditory system.

The question of linearity of cochlear mechanics essentially has been answered.

Improved techniques and instrumentation later showed cochlear mechanics *in vivo* to be much more sharply tuned than the observations of Békésy (Johnstone and Boyle, 1967; Wilson and Johnstone, 1975). Most importantly, Rhode (1971, 1973) showed that the basilar membrane response could be highly nonlinear, and that this nonlinearity was a function of the health of the cochlea. In essence, the nonlinearity sharpens the tuning of the mechanics at low stimulation levels, and broadens the tuning at high levels. The nonlinearity disappears in dead or even slightly damaged cochleas (Rhode 1978, 1980). It is now realized that the high sound levels used in the past to obtain measurements of mechanical tuning probably damaged the nonlinearity to the extent that it was never seen (LePage and Johnstone, 1980).

2. Mechanical versus Neural Tuning

With this knowledge of the vulnerability of cochlear mechanics, can we now answer the question of whether or not a second filter is needed to sharpen the neural tuning? As of this writing, the answer is still unknown. Geisler *et al.* (1974) directly compared single-fiber tuning with the tuning of cochlear mechanics in squirrel monkey, as have Evans and Wilson (1973, 1975) in cat. All such studies seemed to show that a second filter was still needed. The best mechanical curves of Rhode (1980) are still not as sharp as their neural counterparts, as shown in Fig. 7. However, the trend is such that with better and better techniques, allowing more accurate mechanical measurements with less sound pressure, the tuning within the cochlea has become increasingly sharp (e.g., Khanna and Leonard, 1981).

This trend strongly supports the work of Pfeiffer and Kim (973), Kim *et al.* (1973), Kim and Molnar (1975), and, more recently, Kim *et al.* (1980) who have suggested that cochlear nonlinearity not only produces the sharp neural tuning, but also is responsible for two-tone suppression and the generation of distortion products. (Note the term ''suppression'' is used rather than ''inhibition.'' The reasoning behind this substitution is that it implies a nonneural basis for the phenomenon.)

The now classic recordings of the receptor potentials of inner hair cells in guinea pig by Russell and Sellick (1977, 1978) and Sellick and Russell (1979) have demonstrated that sharp tuning and two-tone suppression are present at the inner hair cell level (see Fig. 8). Hair cell tuning seems identical to that of single fibers, at least for high-CF fibers associated with the cochlear base where the inner hair cell recordings were made. Thus, if there is a second filter, it now must be sandwiched between the inner hair cell and the basilar membrane.

On the other hand, in support of some type of additional mechanism for tuning are the results of Weiss *et al.* (1978) and Peake and Ling (1980) in the alligator lizard. Low-CF fibers in the auditory nerve of that lizard show frequency selectivities that are comparable to mammalian fibers, yet mechanical measurements

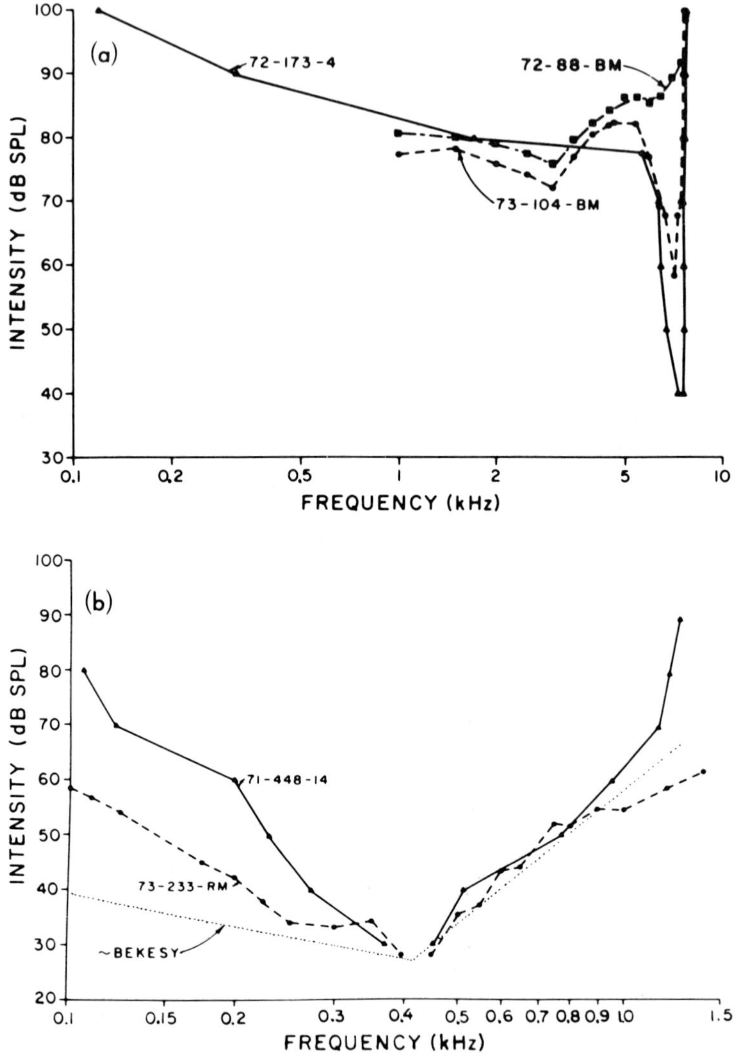

Figure 7 Comparison of the tuning of cochlear mechanics and single auditory nerve fibers in squirrel monkey. Solid lines refer to single-fiber responses; dashed lines to mechanical measurements which have been inverted and normalized to the low-frequency tail of the neural curve. In (a) the broadly tuned 72–88 mechanical curve of the basilar membrane response was taken at high levels (90 dB SPL) at frequencies around the tip, whereas the 73–104 curve was taken at a more moderate level (65 dB SPL) around the tip. Note the difference in sharpness of tuning of the two curves. (b) compares mechanical and neural tuning in the third turn of the squirrel monkey cochlea. In this case, the mechanical curve was derived from measurements on Reissner's membrane. One of Bekesy's measurements of basilar membrane motion in an apical region of the cochlea is shown for comparison (dotted lines). In all cases the mechanical curves are not as sharp as the neural curves. [From Rhode (1980) with permission.]

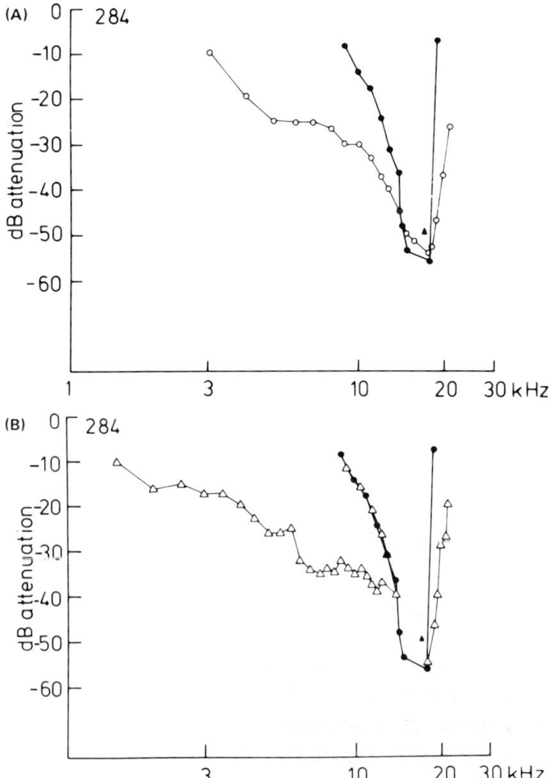

Figure 8 Excitation and suppression areas as measured in the response of the receptor potential of an inner hair cell in the basal turn of a guinea pig cochlea. The excitatory isoresponse curve for the DC component of the depolarization of the receptor potential is shown with the aid of filled circles in (a) and (b). Open symbols outline the boundaries of the two-tone suppression areas corresponding to a 20% reduction of the response to the excitor tone (filled triangles). In (a) the isoinhibitory boundary of the AC component is plotted (open circles); in (b) the isoinhibitory boundary of the DC potential. The resulting curves are very similar to corresponding single-fiber responses in the auditory nerve. [From Sellick and Russell (1979) with permission.]

indicate that the apical papilla (the equivalent of the basilar membrane in mammals) is very broadly tuned, essentially resonating at one frequency, even though the fibers are tuned to different CFs. Various hypotheses have been formulated proposing that the micromechanics of the tectorial membrane–hair cell–sterocilia complex is the site of the additional (second) filter (Allen, 1977, 1980; Duifhuis and Van de Vorst, 1980; Zwislocki and Kletsky, 1979). Other second-filter models include one that incorporates spatial differentiation of a nonlinear traveling wave (Hall, 1977a,b, 1980) and several that operate by means of the electrical currents present within the cochlea (Strelioff *et al.*, 1976; Manley,

1978). Some of these second-filter models are essentially linear operators. Thus, in order to account for nonlinearities, like suppression, they most often depend on a nonlinear damping term that increases with increasing stimulus levels (Kim *et al.*, 1973).

C. Manipulations Affecting Cochlear Tuning

1. Efferent Stimulation and Second Tones

Wiederhold (1970) and Kiang *et al.* (1970) have shown that stimulation of the crossed olivocochlear bundle (COCB) in cat reduces the sensitivities of single auditory nerve fibers. The reduction is greatest at frequencies near the CF of the fiber; at frequencies far below and above CF, COCB stimulation has little effect on fiber threshold. Thus, it is the sensitive tip of the tuning curve that is most shifted when the efferents are excited, as shown in Fig. 9. In the lower part of the

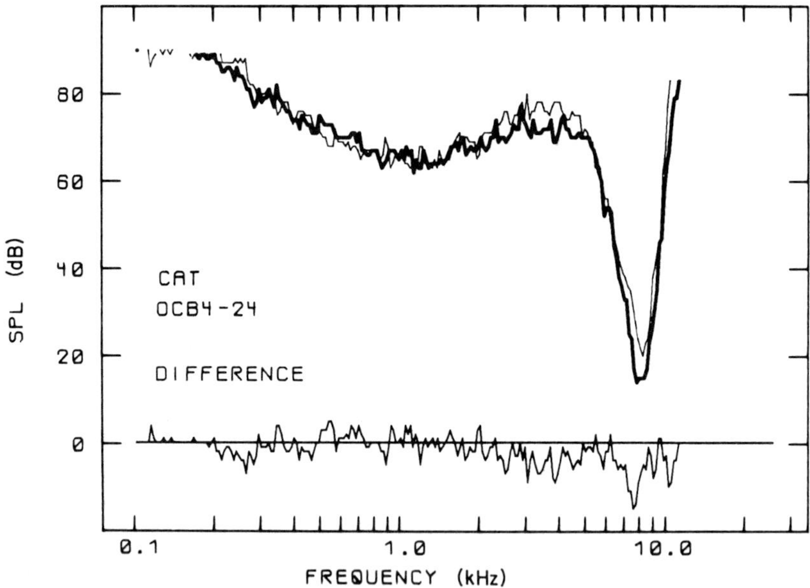

Figure 9 Effects of stimulation of the crossed olivocochlear bundle (COCB) on primary single-fiber tuning curves in cat. The COCB efferents were stimulated electrically at the midline of the brainstem on the floor of the fourth ventricle. The methods followed those of Wiederhold (1970) and Kiang *et al.* (1970). The normal tuning curve is plotted by means of a thick line; the curve associated with efferent stimulation is plotted with a thin line. The decibel difference between the two curves is also graphed at the bottom of the figure with the same ordinal scale. Note the largest effect (15 dB) occurs at frequencies near the fiber CF. The tail is shifted little or not at all. Fiber OCB4-24, spontaneous rate, 50 spikes/sec.

figure is plotted the difference in dB between the two curves. The greatest difference (15 dB) occurs at frequencies around the fiber CF.

Another way of changing the tuning of a primary fiber associated with a normal cochlea is by adding simultaneously a second tone or narrowband noise of constant level and frequency while the tuning curve is being obtained. When the second tone or noise is placed below CF in the tail of the tuning curve, Kiang and Moxon (1974) have shown that only the tip becomes desensitized, very much like the efferent effect shown in Fig. 9. Putting a second tone above CF affects not only the tip, but also can affect the tail of the curve as will be shown in a subsequent section. Kiang and Moxon (1974) also have demonstrated that a tuning curve obtained in the presence of either a white (wideband) noise or a narrowband noise centered at the fiber CF will shift the entire curve, tip and tail, upward by a constant amount. In other words, a white noise will act to desensitize the fiber about equally across all frequencies.

2. Cochlear Injury

Much of the effort in auditory physiology over the past decade has been directed toward examining the activity of primary fibers associated with abnormal cochleas. The usual methods for producing cochlear abnormalities have been by means of treatment with ototoxic drugs (aminoglycosides) (Kiang *et al.*, 1970; Evans, 1975a; Dallos and Harris, 1978; Robertson and Johnstone, 1979; Schmiedt *et al.*, 1980; Schmiedt and Zwislocki, 1980; and Harrison, 1981) or overexposure to noise (Davis *et al.*, 1935; Kiang *et al.*, 1976a; Liberman and Kiang, 1978; Liberman and Mulroy, 1982; Salvi *et al.*, 1982; Schmiedt, 1982c). What happens to the frequency–selectivity of single fibers under circumstances of cochlear injury can be complex, involving at times both the tip and tail of the tuning curve. Figure 10 summarizes some of the tuning curves obtrained from single fibers in cats with chronic theshold shifts due to noise exposure. In Fig. 10A the entire curve has been displaced upward with regard to the curves of normal fibers of similar CF (stippled area). In Fig. 10B, mainly the tip of the curve has been affected, while in Fig. 10C the tail has become hypersensitive in the presence of a hyposensitive tip. Finally, in Fig. 10D, a bowl-shaped curve is plotted which has no assignable CF.

Of interest with respect to assigning CFs to fibers associated with injured cochleas is the work of Robertson and Johnstone (1979). By recording from ganglion cell bodies in the basal turn of the guinea pig cochlea, they were able to show that the best frequencies of tuning curves obtained in cases of injury were shifted down in frequency between one-half and one octave below the expected CFs found in normal cochleas at similar positions along the cochlear turn (see Fig. 11). The key here is that CFs associated with cell bodies at a given position on the cochlear turn are normally quite consistent from cell to cell and from animal to animal. Thus, at least in the basal turn, cochlear damage in terms of

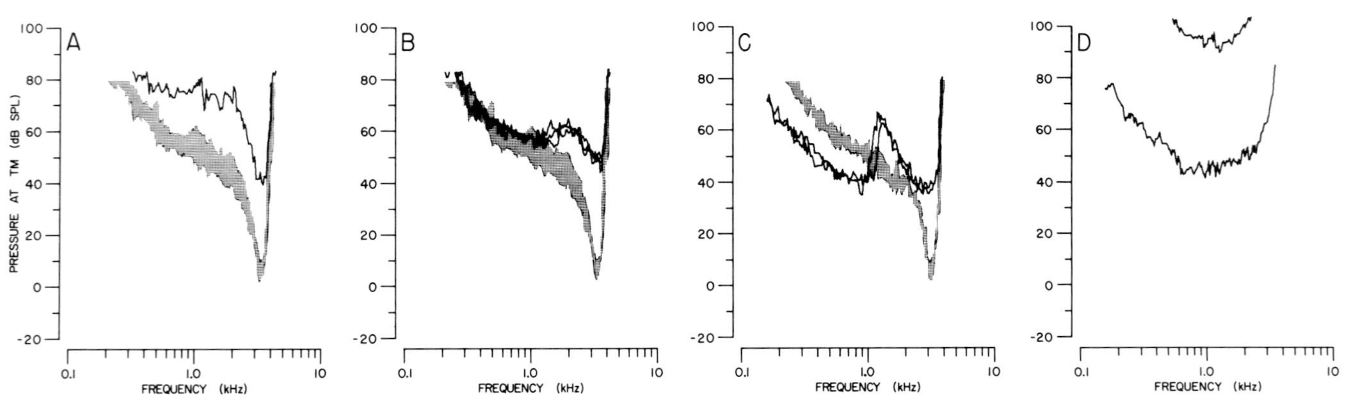

Figure 10 Various changes in tuning curves of single auditory nerve fibers associated with abnormal cochleas. The cochleas were permanently injured by means of exposure to noise. Stippled areas indicate regions of normal thresholds of high-spontaneous fibers with CFs corresponding to the abnormal curves. In D, the fibers have no assignable CFs, so normal curves are shown. Contrast the hyposensitive tip and tail in A with the hyposensitive tip and hypersensitive tail in C. [From Liberman and Mulroy (1982) with permission.]

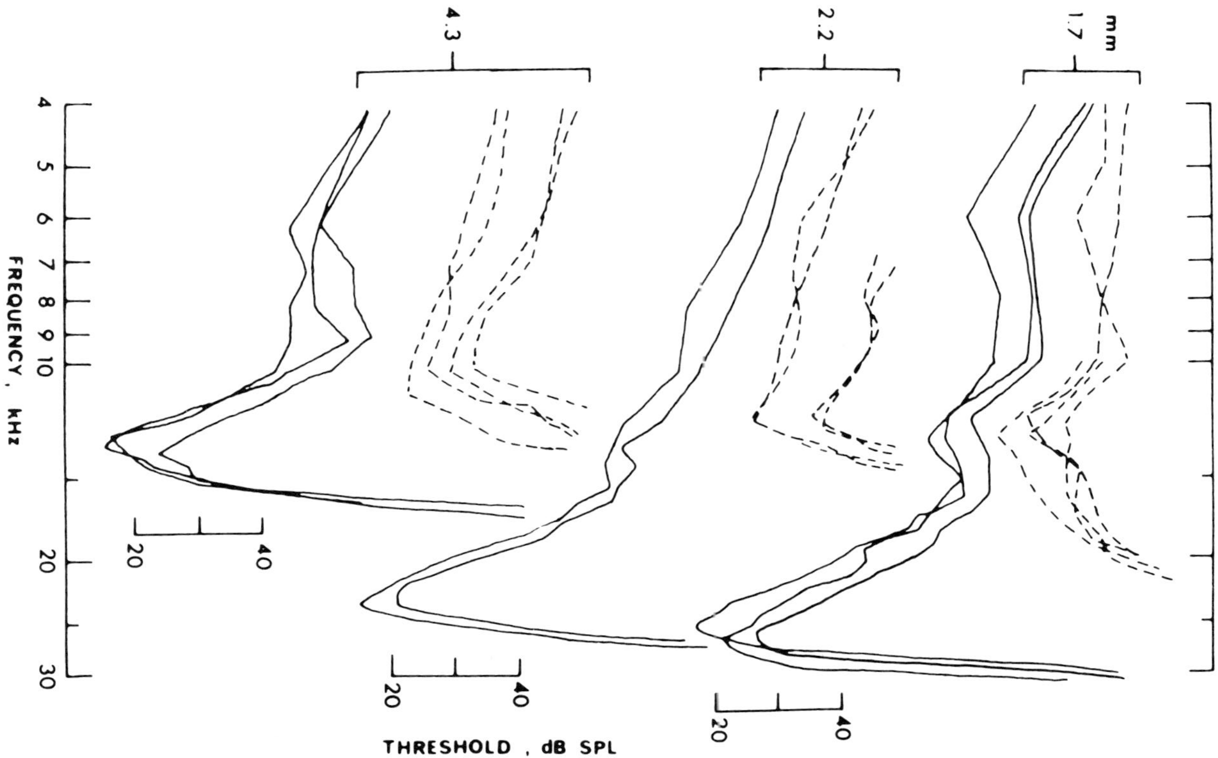

Figure 11 Tuning curves obtained from spiral ganglion cells in Rosenthal's canal in the basal turn of the guinea pig cochlea. The three sets of curves correspond to three locations along the basilar membrane: 1.7, 2.2, and 4.3 mm from the basal end. Solid curves were obtained from normal cochleas, dashed curves, from cochleas devoid of outer hair cells in the basal turn. There is not only a loss of the sharply tuned tip segment in the dashed curves, but also a discrepancy in the apparent best frequency of the neurons as compared to their normal counterparts. Thus, cochlear injury may well alter the tonotopic (frequency–distance) map of the cochlea. [From Robertson and Johnston (1979) with permission.]

hair cell loss seems to correspond to an alteration of cochlear tuning, i.e., the tonotopic map of the cochlea changes. As a result, the apparent CFs of abnormal tuning curves are probably not the true CF of the fiber in terms of its innervation point along the basilar membrane in a normal cochlea.

D. Relationships between Tuning and Suppression

1. Tuning Variabilities in Normal Cochleas

How valid is the assumption that single-fiber tuning is similar for all mammals? Figure 12 compares tuning curves of similar CF and CF threshold from cats (thin line) and gerbils (thick line). All in all, there is little difference. One dichotomy does stand out; the "notch" present between the tip and the tail of the cat curve about an octave below CF is typically absent in gerbil curves. In cats the tip of the tuning curve for high-CF fibers is thereby accentuated by the notch as compared to similar curves obtained from rodents. Otherwise, in a general sense, mammalian curves are fairly similar.

Another question of relevance in our examination of physiological tuning curves is their variability in shape within a given animal or among animals of the same species. Geisler *et al.* (1974) and Liberman (1978) have shown in squirrel

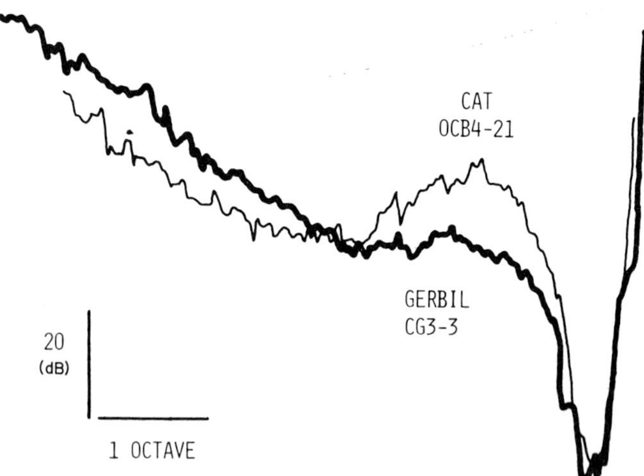

Figure 12   A comparison of the tuning of two high-CF fibers, one from the auditory nerve in cat (thin line) and one from the same nerve in gerbil (thick line). The two curves have been normalized at their tips by aligning their CFs and CF thresholds. Note the typical presence of a notch about an octave below CF in the cat data; tuning curves of gerbil fibers are not usually characterized by such an extensive notch. Fiber, CF, CF threshold, and spontaneous rate are as follows: OCB4-21, 6.683 kHz, 18 dB, 19 spikes/sec; CG3-3, 6.26 kHz, 5 dB, 26 spikes/sec.

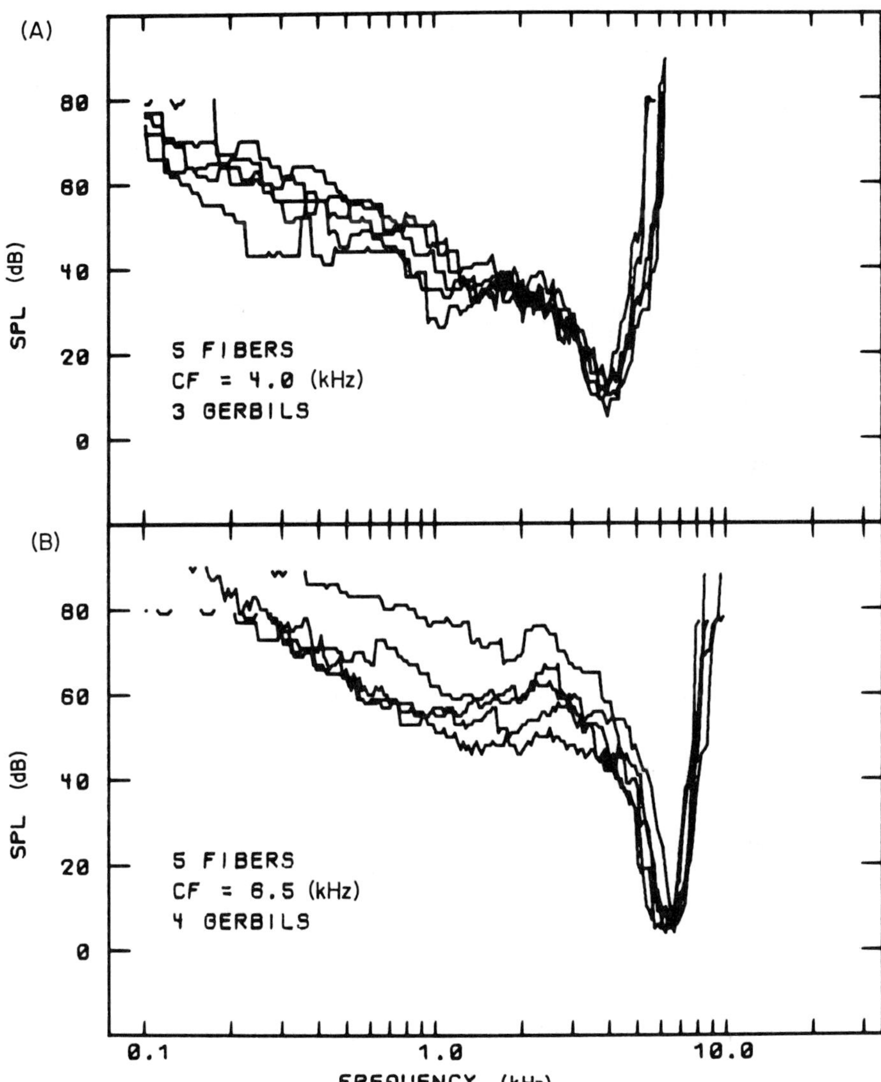

Figure 13 Comparison of tuning curves of single auditory nerve fibers of similar CFs in gerbils. The curves are not normalized, but were selected to correspond closely in CF (± 250 Hz) and CF threshold (± 2 dB); all data were obtained from high-spontaneous fibers. Fibers with CFs around 4.0 kHz are represented in (A), CFs around 6.5 kHz, in (B). Five curves are shown in (A) and in (B). The variability is representative of data from a single animal and among animals. Gerbils, probably because they can be raised easily in controlled environments, have fairly homogeneous fiber characteristics (Schmiedt *et al.*, 1980; Schmiedt, 1982a).

monkey and cat, respectively, that the spontaneous rate (spont) of a fiber is strongly correlated with its CF threshold. In cat, chinchilla (Salvi *et al.*, 1982), and gerbil (Schmiedt, 1982a), fibers can be divided into three groups: high-spont (greater than 18–20 spikes/sec), medium spont (between 0.5 and 18 spikes/sec), and low-spont group (less than 0.5 spikes/sec). The high-spont fibers have the lowest thresholds at CF, the low-spont fibers, the highest. In a given animal, the range between thresholds of high- and low-spont groups is typically 10–20 dB; however, the range can be as large as 60–80 dB. An important finding in this regard is that it is not just the tuning curve tip that is shifted upward in the low-spont fibers relative to the high-spont fibers, but the entire tuning curve.

If fibers are segregated into spont groups, the variability of fiber tuning within a species is reduced considerably. This can be seen in Fig. 10 for cats and Fig. 13 for gerbils. Within a species there is often one CF region that is characterized by more variability in the respective thresholds and tuning than in other regions. For example, in cats, a variable region seems to exist at CFs between 3 and 4 kHz (Liberman, 1978). In gerbils there is an increased variability in thresholds and tuning at CFs between 4 and 6 kHz. As with a physical filter, we can define a quality factor, Q, for fiber tuning such that

$$Q_{10\ \mathrm{dB}} = \frac{\text{Fiber CF}}{\text{Bandwidth at 10 dB above CF threshold}}$$

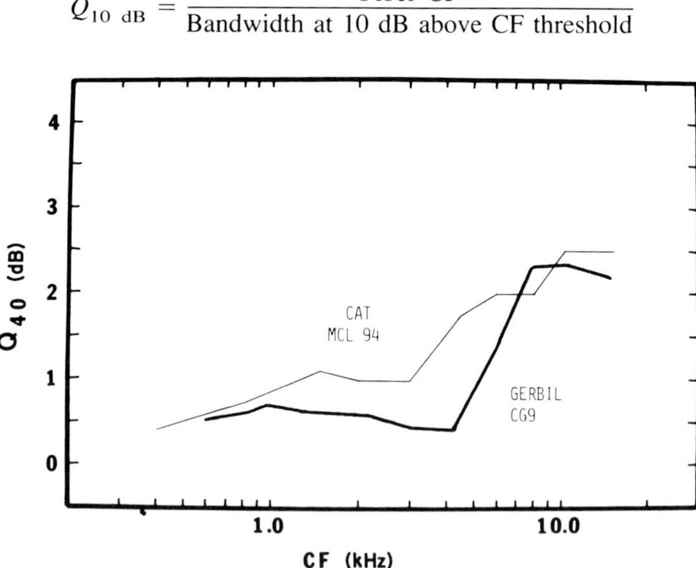

Figure 14   Median curves of a measure of the sharpness of tuning as a function of CF of single fibers in the auditory nerves of one cat and one gerbil. The Q value was calculated from the bandwidth measured at 40 dB above CF threshold. The curves are similar, but are shifted somewhat along the abscissa. This shift may be due in part to the emphasized notch and tip present in the cat single-fiber tuning (see Fig. 12). Cat data are from Liberman (1978).

(Kiang *et al.,* 1965). If we plot Q values as a function of fiber CF, it is a general trend that tuning sharpness increases with CF ($Q_{10\,dB}$ values increase). Figure 14 illustrates this trend for gerbils and cats with a measure of Q taken 40 dB above CF threshold ($Q_{40\,dB}$). Note that there is a breakpoint in the curve at 3 and 4.5 kHz, respectively, for cats and gerbils, the same CF regions where fiber thresholds are the most variable.

2. Suppression Boundaries

Figure 6 illustrates schematically the two-tone suppression (inhibitory) areas associated with primary auditory nerve fibers. The actual lower threshold boundaries of the suppression areas and their relationship to the tuning curve are shown in Fig. 15. These curves were obtained in cats, and data from this fiber are also shown in Fig. 9. The main point is that the boundary of the suppression area below CF follows the shape of the tail of the tuning curve (Schmiedt, 1982b).

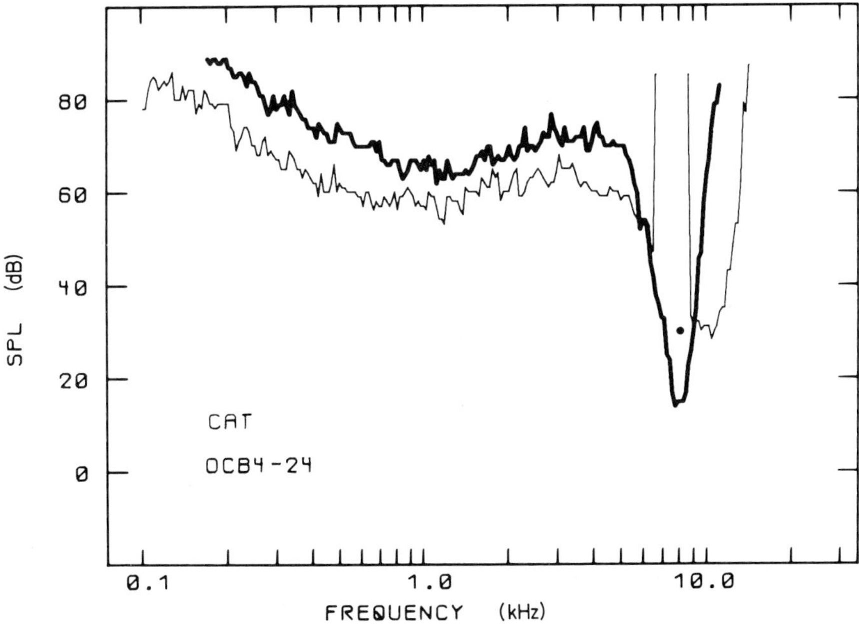

Figure 15 A single-fiber tuning curve and its associated suppression boundaries in cat. The suppression boundaries were tracked with the aid of a modified tuning curve algorithm (Kiang and Moxon, 1974; Holton, 1980). The tracking criterion for the tuning curve and suppression boundaries was a 20–40 spikes/sec rate increase or decrease, respectively, over a control interval. Frequency resolution is 32 points/octave, and the filled circle represents the coordinates of a continuous excitor tone (CTCF) used to obtain the suppression boundaries. Note how the boundary below CF follows the shape of the tail of the tuning curve. Fiber OCB4-24, 8.12 kHz, 15 dB, 52 spikes/sec.

  John H. Mills and Richard A. Schmiedt

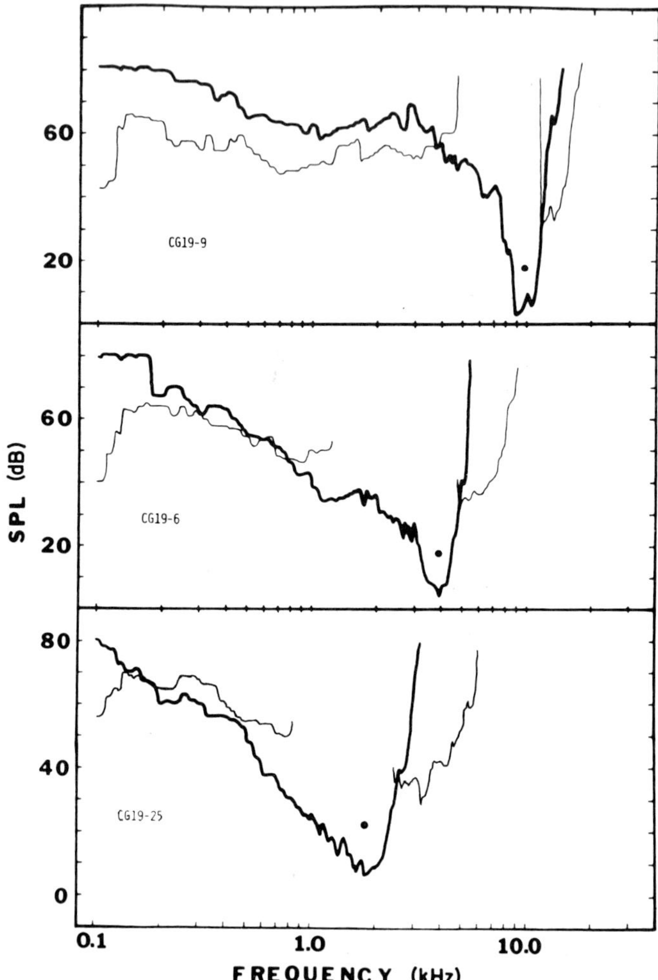

Figure 16 Tuning curves and suppression boundaries from three gerbil auditory nerve fibers. Symbols and curves are described in Fig. 15. Tuning curve tails and suppression boundaries below CF have a frequency resolution of 8 points/octave; in the tip region around CF, the resolution is 32 points/octave. All curves were obtained with a criterion rate increase or decrease of between 0 and 20 spikes/sec over a control interval. The sharp upward slope of the suppression boundary at 0.1 kHz is artifactual due to the constraints of the algorithm and the weak two-tone suppression gradient found at very low frequencies (see text). Note that the shape of the suppression boundary follows that of the tail of the tuning curve; also the suppression boundaries below CF for the three fibers all have similar absolute positions. [From Schmiedt (1982b) with permission.]

That the shape of this suppression boundary essentially follows the tail of the tuning curve is also true in gerbils (Fig. 16). (The deviation of the boundary from the tuning curve at very low frequencies around 100 Hz is an artifact of the tracking algorithm due to the low criterion values used to obtain the curve and the relatively weak gradient of suppression with respect to intensity found at very low frequencies.)

Another property of the suppression boundaries obtained from low, medium, and high-CF fibers in gerbils is shown in Fig. 17. Here, the respective tuning curves have not been plotted. Above about 3 kHz the boundaries of suppression above CF are dominant with slopes between 80 and 300 dB/octave. Below 3 kHz, the boundaries below CF are seen to form a relatively tight distribution. This stability of the position of the suppression boundary below CF is fairly independent of tuning curve shape, CF, and CF threshold. Note that the SPL levels are absolute and are not normalized in any fashion.

Figure 18 illustrates the stability of the suppression boundaries below CF with regard to tuning curve shape. In each of the two panels, two fibers with widely varying tuning curves of similar CF were selected from one gerbil. In both panels the suppression boundaries are similar, even though the tails of the tuning curves differ by up to 30 dB (Schmiedt, 1982b). Thus, the position of the lower threshold boundary of two-tone rate suppression obtained with suppressors

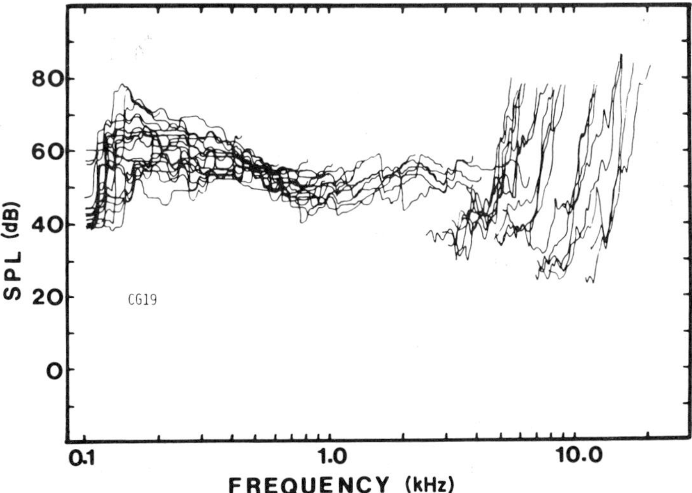

Figure 17 Population plot of suppression boundaries obtained from 27 fibers in one gerbil. Fiber CFs ranged from 1.8 to 16.0 kHz. The technical details of obtaining the boundaries are described in Fig. 16. The steep curves above about 3 kHz are the suppression boundaries found above CF. The approximately horizontal contours below 3 kHz are those obtained with suppressors below CF. Normalization of any type was not performed. [From Schmiedt (1982b) with permission.]

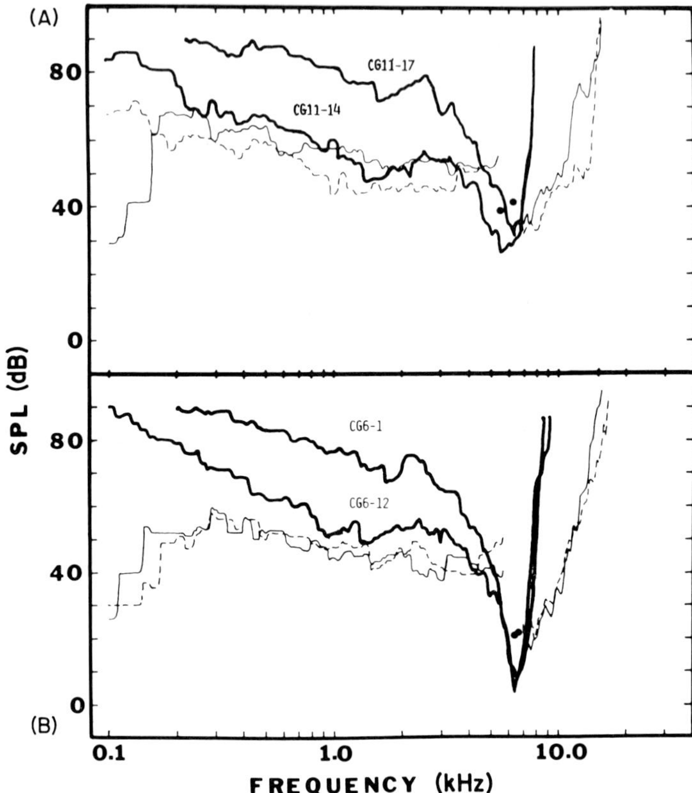

Figure 18 Comparison of tuning curves and suppression boundaries obtained from fibers innervating the same cochleas. Plots are similar to those in Fig. 16 and are not normalized. Thin dashed lines represent suppression boundaries associated with the tuning curves having the smaller tip-to-tail ratio of thresholds; thin solid lines are associated with the fibers having the larger ratio. Note that the shapes of the tuning curves can differ substantially, yet the suppression boundaries below stay constant in absolute position. [From Schmiedt (1982b) with permission.]

placed below CF is fairly independent of the shape, CF, and CF threshold of the tuning curve.

3. Two-Tone Tuning Curve

Previously we mentioned the work of Kiang and Moxon (1974) wherein tuning curves were obtained from primary fibers in the presence of white noise or a narrowband noise placed at or below CF. In those respective cases, the entire curve or just the tip became desensitized. What happens to the tuning curve when a second tone is placed in the suppression area above CF? Results obtained under such conditions are shown in Fig. 19. Fig. 19A and B, the normal tuning curves are plotted as thick lines, the two-tone curves taken in the presence of a 70 dB SPL tone placed above CF (triangle) are plotted as thin lines. The second tone by itself was not excitatory. The dotted lines are the suppression boundaries. The minima present above CF in the two-tone curves are due to the distortion products, f_2-f_1, and $2f_1-f_2$, falling near the fiber CF. The influence of the second tone is present in the desensitized tip of the two-tone curve and, in the upper panel, a hypersensitive tail. The tip is desensitized because the second tone was placed in the upper suppression area, indicating that rate suppression has its strongest influence at frequencies around fiber CF, as also found by Kiang and

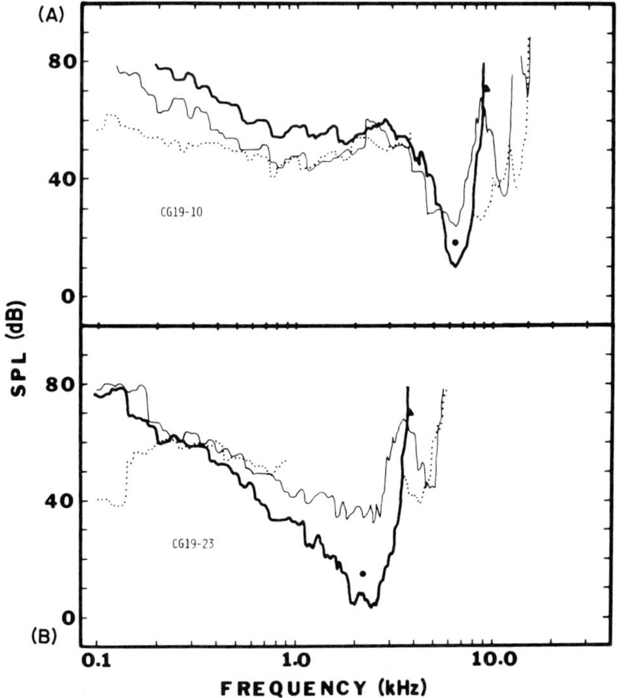

Figure 19 Effect on the tuning curve of a continuous tone placed in the suppression area above CF; the tone by itself was not excitatory. Normal tuning curves are plotted with thick lines, tuning curves taken in the presence of the second tone are plotted with thin lines. Suppression boundaries are represented with dotted lines. Coordinates of the excitor tone at CF used to obtain suppression measures and the second tone above CF are indicated by filled circles and triangles, respectively. Methods used are similar to those described in Fig. 16. The secondary minima closest to the edge of the tuning curves with thin lines result from the $2f_1-f_2$ distortion products. In (A) another minimum is present around 13 kHz and is due to the f_2-f_1 distortion product. Note how the tails of the two-tone tuning curves shift to coincide with the suppression boundaries below CF, making the high-CF fiber hypersensitive at low frequencies. [From Schmiedt (1982b) with permission.]

Moxon (1974). The hypersensitive tail of the two-tone curve in Fig. 19A is the result of the tail shifting to the position of the boundary of the suppression area below CF. In Fig. 19B, the tail of the two-tone curve also shifts to the suppression boundary, but because the boundary is above the tail of the normal curve, the end result is a two-tone curve with a hyposensitive tail.

4. Abnormal Cochleas

Experiments with abnormal cochleas allow further examinations of the relationships between tuning curves and their associated suppression areas. Again, we find that tuning is only loosely coupled to the presence or absence of two-tone rate suppression. Figure 20 demonstrates this point. In this experiment, Robertson and Johnstone (1981) obtained tuning curves and suppression boundaries from single primary neurons (solid symbols). After the normal data were taken, the animal was exposed to a 110-dB tone continuously for about 1 min. This

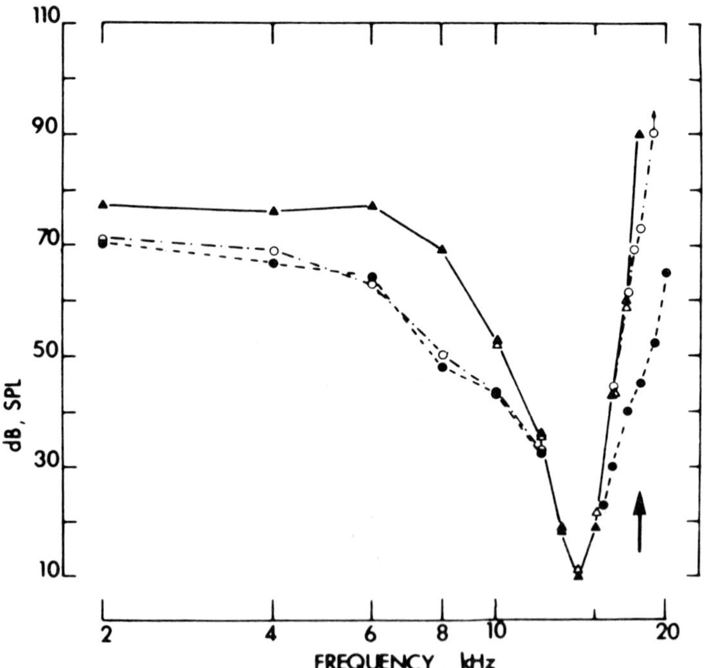

Figure 20 Effects of a high-level fatiguing tone on tuning and suppression in primary neurons in the guinea pig cochlea. Closed triangles and circles represent, respectively, tuning curves and suppression boundaries before fatigue, corresponding open symbols, after fatigue. Fatiguing tone was placed at the arrow at 110 dB SPL for 1 min. The tuning curve and the suppression boundary below CF remain essentially unchanged by the fatiguer. The suppression above CF is largely, but not totally, eliminated. [From Robertson and Johnson (1981) with permission.]

fatiguing tone was placed above CF outside the response area of the neuron, so the neuron was not itself fatigued. After fatiguing, the two-tone suppression above CF was largely, but not totally, absent, whereas the suppression boundary below CF and the tuning curve showed little change. Note that this effect was temporary, and some residual suppression above CF was always present. Another point of interest in the results of Robertson and Johnstone was that the large loss of suppression also was correlated with a decrease in the level of fiber excitation due to the distortion components, f_2-f_1 and $2f_1-f_2$, generated by two tones above CF (see also Dallos *et al.*, 1980). It would seem that the mechanism of suppression above CF may be responsible for distortion product generation in the cochlea.

Data along these same lines showing a large degree of independence between suppression and tuning have been obtained in permanently injured cochleas by Schmiedt and Zwislocki (1980) and Schmiedt (1982c). They found that under conditions of permanent damage, two-tone suppression was sometimes completely lost on the high-frequency side of the tuning curve. Under these conditions, the gross shape of the tuning curve was little affected, as Robertson and Johnstone (1981) found. However, the slope of the high-frequency leg of the tuning curve was always less steep than normal (70–200 dB/octave as compared

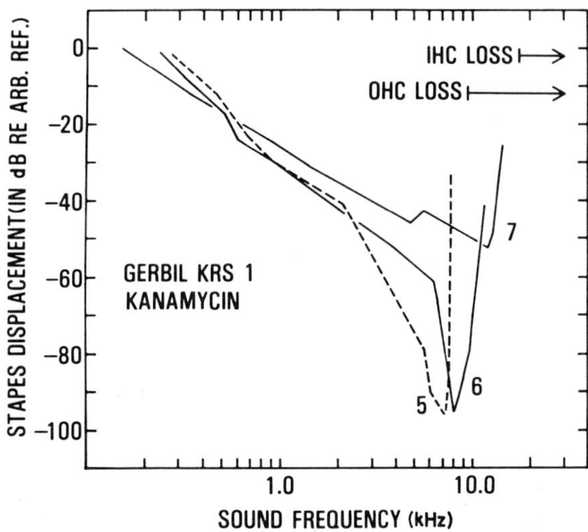

Figure 21 Tuning curves of three fibers from a gerbil treated with the ototoxin, kanamycin. Fiber 5 (dashed line) was about normal in threshold at CF and exhibited substantial two-tone suppression above CF. Fibers 6 and 7 had a complete loss of suppression above CF. Compare the high-frequency slopes of the dashed curve (about 1100 dB/octave) with the slopes of the fibers without suppression (about 180 dB/octave). [From Schmiedt (1982c) with permission. Copyright 1983, American Medical Association.]

to 300–1100 dB/octave). This slope change is shown in Fig. 21. Another correlation with the loss of two-tone suppression above CF was the loss of the frequency-dependent nonlinearity present in the intensity (rate-level) functions obtained with tones above CF. This nonlinearity is always present in normal cochleas and causes intensity functions to have lowered slopes and saturation rates as tones are placed increasingly further above CF. Thus, complete loss of suppression above CF is reflected in the tuning curve as a decreased high-frequency slope. It has also been shown that tuning curves with hypersensitive tails have no suppression areas below CF. The converse, however, seems not to be true: a lack of suppression below CF does not necessarily imply hypersensitivity to low-frequency stimuli (Schmiedt and Zwislocki, 1980).

In Figure 22 are shown two-tone suppression boundaries and tuning curves obtained from two fibers in the same gerbil. The cochlea was permanently damaged by means of a low-frequency noise exposure. Again, as in Fig. 20, we see some independence between suppression and tuning, as well as independence between the presence or absence of suppression areas above and below CF. In Fig. 22A, a sharply tuned fiber is seen to have suppression below CF but none above. However, the high-frequency slope of the tuning curve is about 180 dB/octave in agreement with Schmiedt and Zwislocki (1980). In Fig. 22B, the tuning curve has lost its tip and has little or no suppression below CF, yet still has suppression above CF. In this case, the high-frequency slope of the tuning curve is about 430 dB/octave. The point is, then, tuning and suppression are loosely coupled phenomena in single, primary-fiber responses. Indeed, even two-tone suppression above and below CF seem to have a large degree of independence.

E. Tuning Assessed by Masking Procedures

In the previous sections, cochlear and fiber tuning have been measured directly, typically in terms of a criterion response to a single tone. Psychophysical procedures, in the context of obtaining tuning curves, demand a different paradigm using forward or simultaneous masking. Complications arise with simultaneous procedures applied to single-fiber responses because of the resulting two-tone suppression and generation of distortion products. Forward-masking procedures have been used with single fibers to analyze just how well the comparable psychophysical methods can be expected to measure auditory frequency selectivity in the periphery (Bauer, 1978; Harris and Dallos, 1979). The stimulus paradigm consists of a masker and probe like those shown in Fig. 36; however, the criterion measure is in the form of a constant reduction in the peri-stimulus time (PST) histogram of the response of the fiber to just the probe signal. In other words, the masking of the response of a fiber is defined as a criterion reduction of the probe-evoked response by the addition of the masker. What is really being studied in this paradigm is the effect of short-term recovery in single fibers (see Smith, 1977, 1979; Harris and Dallos, 1979). Smith as well as Harris and Dallos

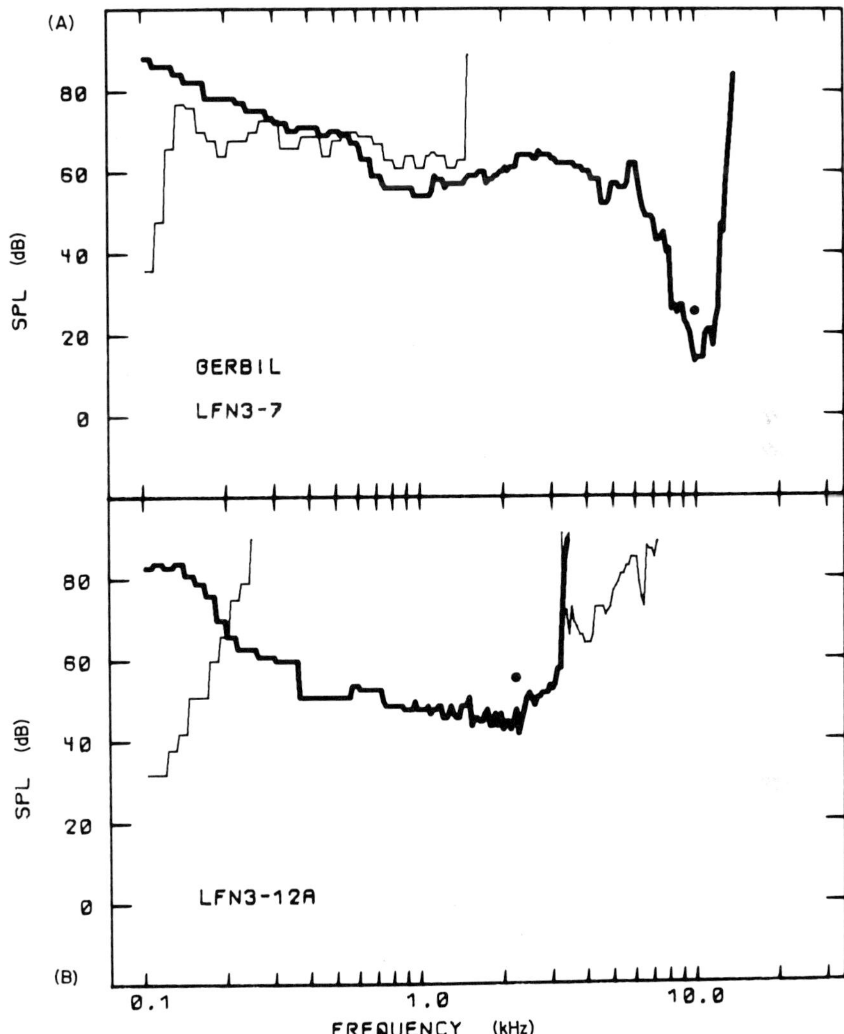

Figure 22 Tuning and suppression characteristics of two fibers from a cochlea permanently damaged by exposure to an octave band of noise centered at 63 Hz at 120 dB SPL for 7 days. Curves and symbols are explained in Fig. 16. In (A) the fiber has sharp tuning, a normal CF threshold, and suppression below CF even though there is a complete lack of suppression above CF (suppression boundaries were tracked twice for verification). In (B) the fiber has lost its sensitivity and sharp tuning around CF and has lost suppression below CF; however, the suppression area above CF is still present, though decreased from normal. High-frequency slopes of the tuning curves are 180 and 430 dB/octave (A) and (B), respectively.

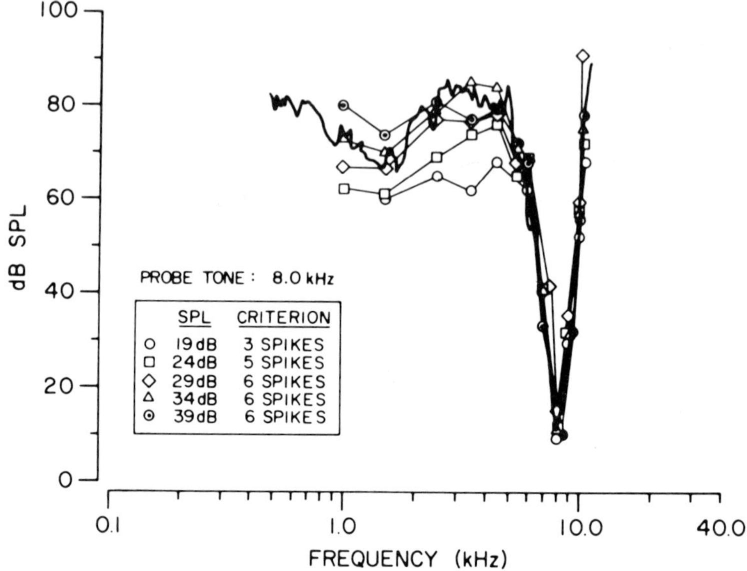

Figure 23 Effects of five probe levels on fiber-masking functions of a high-CF fiber in cat. The normal tuning curve is shown as a thick line. The response criteria for the masked-threshold functions were chosen to bring the tips of the masking functions into agreement with the actual tuning curve. Note that low probe levels tend to underestimate the true tail threshold, whereas higher level probes yield functions that agree well with the tuning curve. [From Bauer (1978) with permission.]

have shown that the recovery process after a tone burst is independent of the frequency of the excitor tone. What matters is only the amount of fiber excitation caused by the tone burst. Thus, because the tuning curve is by definition a criterion boundary in terms of fiber excitation, the amount of "masking" seen in the probe-evoked response as a function of masker frequency will be a reflection of the tuning curve. Typically, the probe stimulus is placed at the CF of the fiber to mimic the psychophysical paradigm. Results from such a study are shown in Fig. 23 for a high-CF fiber. At low probe levels, the masker-defined tail of the tuning curve falls below the actual tuning curve. At high probe levels, between 25 and 35 dB above CF threshold, the masker and actual tuning curve tails line up fairly well. The tip is accurately defined at all probe levels. [Note here that Harris and Dallos (1979) found that an accurate tail could be obtained with probes at 15 dB above CF threshold in chinchilla. This dichotomy may be due to slight differences in their stimulus paradigms.]

Evoked-Potential Masking Curves

The above forward masking paradigm used with fibers also has been successfully used with evoked potentials, like the whole-nerve action potential (AP) of the auditory nerve and the brainstem response (Dallos and Cheatham, 1976). Furthermore, as in psychophysics, suppression characteristics may be assessed with a third tone introduced to suppress the effect of the masker, thereby producing "unmasking" (Dallos and Cheatham, 1977; Harris, 1979).

The AP can be elicited by a brief tonal probe; however, as with all neural-

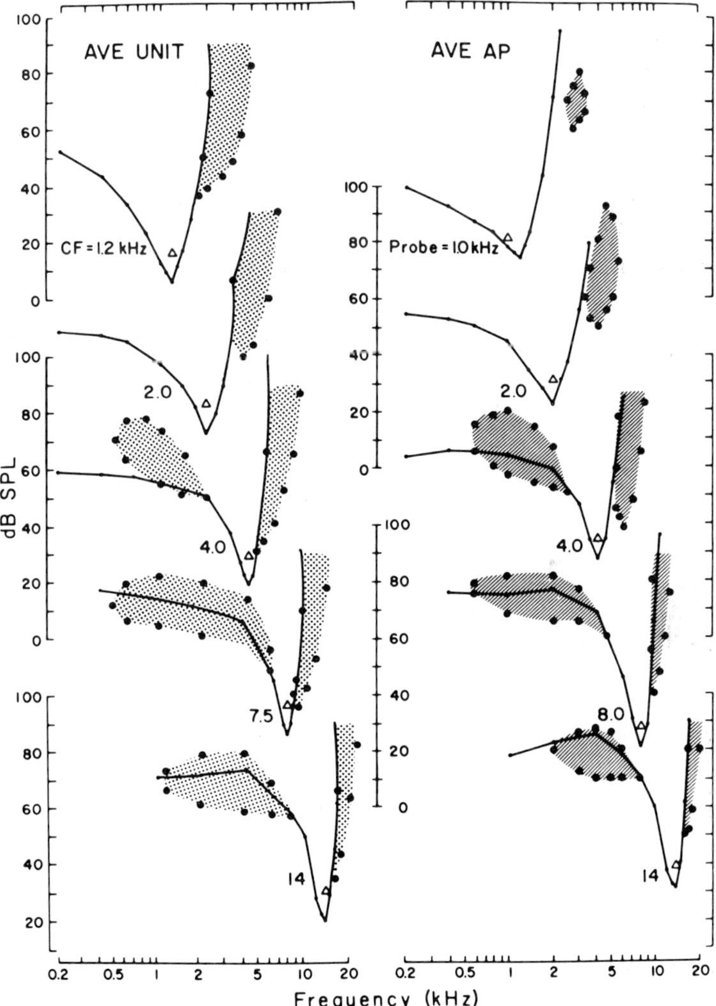

Figure 24 Comparison of averaged single-fiber tuning curves (left) and averaged masked AP (evoked-response) curves (right). Shaded areas represent the two-tone suppression boundaries in the case of the fibers, and the areas of unmaking with the AP data. There is a strong similarity between the fiber and AP data. [From Harris (1979) with permission.]

evoked potentials, the AP is dependent on the synchronous discharge of many neurons (Kiang *et al.*, 1976b). Synchrony is best achieved with short, sharply defined stimuli in the time domain. Remembering the Fourier transform (see Fig. 1), we know these brief stimuli will have associated with them broad spectra. Thus, a compromise must be struck between synchrony and frequency-selectivity. Typically the probe signal used to evoke the AP and brainstem potentials is 2 to 10 msec in duration with rise–fall envelopes of between 0.5 and 2 msec.

A comparison between averaged neural tuning curves and suppression areas obtained in the usual fashion and AP tuning curves and their associated suppression areas is shown in Fig. 24. These data were obtained by Harris (1979) in the chinchilla. The correspondence between the single-fiber and AP curves is rather striking. Other studies of the tuned AP response have shown it to be a valuable indicator of cochlear injury (Henderson *et al.*, 1969; Eggermont, 1977; Dallos *et al.*, 1977, 1978; Robertson *et al.*, 1980).

Another evoked potential of great interest at present is the brainstem potential,

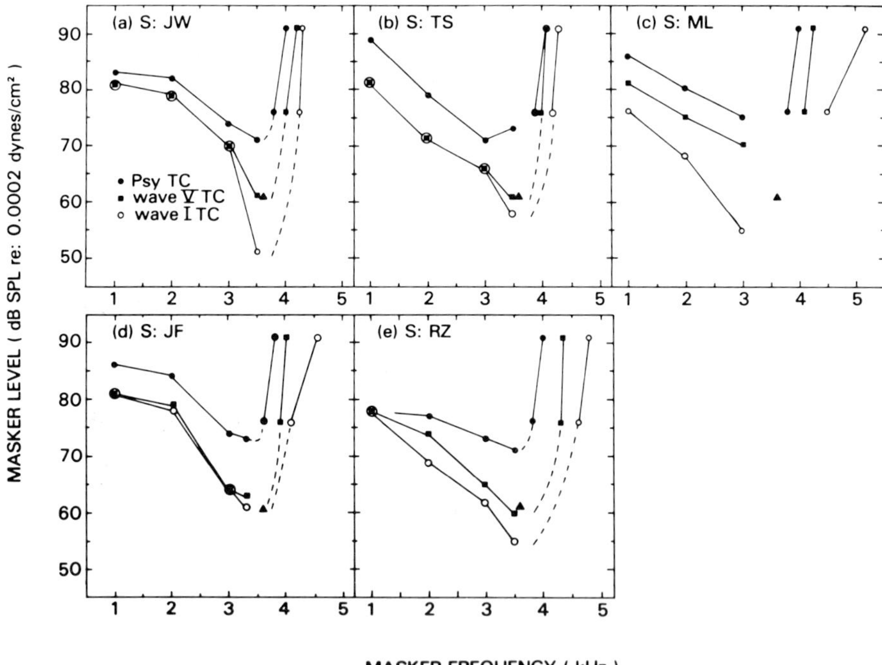

Figure 25 Comparison of psychophysical and physiological (waves I and V) tuning curves from five normal human subjects (a–e). Masking criterion used to obtain the psysiological curves was one-half the unmasked amplitude of the probe-evoked response (see text). Filled triangles represent the probe-tone frequency and level. [From Klein and Mills (1981a) with permission.]

specifically waves I and V (Jewitt and Williston, 1971; Davis, 1976). Wave I is the analog of the AP waveform originating from the depolarization of the auditory nerve; wave V is a more complex potential probably arising from the inferior colliculus in humans. Klein and Mills (1981a,b) and Klein (1982a,b) have recently explored the tuning properties of these potentials in humans with and without temporary threshold shifts (TTS) caused by noise exposure. In these brainstem experiments it should be noted that the masker was a continuous tone; thus, a simultaneous procedure was used rather than forward masking, as in the AP tuning curves discussed above. Klein and Mills (1981a) have shown that the tuning is similar for both the psychophysical and physiological measures obtained with the same methods (Fig. 25). The psychophysical curves always required the strongest masker, whereas the wave I curves often required the least masking.

Another measure of physiological tuning in the brainstem response is shown in Fig. 26. Here, as before, a simultaneous procedure was used to mask the probe-evoked response. In this case, however, the specific potential masked was the slow negative potential appearing just after wave V. Davis and Hirsh (1979) have termed this wave SN_{10} because it has about a 10 msec latency. Of interest is the tuning of this potential at frequencies as low as 250 Hz (Fig. 26A). It is apparent that with a 250-Hz probe, the most effective masking is displaced from the probe frequency and occurs at 350 Hz. This frequency shift is probably due to the

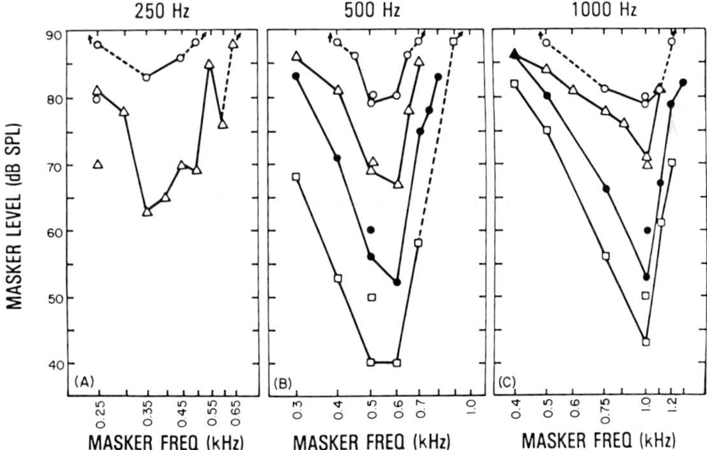

Figure 26 Brainstem–response tuning curves obtained at low frequencies with the SN_{10} potential in human subjects. Probe levels and frequencies are indicated by the isolated open and closed symbols. At 250 Hz the tips of the curves are shifted away from the probe frequency; the shift is probably caused by frequency splatter of the probe spectrum and the relative insensitivity of the ear to frequencies below 250 Hz. The V shape of the curves agree well with the shape of single-fiber curves with corresponding CFs. [From Klein (1982b) with permission.]

frequency splatter (large bandwidth) of the probe coupled with the steeply rising threshold of the human audibility curve below 250 Hz. The 500 and 1000 Hz curves, however, are strikingly similar to the tuning of auditory nerve fibers with low CFs, i.e. typically V-shaped (see Fig. 5). Additional discussion of evoked-response curves can be found in later sections of this article.

F. Acoustic Emissions

So far in our examination of physiological tuning we have gone from cochlear mechanics, to primary fibers, to peripheral-evoked potentials, and to brainstem-evoked potentials. Let us now retrace our path back to the ear canal. In 1978 Kemp changed the way physiologists think about cochlear mechanics by describing an echo phenomenon present acoustically in the outer ear. Simply put, the cochlea in a human subject often responds to brief acoustic stimuli with acoustic emissions that are delayed from the signal onset. In humans, the delay is on the order of 5 to 15 msec (Kemp, 1978, 1979, 1982); in lower animals, the delay is much shorter, if the echo is present at all (Anderson and Kemp, 1979; Zwicker and Manley, 1981; Schmiedt and Adams, 1981).

A property of these acoustic echoes is that they often resemble the ringing of a filter sharply tuned to a specific frequency (for example, see Fig. 3). Kemp (1979) demonstrated that the major frequency components in the echo could be suppressed with a continuous masker, very much like the procedure described above for brainstem potentials. Figure 27 illustrates that the masking function does indeed resemble psychophysical and evoked-potential tuning curves. Be-

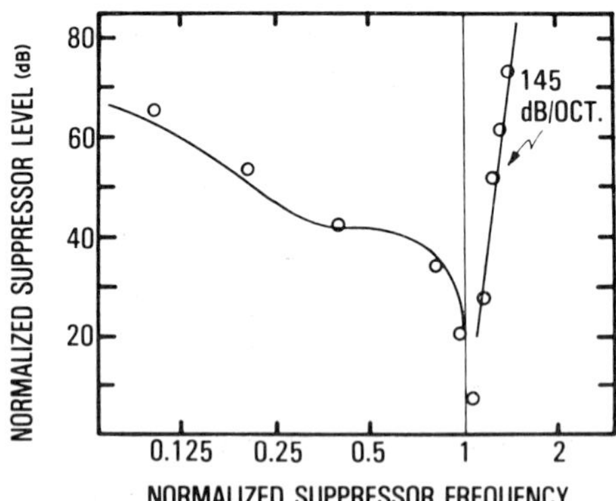

Figure 27   An average tuning curve derived from the acoustic echo response measured in three ears of human subjects at five separate frequencies. The curves were obtained by adjusting the level of a continuous masking tone so as to just suppress a given frequency component of the echo response to a brief tone pip. Echo frequencies ranged from about 1200 to 2200 Hz. Data from one subject are shown with the aid of open circles. The frequency scale has been normalized to the respective component frequencies. [Adapted from Kemp (1979).]

cause the best ringing frequency varies with the individual ear, the frequency of the excitor probe must be adjusted for each subject to yield the optimum echo. Thus, the abscissa in Fig. 27 is normalized to individual probe frequencies.

Along with Kemp's echo have come the rediscoveries of two other types of acoustic emissions in the ear canal, both of which arise within the cochlea: spontaneous emissions (Zurek, 1981) and distortion-product emissions generated by two continuous primary tones (Kim *et al.*, 1980; Schmiedt and Adams, 1981). In the latter case, a wave analyzer (tuned voltmeter) is needed to separate the distortion component from the two primary frequencies. We can add a third signal (suppressor) to the two primaries, that will decrease the level of the distortion product by a criterion amount (3 dB) and map out a suppression curve. This simultaneous paradigm is similar to the procedures previously described for

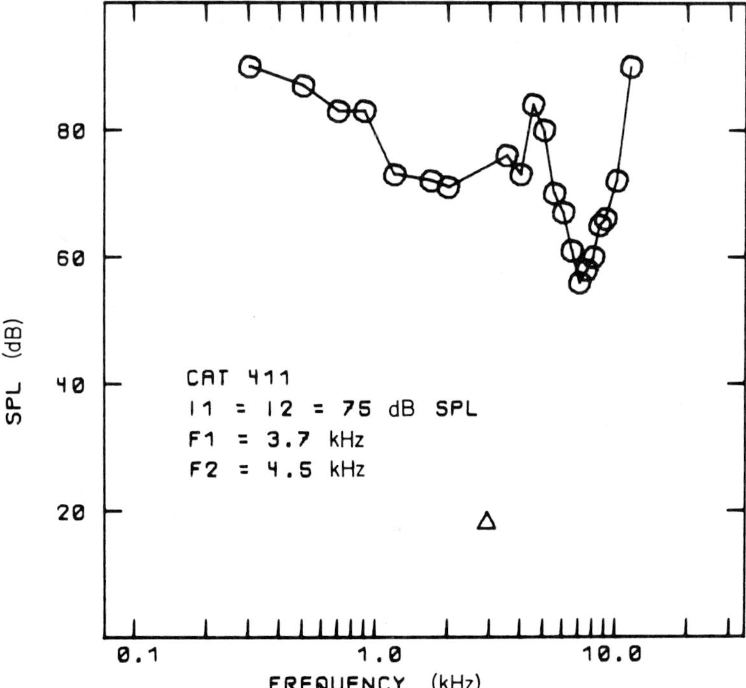

Figure 28 Isosuppression function of the acoustic emission of the $2f_1-f_2$ distortion product generated by two continuous primaries in the ear canal of a cat. The ordinate is SPL of the suppression, and the abscissa is the frequency of the suppressor. The unsuppressed level and frequency of the $2f_1-f_2$ component is indicated by the open triangle. Primary frequencies were 3.7 and 4.5 kHz, and both were presented at a level of 75 dB SPL. A third tone was used as the suppressor. Open circles indicate the levels and frequencies of the suppressor needed to reduce the distortion magnitude by 3 dB as measured on a wave analyzer. Maximum suppression of the distortion product occurs about an octave above the frequency of the $2f_1-f_2$ component. In this respect, the suppression function is more like the outline of two-tone suppression areas in single fibers than a tuning curve as such.

the evoked potentials and acoustic echoes. However, the resulting curve, shown in Fig. 28, is more like the boundary of single-fiber suppression than a tuning curve. The maximum suppression occurs about an octave above the probe (distortion-component) frequency, and has a relatively flat "tail" at low frequencies. The suppressor here also may be acting on the primary tones and not on the distortion product.

G. Discussion of Physiological Results

A central theme throughout the above results is that tonotopic organization exists at all physiological levels from acoustic emissions in the ear canal to the brainstem potentials. Moreover, there is a strong similarity in the tuning characteristics at and among the various levels of the auditory system.

With regard to mechanisms of tuning and suppression, the relation between the boundary of the response area and the boundaries of the suppression area is of particular interest. To a large extent, it has been found that tuning and suppression characteristics are independent entities that are only loosely coupled (Schmiedt and Zwislocki, 1980; Schmiedt, 1982b,c; Robertson and Johnstone, 1981). This concept of independence argues against models incorporating the same nonlinearity to both sharpen the mechanical tuning and account for suppression and distortion phenomena (for example, Kim *et al.*, 1980). The degree of independence between sharp tuning and two-tone suppression strongly implies that their respective mechanisms are also somewhat independent. Thus, there may be at least two major nonlinearities, one to sharpen cochlear tuning, the other to add suppression and, as a possible consequence, generate distortion products. On the other hand, it is apparent that a total loss of suppression above CF is reflected in a shallow slope of the high-frequency leg of the tuning curve. The suppression nonlinearity above CF therefore seems to increase the rejection rate of the neural filter, especially at high stimulus levels. If the high-frequency slope of the tuning curve is important to psychophysical measurements of frequency selectivity, then a total loss of suppression above CF may drastically reduce the frequency resolving power of an observer.

Another line of reasoning follows from the physiological and anatomical studies of Liberman (1978, 1982). As stated in a previous section, Liberman (1978) has shown that low-spont fibers are associated with tuning curves that are raised in threshold with respect to high-spont fibers, but at the same time the low-spont curves are as sharp or sharper than their more sensitive counterparts. Liberman (1980, 1982) has recently traced low- and high-spont fibers to their respective origins on the bodies of inner hair cells. The synapses of the high-spont group are preferentially located on the modiolor side of the cell body, whereas the synapses of the low-spont group cluster on the opposite side. The point here is that the low- and high-spont fibers seem likely to arise from the same hair cell. How is it possible, then, with all the various nonlinearities present in cochlear mechanics, that the low-spont fibers are so sharply tuned? Because the low-spont curves are obtained at higher stimulus levels, should they not be broader than their more sensitive counterparts? It is conceivable that the tuning mechanism is a fairly linear one operating in a somewhat independent fashion with another nonlinear mechanism which forms the basis of suppression.

At present, the above speculation is just that: speculation. Certainly the mechanics of the basilar membrane are nonlinear and are extremely vulnerable to any type of trauma. It can also be envisioned that two or more nonlinearities work in concert to enable the tuning of the low-spont fibers to stay sharp even at high stimulus levels, or that a second filter is involved in the transduction process. Whatever their underlying mechanisms, tuning and suppression phenomena together form the basis of much of our understanding of how frequency selectivity is accomplished by the ear. As we shall see in the following sections, sometimes psychophysical results parallel those obtained by means of physiological measures, and sometimes there is little correspondence.

IV. FREQUENCY SELECTIVITY: PSYCHOPHYSICAL TUNING CURVES

A. Introduction

The term "frequency selectivity" is used to refer to the ability of the ear to analyze complex sounds with respect to frequency (spectral) information. One way of examining frequency selectivity is by means of masking experiments. Indeed, there are probably more experiments on masking than on any other auditory phenomenon. This experimental devotion to the topic of masking reflects the belief that many of the facts of masking are direct indicators of the facts of the operation of the auditory system, and that any comprehensive model or theory of hearing must account for the facts of masking. Of course, masking data relate to issues concerning the absolute sensitivity of the ear as well as the differential sensitivity of the ear with respect to intensity and frequency. Masking data are also used in applied acoustics, for example, speech-interference levels, community responses to noise, clinical audiology, etc.; however, the focus here is on issues related to frequency-resolving power of the ear, particularly psychophysical tuning curves, their counterparts in physiology, and the ramifications for auditory theory and practical applications.

Prior to the 1950s data on the masking of a pure tone by a pure tone were the property of Wegel and Lane (1924). In their classic experiment, masking patterns [SPL (dB) of the signal required for detection as a function of the frequency of the signal with masker frequency and level as parameters] were shown to be asymmetrical, whereby low-frequency sounds masked higher frequency sounds more than high-frequency sounds masked low-frequency sounds. There were interactions (beats) between the signal and the masker when the signal and masker were nearly identical in frequency. Also, masking patterns reflected nonlinearities, particular harmonic and intermodulation distortion products. Wegel and Lane discussed their data in terms of basilar membrane mechanics. Following Wegel and Lane, most studies of simultaneous masking were directly or indirectly related to the concept of "the critical band" as detailed by Fletcher (1940). Many of these studies have been reviewed elsewhere and will not be reviewed here (for excellent reviews see Zwislocki, 1978; Green, 1976; Scharf, 1970).

For reasons unknown, the masking of a pure tone by a pure tone received little further attention until Chistovich (1957), Small (1959), and Ehmer (1959). Small (1959) changed the masking paradigm so that the dependent variable was the level of the masker, the independent variable was the frequency of the masker, and the parameters were the level and frequency of the signal. Thus, the psychophysical tuning curve was born. The "masking patterns" observed bore a striking resemblance to the tuning curves of the physiologist—high-frequency skirts with slopes of 150 dB/octave, sharply tuned tips, and a low-frequency "tail" segment. In addition to confirming many of the observations of Wegel and Lane, Small observed irregularities in the tuning curves when the frequency of the masker was about 0.85 that of the signal. It is interesting to note that both Small (1959) and Chistovitch (1957) made comparisons between psychophysical tuning curves and tuning curves at the level of the basilar membrane, auditory nerve, cochlear nucleus, and higher levels. These comparisons of psychophysical and physiological data suggested that tuning of the auditory system increases as the auditory system is ascended—a notion that is still offered and debated today (see Dallos *et al.*, 1977).

For reasons unknown to us psychophysical tuning curves were ignored for the next 10 years or so, perhaps until interest arose in the apparent absence of the effects of lateral inhibition in auditory psychophysical data. Carterette *et al.* (1969) surveyed the literature and attempted to show data that were explainable in terms of lateral inhibition. They also conducted masking studies using a masking noise with unusually steep skirts, and showed small changes in masked thresholds near the edges of the masking noise. These small effects were attributed to lateral inhibition, and it was considered to be the first demonstration of this phenomenon in audition. Previously, lateral inhibition had been demonstrated conclusively in vision (Ratliff, 1965) and the skin (Békésy, 1958). However, Houtgast (1972) suggested that the threshold of a test signal which is presented simultaneously with a masker cannot show lateral inhibition effects since both the test tone and the masker will be affected. In a series of experiments Houtgast (1972, 1973, 1974) measured nonsimultaneous masking (forward masking), gap masking (a combination of forward and backward masking), and "pulsation threshold." These data were definitive in their demonstration of "lateral suppression" in audition and in providing a strong psychophysical correlate of two-tone rate suppression as found at the level of the auditory nerve

(Nomoto *et al.*, 1964; Sachs and Kiang, 1968), cochlear nucleus (Galambos and Davis, 1944), and higher levels. Given the papers of Houtgast and the masking paradigm developed by Small (1959), it comes as no surprise to see psychophysical tuning curves measured using nonsimultaneous masking techniques.

Some of the first papers on nonsimultaneous masking (Luscher and Zwislocki, 1947, 1949; Gardner, 1947; Harris *et al.*, 1951; Munson and Gardner, 1950; Harris and Rawnsley, 1953) involved what has been called forward masking. In these and later experiments, a test signal of a few milliseconds duration followed a 200–400 msec masker. The interval between masker offset and signal offset is usually varied from about 10 to less than 100 msec. Results of earlier experiments have been summarized by Zwislocki (1978). With respect to frequency selectivity in forward masking results of Gardner (1947), Munson and Gardner (1950), and Zwislocki and Pirodda (1952) show that at low and moderate masker levels, masking is largest at the masker frequency, and that the masking pattern is asymmetric as it is in simultaneous masking. At masking levels greater than 80 dB SPL, masking is greatest about one-half octave above the frequency of the masker. Masking at the one-half octave frequency also behaves differently with respect to masker intensity and decay than masking at the primary frequency. Zwislocki and Pirodda (1952) attribute this one-half octave shift to a different mechanism than that associated with the masking observed at the masker frequency. As noted by Zwislocki the correspondence between forward masking data at a test frequency one-half octave above the masker and data on temporary threshold shifts (TTSs) produced by minutes or hours of exposure to loud sounds (Hirsh and Bilger, 1955) is striking.

The forward masking paradigm is now used frequently to measure psychophysical tuning curves. Indeed, between 1974 and 1982, psychophysical tuning curves and psychophysically measured suppression (see Jesteadt *et al.*, 1982, and the references therein) have attained a popularity rivaling masking level differences and signal detection experiments in the 1960s. Part of this popularity reflects the assumed correspondence between psychophysical and physiological tuning curves, and psychophysically measured suppression and physiologically measured suppression. Physiological suppression is used by most psychophysicists to refer to two-tone rate suppression and in some instances synchrony suppression. It does not refer to the suppression or reduction of spontaneous neural activity by means of a single tone.

While most of the current efforts on psychophysical tuning curves and suppression use nonsimultaneous masking (for example, see Moore, 1978, 1980a,b; Weber and Green, 1978, 1979; Weber and Moore, 1981), our first experiments on psychophysical tuning curves involved simultaneous masking. We proceeded with simultaneous masking even though there is a problem with beats, confounding by combination tones, and suppression effects are not directly measurable. It was our belief then and it is our belief now that there is room for simultaneous masking in a clinical audiological work-up and that there is theoretically applicable knowledge to be gained as well. Moreover, the difficulty of the task for the listener in simultaneous masking is trivial relative to the difficulty of the task in forward masking. Thus, we see applications of the simultaneous masking paradigm that are realistic for hearing-impaired persons which can provide information pertinent to frequency selectivity, intensity discrimination, and combination tones.

B. Simultaneous Masking

Great care was exercised in the selection of subjects, especially with regard to excluding those persons with history of ear disease, hearing levels in excess of 10 dB HL (re ANSI S3-1969) from 250 to 8000 Hz, and a history of noise exposure. Potential subjects were required to deny the use of medicinal drugs (including histamines, analgesics, aspirin, etc.) and recreational drugs. Most subjects were between the ages of 18 and 22 years, although on occasion a 23–25 year old was used. In addition, reliability in judgments and in keeping appointments was required. Subjects were paid an hourly wage and received at least 2 hours training in each listening task. Most subjects showed little improvement after the first and second 30-min practice session. To obtain one subject for the masking experiments approximately four had to be screened. The most common reason for rejection of a subject was a 10–15 dB notch in the audiogram at 4.0 or 6.0 kHz.

The method of adjustment was used. This fact will be a source of chagrin to many psychophysicists and will be regarded as blasphemy by many others. However, we were faced with conflicting demands. On the one hand, there was the need to control for the criterion used by the observer and therefore the need for signal detection paradigm. On the other hand, in the planned experiments we would have auditory sensitivity changing by as much as 20 dB in 1–2 hours. Indeed, later we will show suppression and tuning curve changes of 40–50 dB occurring in a 2-hour period. The need for a rapid measurement was essential. For these reasons, the method of adjustment was selected. Adaptive forced-choice psychophysical methods are still too slow. Specific details of our methods changed as our experiments progressed and these are discussed throughout this article when appropriate. With our current methods and trained subjects we can obtain an entire tuning curve in less than 15 min and have excellent repeatability. (In forward masking, about 20–25 min are required for a tuning curve and suppression.)

Simultaneous masking data are given in Figs. 29 and 30 (for probe tones) of 4.0 and 1.0 kHz. These data are for two individual subjects whose audiograms were indistinguishable but who demonstrated subtle and not so subtle differences

Figure 29 Psychophysical tuning curves at 4.0 kHz in simultaneous masking for two observers. Level of the signal is varied from 20 to 50 dB SPL in 10-dB steps. Note the similarity of the tuning curves for the two subjects, and that the most obvious difference is the presence or absence of the irregularity at a masker frequency of 3.2 kHz. This irregularity which occurs at about 0.85 probe frequency is due to the presence of a combination tone, the cubic tone.

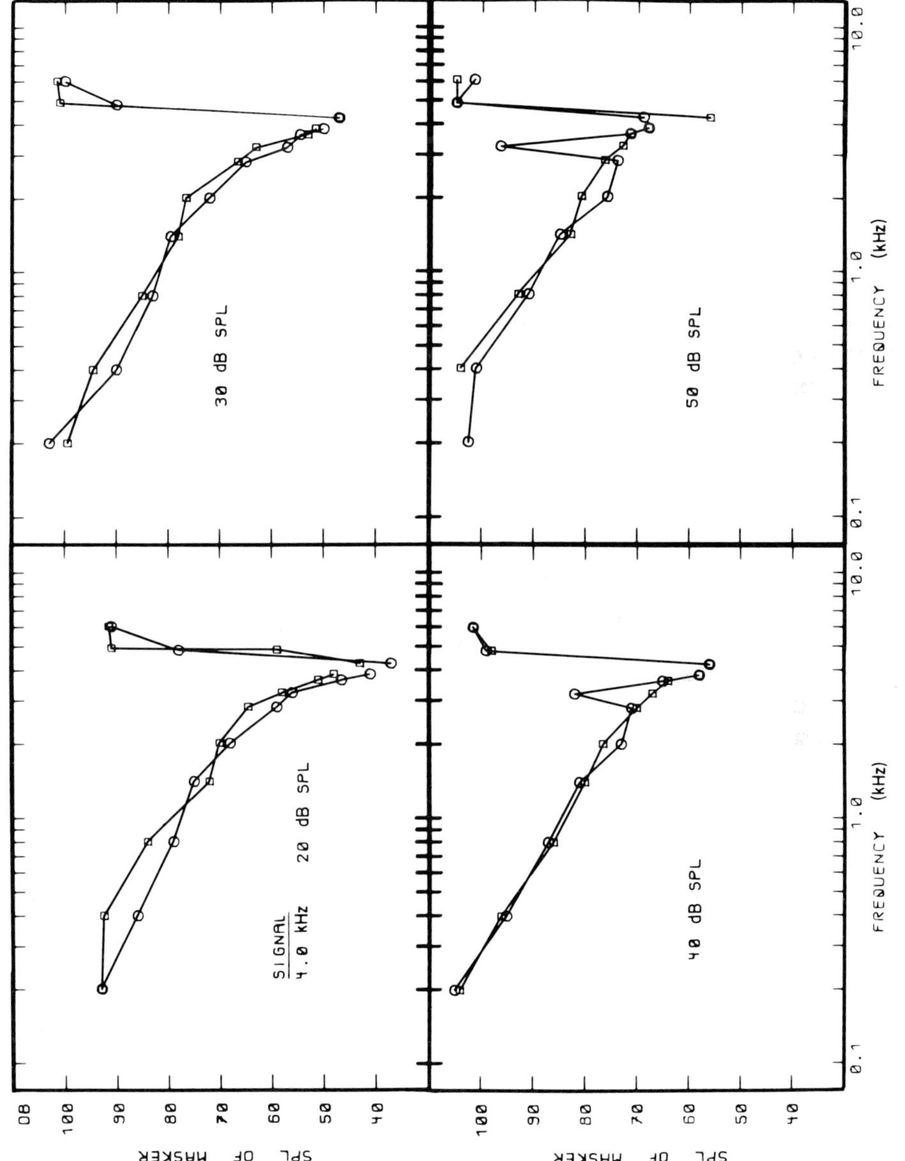

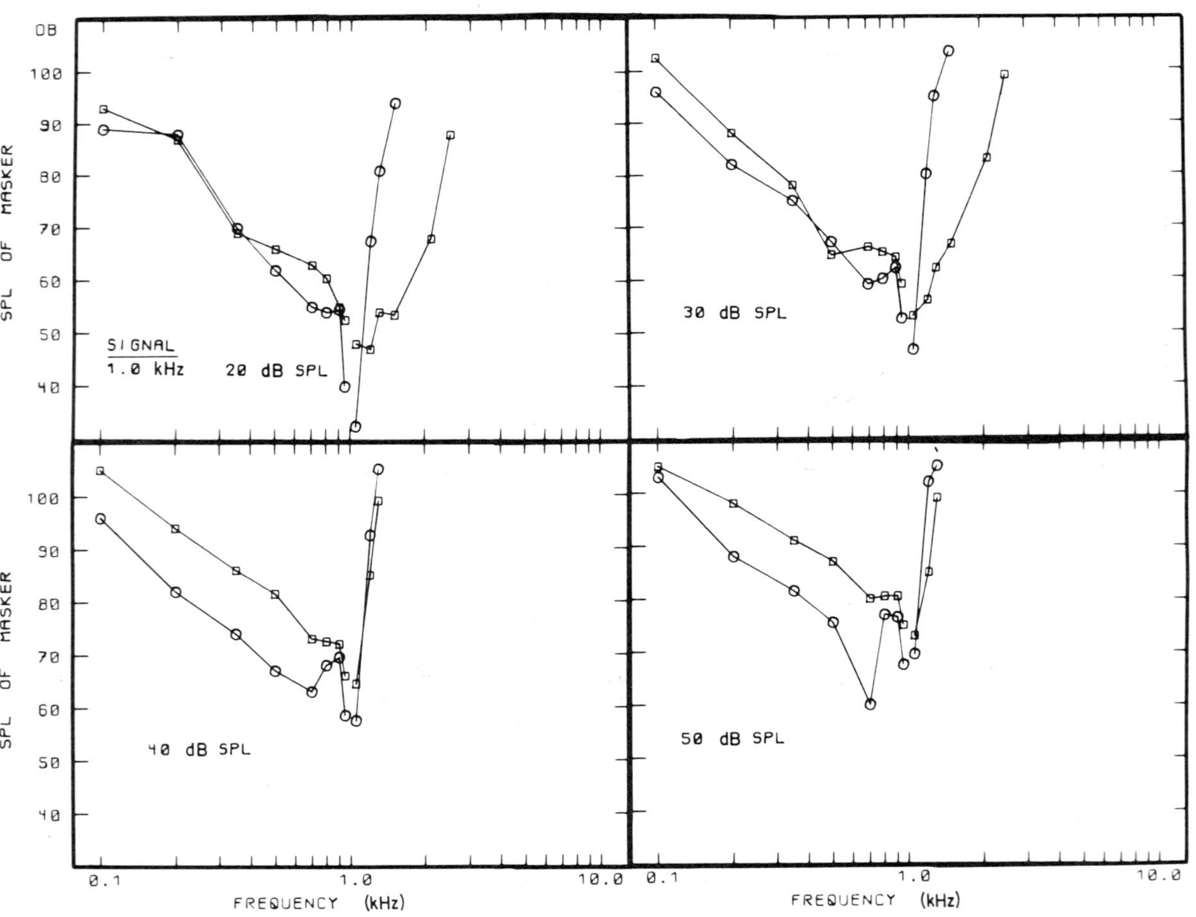

SPL OF MASKER
SIGNAL
1.0 kHz
20 dB SPL
30 dB SPL
40 dB SPL
50 dB SPL
FREQUENCY (kHz)
0.1
1.0
10.0

in their psychophysical tuning curves. They have been selected from a group of 12 subjects. Data for a probe tone of 4.0 kHz at levels of 20, 30, 40, and 50 dB SPL are given on Fig. 29. Comparisons of the high side of the tuning curves for the two subjects in Fig. 29 show they are identical in some regions and highly similar in others. Likewise, the low sides of the tuning curves are striking in their similarity with one exception, namely, the peak at 3.2 kHz for one subject at probe levels of 40 and 50 dB (Fig. 29). This peak or irregularity at 3.2 kHz (or 0.8 × 4.0 kHz) is identical in its frequency location to those irregularities noted by Chistovitch (1957) and Small (1959). For several years this irregularity remained a puzzle. Greenwood (1971) studied it in great detail and attributes it to the detection of a distortion product, namely, the cubic combination tone $(2f_1 - f_2)$. The subject, according to Greenwood, detects the cubic tone rather than the probe tone, and thus must increase the level of the masker. The exact increase in the level of the masker needed to mask both the probe and cubic tones reflects an interaction between the effectiveness of the masker as its frequency and level are changed and as the amplitude of the combination tone changes (see also Zwislocki, 1978; Green, 1976).

While we are comfortable with Greenwoods's explanation of this irregularity in "masked audiograms" at about 1.6 times the probe frequency and in psychophysical tuning curves at about 0.85 probe frequency, we are puzzled by its prominence in one subject and its absence in others. Examination of all of our subjects shows the presence of the irregularity for 10 of 12 subjects. The magnitude of the irregularity, however, varies from 0 to 20 dB depending on probe level and the individual. Explanations for the absence of the effects of the cubic tone in simultaneous masking probably have to include "subject criterion effects," and the possibility that the subjects are using different information or cues in the detection task. Another possibility is that the ears of the subjects are different, and that this difference is not reflected in the gross shape of the psychophysical tuning curve but in the effects of the cubic tone or in the mechanisms which produce the cubic tone. We prefer the latter possibility, particularly because of the data for these same two subjects at 1.0 kHz which are shown in Fig. 30. Irregularities in the tuning curves in Fig. 30 at or near 800 Hz are most pronounced for probe levels of 30, 40, and 50 dB, and are larger for one subject than the other.

Figure 30 shows psychophysical tuning curves for a probe of 1.0 kHz at levels of 20, 30, 40, and 50 dB SPL. The subjects are the same as in Fig. 29. Note the high side of the tuning curves. At low probe levels, 20 and 30 dB SPL, one

---

Figure 30 Psychophysical tuning curves at 1.0 kHz obtained with simultaneous masking for the two observers of Fig. 29. Level of the signal is varied from 20 to 50 dB SPL in 10-dB steps. Note the lack of similarity in the tuning curves on their high sides at probe levels of 20 and 30 dB. At higher probe levels, the tuning curves are similar on the high side and differ on the low side. Observe also that the effects of the cubic tone are now present for both subjects at 1.0 kHz although they were observed only for one subject (○) at 4.0 kHz.

subject is significantly different from the other whereas at probe levels of 40 and 50 dB SPL, the tuning curves in the high side are nearly identical. Similarly, on the low side at 20 dB SPL the two subjects are identical at some masker frequencies and similar at others. When the level of the probe is increased from 20 to 30, 40, and 50 dB SPL there are large (15–20 dB) differences between the two subjects on the low side of the tuning curve. It would seem, therefore, that either the ears of these subjects are different or one subject changes criterion and strategy when the probe tone is changed from 1.0 to 4.0 kHz.

The points which we should like to emphasize about Figs. 29 and 30 involve aspects of tuning curves and individual differences. Recall the fact that the audiograms of the two individuals on Figs. 29 and 30 are nearly identical from 0.25 to 6.0 kHz. Also, on standard clinical tests of hearing (SRT, acoustic reflex, tympanograms, speech discrimination in quiet) as well as on brainstem-evoked responses neither subject gave results that would be considered even slightly abnormal. Thus, we were at first suspect of some of these results, and therefore made a large number of measurements per condition (10–25 measurements/datum point/subject). Repeatability is impressive. For example, on the low side of a tuning curve where the subject adjusts the intensity of the masker which is fixed at a given frequency, the range of judgments is 4 dB (± 2 dB of the median). On the high side of the tuning curve where the subject adjusts the frequency of the fixed-level masker, the range of judgments for a 1.0-kHz probe is about 30 Hz (± 15 Hz of the median) and about 150 Hz (± 75 Hz of the median) for a 4.0-kHz probe. On the high side variability is slightly larger near the tip of the tuning curve and decreases at higher levels. In other words, we have no doubts about the repeatability of the data in Figs. 29 and 30. The possibility remains that each subject uses a different criterion in making the judgments. We have not controlled for criterion effects as rigorously as is possible because we used the method of adjustment rather than a signal-detection paradigm. If the differences between subjects reported in Figs. 1 and 2 are due to criterion effects then one has to argue that these criterion effects are dependent upon the frequency of the probe tone, the level of the probe tone, the frequency of the masker, and the level of the masker. It strikes us that criterion effects are more likely to be manifest as constant errors, and are much more likely to change a datum point by a "few dB." Another explanation is that one subject uses different cues than the other to make the decision (pitch vs loudness, quality vs pitch, etc.). We cannot eliminate this possibility, but neither can it be eliminated by other psychophysical methods. We assume in the discussion that follows that the observations reported in Figs. 29 and 30 represent internal characteristics of the auditory system. This assumption is common to masking studies.

Perhaps the most unusual aspects of the data are the striking similarities of the tuning curves at 4.0 kHz and the striking dissimilarities of the tuning curves at 1.0 kHz. Stated differently, given the similarity of the audiometric data for the two subjects from 250 to 800 Hz and the similarity of the tuning curves at 4.0 kHz (except the irregularity due to the combination tone), the disparities of the tuning curves observed at 1.0 kHz thus were unpredictable. Likewise, given the tuning curves at 1.0 kHz for probe levels of 40 and 50 dB SPL, one would not be able to predict the tuning curves at 1.0 kHz for probe levels of 20 and 30 dB SPL. Some tentative conclusions are that the low side of a tuning cannot be predicted accurately given the high side of a tuning curve and vice versa. Similarly, differences between an individual's tuning curves exist and these differences can be independent of auditory sensitivity at the probe frequency and adjacent frequencies. Lastly, normal tuning curves in one frequency region are not predictive of tuning curves at other frequency regions although auditory sensitivity may be "perfectly normal" in all frequency regions.

In regard to the irregularities in the tuning curves at 0.8 of probe frequency, both subjects had the irregularity at 1.0 where the tuning curves were strikingly dissimilar; however, at 4.0 kHz when the tuning curves were strikingly similar, only one subject showed the presumed effects of the cubic combination tone. It would thus seem possible that the effects of the cubic combination tone occur independently, or nearly so, of the shape of the tuning curves.

While there are very many studies showing unusual masking patterns and distortion products in persons and animals with hearing impairments (deBoer and Bouwmeester, 1974; Florentine *et al.*, 1980; Jerger *et al.*, 1960; Leshowitz and Lindstrom, 1977; Martin and Picket, 1970; Margolis and Goldberg, 1980; McGee *et al.*, 1976; Nelson and Turner, 1980; Pick *et al.*, 1977; Rabinowitz *et al.*, 1980; Salvi *et al.*, 1982; Smoorenburg, 1980; Thornton and Abbas, 1980; Wightman *et al.*, 1977; Wightman, 1982) comparison to the data in Figs. 29 and 30 is not straightforward. It must be kept in mind that our data and effects occur in persons with excellent auditory sensitivity and other perfectly normal auditory functions, whereas in most of the studies cited hearing losses of 30–60 dB are the rule. Notable exceptions are Martin and Pickett (1970) and Rabinowitz *et al.* (1980) who demonstrated wide variations in masking among persons with identical hearing threshold levels.

So far in discussing the tuning curves obtained in simultaneous masking the tip of the tuning curve has not been mentioned. One reason is that measurements were not made when the frequency of the signal was within 100 Hz of the frequency of the masker. Such measures are confounded by beats and, in addition, increase the data collection time considerably. In the interests of efficiency these measures were discontinued and tips of the tuning curves were estimated by extrapolation from the low and high sides of the tuning curves. Extrapolations made from the data in Figs. 29 and 30 suggest that the tips for both subjects are equal or nearly so (+2 dB) at 4.0 kHz, but differ by as much as 5–10 at 1.0 kHz. The possible disparity in the absolute value of the tips of the tuning curves at 1.0 kHz is not sufficient to account for the gross disparities of the tuning curves. For example, if in Fig. 2 one "normalizes" the tuning curves at the tips or by the low-frequency sides, the high-frequency slopes are still unusual and, indeed, become even more disparate in some instances.

The most common criticism of the simultaneous masking paradigm is the confounding effects of masker–signal interactions which produce beats and harmonic and intermodulation distortion products. A second and less common criticism of simultaneous masking studies is energy splatter of the probe signal. In most simultaneous masking studies, including ours, the probe signal has relatively long rise–decay times (5–25 msec) and duration (50–250 msec). Usually, energy splatter is viewed as a serious problem for such signals only at low frequencies or high frequencies where the shape of the audibility curve becomes steep. In these instances, energy spreads from one region of sensitivity to an adjacent but much more sensitive region. At signals frequencies of 2.0 kHz, for example, energy splatter of a 200 msec tone with rise–decay times of 10 msec or so should not be a problem, or should it?

Johnson-Davies and Patterson (1979) addressed all of the issues mentioned in the preceding paragraph. In this very clever study of tuning curves at 2.0 kHz (simultaneous masking) beats were eliminated by the use of a narrow and steep band of noise as the masker, the effects of the cubic tone were eliminated by the use of a low-pass filtered noise, and energy splatter was reduced by the insertion of a 1.8-kHz tone or a 2.2-kHz tone. The level of the 1.8- or 2.2-kHz tones was 10 or 15 dB below the level needed to mask the 2.0-kHz signal. For all three of their subjects the insertion of the 1.8-kHz tone affected the high side of the tuning curve, i.e., masker levels were reduced in level by as much as 20 dB. Insertion of the 2.2-kHz tone, according to Johnson-Davies and Patterson, depressed the low side of the tuning curve and had little effect on the high side of the tuning curve. They explain these results in terms of residual excitation patterns. That is, when the masker is greater in frequency than the signal, the residual excitation pattern (excitation pattern of the masker minus excitation pattern of the signal) is below signal frequency. Thus, the insertion of the 1.8-kHz tone should depress the high side of the tuning curve. Similarly, when the masker frequency is less than signal frequency, the residual excitation pattern is above the signal frequency. Thus, the insertion of the 2.2-kHz tone should depress the low side of the tuning curve. While we are impressed with the correspondence between their data and their predictions for the effects of the 1.8-kHz tone, we are less impressed with the correspondence between their data and their predictions for the insertion of the 2.2-kHz tone. Indeed, to us the most impressive feature (see their Fig. 3) is the difference between individuals. It looks as if the tuning curve for two or three subjects is depressed on both the high- and low-frequency sides and at the tip. For the third subject (RM, see their Fig. 3) the 2.2-kHz tone seems to have depressed both the high and low sides, but elevated the tip by 3dB or so. In other words, we believe support of residual excitation pattern hypothesis is strong for the 1.8-kHz condition and equivocal at best for the 2.2-kHz condition. It should be noted that Green *et al.* (1981) applied the two-tone strategy of Johnson-Davies and Patterson in forward masking. Predictions of the residual excitation pattern hypothesis were supported for two of four subjects.

The Johnson-Davies and Patterson study is provocative and one wonders about the effects of restricting the frequency region available to listeners (effectively narrowing the spectrum of the signal) in other studies of temporal integration, frequency discrimination, etc. Also, one wonders about the calculation of excitation areas and their residuals. What level of the auditory system should be used? Mechanical data at the level of the basilar membrane? Spatial excitation patterns in the primary auditory cortex? What is the appropriate criterion measure of response areas? The population response of the auditory nerve as defined by Pfeiffer and Kim (1975) and Kim and Molnar (1979)? If so, which of five measures of population response is most appropriate? As far as we can tell, these issues are open. Kim and Molnar report that spatial distributions of single units are level and frequency dependent, and that measures of excitation that appear appropriate at one frequency and level are inappropriate at others. Indeed, the definition of response area is so complicated that Kim and Molnar urge caution in comparing neural and mechanical measures of frequency selectivity. Of course, if caution should be exercised in comparing mechanical excitation patterns with neural patterns at the periphery of the auditory system, what should be exercised in discussing psychophysical tuning curves?

C. Effects of TTS on Tuning Curves in Simultaneous Masking

At the onset of these experiments in 1975 we were unaware of studies on the effects of TTS on psychophysical tuning curves obtained in a simultaneous masking paradigm. At that time, papers by Zwicker (1974) and Vogten (1974) using normal and abnormal hearing subjects became available as did the works of others (Leshowitz and Lindstrom, 1977; Wightman *et al.*, 1977). Our strategy was to use subjects with normal hearing and with a form of sensorineural hearing loss, noise-induced temporary threshold shift (TTS), that could be produced under the control of the experimenter. By a judicious selection of exposure signals the magnitude and frequency location of the temporary hearing loss can be controlled. The magnitude of the hearing loss can be estimated (± 5 dB) by knowing the spectrum and level of the noise (see Mills *et al.*, 1979, 1981) whereas the frequency location can be controlled by the spectrum of the noise.

The ability to control the frequency location of TTS supports the application of critical band theory to TTS (Weissing, 1968; Yamamoto *et al.*, 1970). Our data support the observations of Weissing and Yamamoto and their estimates of a critical band at high levels of stimulation. Figure 31 shows the TTS audiogram for one subject who was exposed for 24 hours to a wide-band noise which was produced by combining four separate octave bands (CF = 0.5, 1, 2, and 4 kHz).

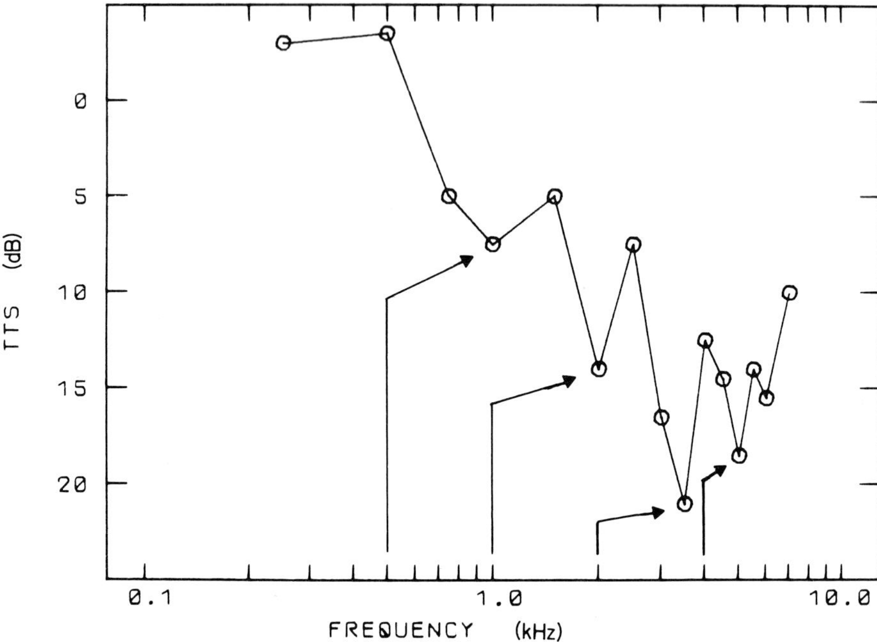

Figure 31   TTS as a function of test frequency after 24-hour exposure to a wide-band noise. This noise had peaks in the spectrum at 0.5, 1, 2, and 4 kHz. Note the corresponding four peaks in the TTS audiogram are one-half to one octave above the spectral peaks.

Note the four maxima in the TTS audiogram and that each maximum is about one-half to one octave above the center frequency of the noise. Thus, for this subject (and eight others) the four maxima in the TTS audiogram suggest that the octave bands of the exposure noise were separated by more than a critical band. For seven others subjects and the group median TTS, the TTS audiogram does not show four maxima. Thus, for these seven subjects the octave bands of the exposure noise are separated by less than one critical band. In addition to showing critical bands in TTS that are dependent on individual differences, these data imply that by selecting the spectra of the noise exposure in a careful manner, one can produce frequency selective TTSs. This ability is exploited as shall be shown later.

Another advantage of the TTS paradigm is that the exposure can be monaural and the "nonexposed ear" can serve as a control. In addition, changes in tuning curves can be measured as a function of the duration of exposure and as a function of the time after cessation of the exposure. Lastly, using the TTS paradigm we are certain of the cause of the hearing loss, and of the specific details of the causal agent (duration, level, and spectrum of the noise).

In the first experiment three subjects were exposed for 24 hours to an octave band noise centered at 4.0 kHz. The level of the noise was 75 dB SPL. The strategy was to have the noise as intense as possible but not intense enough to produce a measureable TTS. Subjects were trained in the simultaneous masking task using the method of adjustment. The probe signal was a 3.0-kHz pure tone with a duration of 250 msec and rise–decay times of 25 msec. The masker was continuous. In this pilot study subjects adjusted the level of the masker and the experimenter varied the frequency of the masker. About 10 min after the 24-hour exposure the subjects had no measurable TTS from 250 to 6.0 kHz. Pre- and postexposure tuning curves are shown in Fig. 32 for individual subjects. Preexposure data are shown by open symbols, and a solid line joins the median points. The shape of the tuning curve in Fig. 32 is similar to those described previously—a steep (105 dB/octave) high-frequency side, a tip, and a more gradual low-frequency side where the tip-to-tail ratio is 40–50 dB. Postexposure data are shown by the filled datum points, and a dashed line joins the median postexposure points. The median data suggest that the noise exposure produced mini-

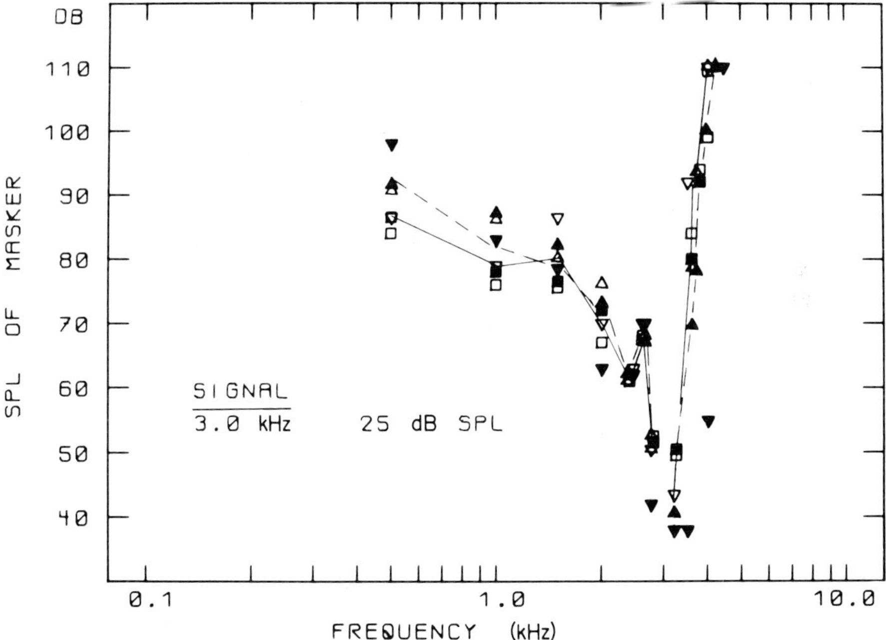

Figure 32 Psychophysical tuning curves at 3.0 kHz in simultaneous masking for three observers prior to exposure (open symbols) to noise and 10–30 min after (filled symbols) a 24-hour exposure to an octave-band noise centered at 4.0 kHz. The level of the probe was 25 dB SPL for all measurements. The noise exposure did not produce any measurable TTS. Preexposure median data points are joined by a solid line. A dashed line joins postexposure medians.

mal effects on the low-frequency side and at the tip, but shifted the high-frequency side by 100 Hz or so in terms of masker frequency, or about 10 dB in terms of masker level. In either case, we were not impressed by the magnitude of the changes in tuning produced by the noise exposure. On the other hand, one of the subjects (▼) showed small changes (<10 dB) on the low side and at the tip, but had changes in masker level on the high side in excess of 50 dB. We were unable to resolve the sizable differences between the subjects. Also, we were concerned about the validity of the data on the high side of the tuning curve. Subjects encountered difficulty in making postexposure judgments. Several minutes (2–5) were often required. Thus, on the one hand it appeared that when subjects were exposed to noise that produced nonmeasurable TTSs, the tuning curves were minimally affected. On the other hand, when individual data were examined it appeared that the high side of the tuning curve could be altered by as much as 50 dB in masking level even though TTS was not measurable. Thus, it was not clear whether the observed changes in the high side of the tuning curve were indicative of the effects of the noise or to random individual variations. It was decided to repeat the experiment.

In the repetition, four subjects were exposed for 24 hours to an octave band noise centered at 4.0 kHz. Its level was 75 dB SPL. The rejection rate (skirt of the noise) was 24 dB/octave. Psychophysical tuning curves in a simultaneous masking paradigm were measured as previously described with two significant exceptions. The first exception was that on the high side of the tuning curve the subject adjusted the frequency of the masker, and the experimenter set the level of the masker. The second exception was the use of both ears of the subject. That is, one ear served as the test ear and the other served as control. During the noise exposure the subject wore an ear plug (EAR) in the control ear. This plug provided about 50–60 dB attenuation at 4.0 kHz. By having the subject adjust the frequency of the masker on the high side of the tuning curve, variability was reduced and the time required to make a judgment was shortened from as long as 5 min to as short as 30 sec. In other words, by having subjects adjust the *frequency* of the masker, rather than the *level* of the masker, a difficult listening task was transformed to a judgment that could be performed quickly and "easily." Of course, it is difficult to directly compare variability in Hz with variability in dB SPL. In the latter case the range of judgments for individual subjects was as large as 20 dB whereas in the former case the range of judgment was about 200 Hz.

Figure 33 shows pre- and postexposure tuning curves for two of four subjects. These two subjects were selected because of the systematic changes produced by exposure to noise on the high side of the psychophysical tuning curves and because of the similarity of their pre- and postexposure tuning curves. The tuning curves of the other two subjects were not changed by the noise experiment. As shown in Fig. 33 the low side and tip of the tuning curve is unaffected by the

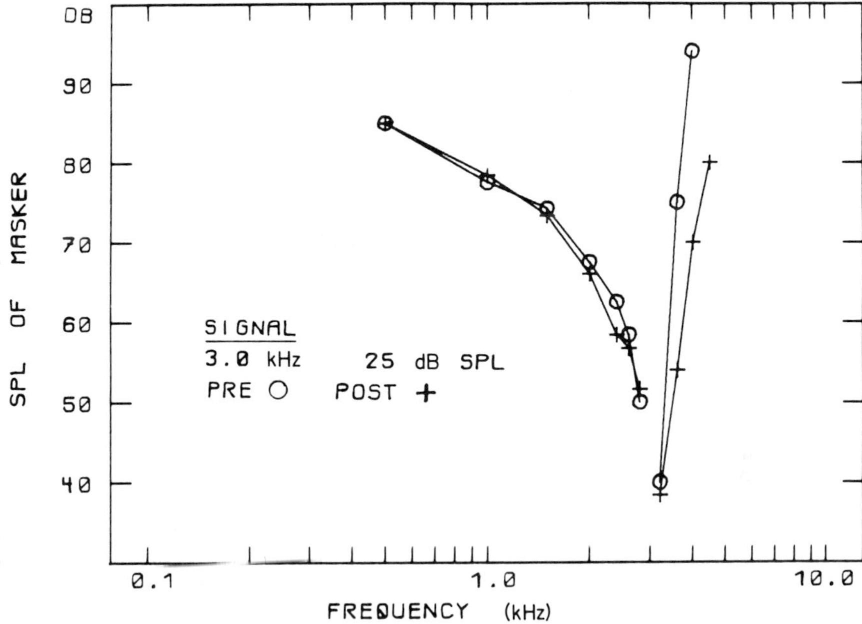

Figure 33 Mean psychophysical tuning curves at 3.0 kHz obtained by simultaneous masking for two observers prior and 10–20 min after exposure to noise. The noise exposure lasted 24 hours. The noise was an octave band centered at 4.0 kHz and presented at a level of 75 dB SPL. The level of the probe was 25 dB SPL. No TTS was measurable 3–5 min after termination of the exposure. Note the changes on the high side of the tuning curve after the noise exposure.

noise exposure, whereas the high side is increased with respect to masker frequency and decreased with respect to the slope of the tuning curve. It appeared, therefore, that the high side of a tuning curve can be altered without affecting the tip and low-frequency side, and that these alterations could occur in the absence of measurable changes in auditory sensitivity.

To increase the validity of the data in Fig. 33, measurements at a masker level of 70 dB SPL were made in the test ear and control ear immediately after 8 and 24 hours of exposure, and 1, 2, 4, and 24 hours after the noise exposure had been terminated. Results for the test ear and control ear are shown on Fig. 34. The tuning curve in the control ear was unaffected by the noise exposure whereas in the test ear the tuning curve on the high side returned to preexposure values between 4 and 24 hours. Given these systematic results for two of four subjects we concluded that exposure to a noise that produces no measurable TTS can nevertheless affect the high side of a psychophysical tuning curve. We have found that most of the changes in the high side occur after 8 hours of noise exposure and do not increase between 8 and 24 hours of exposure. Recovery of

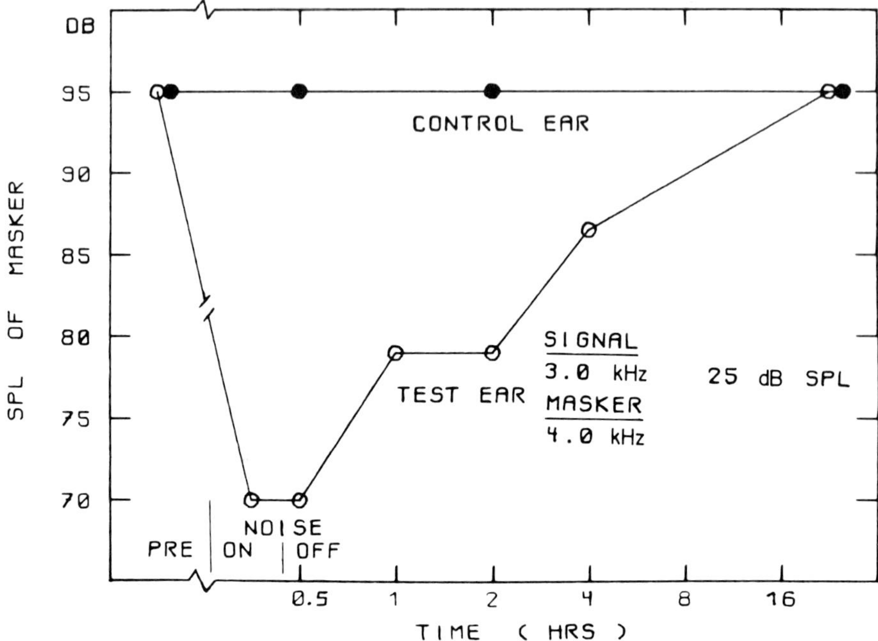

Figure 34 Recovery of the threshold of the high side of the tuning curve after exposure to noise for the two subjects of Fig. 32. These mean data are for a masker level of 70 dB SPL. Note that the control ear (non-noise-exposed ear) is unaffected by the noise exposure. The measurements in the test ear were made prior to exposure, about 5 min after an 8-hour exposure to 4 kHz noise, about 5 min after a 24-hour exposure, and then 1, 2, 4, and 24 hours after a 24-hour exposure.

the tuning curve requires about 4–24 hours. The data indicate also that the high side of a tuning curve can be affected in the absence of any measurable changes near the tip or on the low side of the tuning curve. Thus, it would seem that the high side of a tuning curve can be independent or nearly so of the tip and the low-frequency side, and of auditory sensitivity at the probe and adjacent frequencies.

The purpose in the next experiment was to produce a small TTS (<10 dB) at and near the frequency of the probe signal and measure its effects on the psychophysical tuning curve (simultaneous masking). Four subjects were exposed for 1 hour to wide-band noise presented at 95 dB SPL. Psychophysical tuning curves were measured using the method of adjustment. As previously, on the high side the subject adjusted the frequency of the masker which was fixed in level by the experimenter. On the low side of the tuning curve the subject adjusted the intensity of the masker which was fixed in frequency by the experimenter. Recovery of auditory sensitivity after a 1-hour noise exposure is rapid in the first hour. In other words, measurements of tuning curves during a time when auditory sensitivity is changing by 15–20 dB are difficult to do and nearly impossible to interpret. Accordingly, our measurements were made at a postexposure time of 1 hour. About 10–15 min were required to obtain a tuning curve for each subject. The amount of recovery between 1 hour and 1 hour and 15 min was less than 3 dB. Results for two subjects are shown in Fig. 35. These two subjects are reported here because they were virtually identical in preexposure hearing levels and in TTS at 1 hr postexposure. Preexposure data (open circles) are unremarkable. Postexposure tuning curves (crosses) were made when TTS was 0 dB at 3.0 kHz, 14 dB at 4.0 kHz, and 17 dB at 5.0 and 6.0 kHz. For both subjects in Fig. 35 the postexposure tuning curves are wider. The widening of the tuning curve can be attributed to changes in the high side and low side of the tuning curve. It is important to note that the level of the probe tone was fixed at 25 dB SPL for both the preexposure and postexposure tuning curves. Thus, the sensation level of the probe was about 14 dB lower in the postexposure mesurements than in the preexposure measurements. We believe that a large portion of the changes in the tuning curves of Fig. 35 reflects little more than the reduced sensation level of the probe tone and that the postexposure tuning curves of Fig. 35 could be duplicated by preexposure tuning curves with a probe of about 10–12 dB SPL. There is the possibility of some exceptions. One is the irregularity in the tuning curve at 0.85 of the probe tone. Note the prominence of this irregularity in the postexposure tuning curve (left-hand side of Fig. 35) and the absence of this irregularity becomes more prominent as the SPL or sensation level of the probe increases. Others (Small, 1959) have made similar observations. It is not clear why the effects of a distortion product would become more prominent when the sensitivity of the system is decreased unless the mechanism of sensitivity is independent or nearly so of the mechanism for distortion products.

Another possibly confounding factor to the data in Fig. 35 involves the phenomenon of temporal integration. It is well documented that the detectability of a tone increases as the duration of the tone is increased to about 200 msec (Zwislocki, 1960). The effects of TTS on temporal integration are well documented also (Jerger, 1955; Henderson *et al.*, 1969; Mills *et al.*, 1970). For example, if detection improves by about 10 dB as the duration of a tone is increased from 16 to 256 msec, the effects of TTS will be to reduce temporal integration. These reductions in temporal integration can be dramatic. As shown in Fig. 36 temporal integration decreases from 12 to about 2 dB at 4.0 kHz during an 8-hour noise exposure at levels ranging from 76 to 81 dB(A). At 500 Hz where TTS=0, temporal integration was unaffected. Similarly, temporal integration in the control ear was unaffected. Thus, the mechanisms responsible for temporal integration can be rendered nearly totally ineffectual by TTS. When TTS is calculated for the subject of Fig. 36 using a 16-msec tone, it is equal to 23 dB. When TTS is calculated using a 512-msec tone, it is 31–33 dB. With these facts in mind how then does one measure the effects of TTS on psychophysical tuning curves? How does one separate the effects of temporal integration on

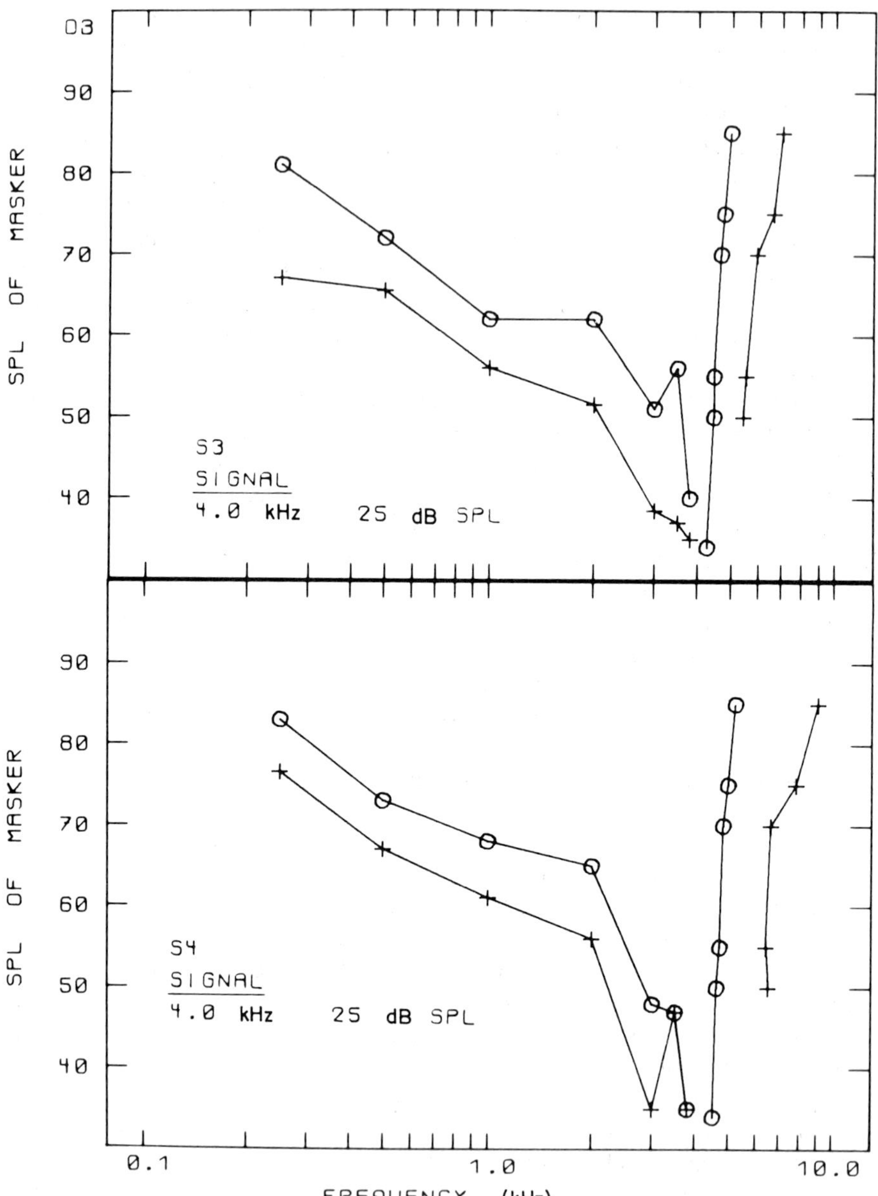

Figure 35 Psychophysical tuning curves at 1.0 kHz obtained by simultaneous masking for two observers prior to (circles) and after (crosses) a 1-hour exposure to noise. The noise was wide band (500–4000 Hz) at 95 dB SPL.

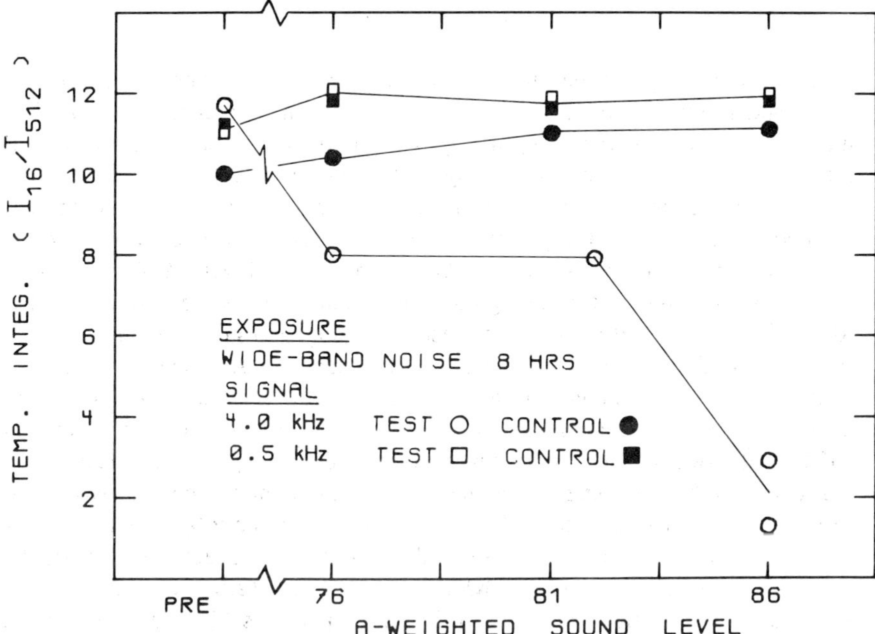

Figure 36 Temporal integration prior to exposure, and about 5 min after an 8-hour exposure to a wide-band noise. Level of the wide-band noise is given on the abscissa. The ordinate is the ratio of the threshold for a 16-msec signal to the threshold for a 512-msec signal in decibels. Note that temporal integration is affected minimally, if at all, at 4.0 kHz in the control ear and at 500 Hz in either ear. In the test ear temporal integration decreases at 4 kHz from about 12 to 2 dB as noise level increased to 86 dB(A).

tuning from the effects of the loss of auditory sensitivity which are independent of temporal integration? One solution is to use very short-duration signals (5–10 msec) to measure TTS and tuning curves. Of course one is then confronted with the problems of the energy splatter which accompanies short-duration signals. (In a later portion of this manuscript the effects of TTS on tuning curves obtained under conditions of forward and simultaneous masking with short-duration probes are reported.) For now, we believe the changes in tuning noted in Fig. 35 are probably largely attributable to the loss of auditory sensitivity at the probe frequency and at adjacent frequency regions, although we cannot support this conclusion rigorously because of confounding by energy splatter and because of the loss of temporal integration. Electrophysiological results with human subjects (Klein and Mills, 1981a,b), in which a ''short-duration'' signal was used, corroborate our psychophysical results, but they do not solve many of the difficulties.

D. Electrophysiological Results with Humans

A major advantage of the tuning curve paradigm is that it can be duplicated exactly and a number of physiological responses can be recorded and used to supplement and complement psychophysical judgments. In papers by Klein and Mills (1981a,b) there were three purposes. One was to develop a procedure that would permit the simultaneous measurement of a tuning curve of the compound action potential of the auditory nerve and the response (so-called wave V or P6) of the auditory brainstem (Jewitt and Williston, 1971; Davis, 1976). A second purpose was to compare the tuning curve of the auditory nerve with that of the auditory brainstem, and to compare these physiological tuning curves with psychophysical tuning curves. Of course, these comparisons become more meaningful when the identical signals are used for all criterion measures and when each subject serves as his/her own control. A third purpose was to measure the effects of TTS on the two physiological tuning curves and on the psychophysical curve.

In regard to the first purpose, namely, a suitable methodology, it was found that an ear canal electrode could be used and excellent simultaneous recordings of the auditory nerve and brainstem could be obtained. Specific details of the recording procedures are given in Klein and Mills (1981a,b). It is important to stress, however, that the procedure works only for some subjects and only when they are relaxed or asleep. Small but frequent movements by the subjects, alpha waves, apnea, and other factors decrease the signal-to-rise noise ratio during data collection. The result is a poorly defined or unreliable physiological response. In other subjects, recording conditions appeared to be excellent, but physiological responses were of poor quality (wave shape) or unreliable. Each data collection session lasted as long as 4 hours, and most of these sessions were held after midnight when subjects were able to sleep. In other words, these physiological responses are recorded with great difficulty, especially for probe levels less than 20 dB SL.

Figure 25 shows tuning curves of the compound action potential of the auditory nerve (wave I) and auditory brainstem (wave V or P_6). Psychophysical tuning curves are shown also. All curves were qualitatively similar across subjects; however, individual differences were quantitatively large. At masker frequencies of 1, 2, and 3 kHz, the psychophysical tuning curves parallel both of the physiological tuning curves for all subjects except RZ. The psychophysical tuning curves almost always require more intense maskers than the physiological curves do. At 3.3 or 3.5 kHz the differences between psychophysical and physiological tuning curves become larger. The result is a greater range between the lowest and highest points on the low-frequency side of the physiological curves than on the psychophysical curve. That is, the tip to low-frequency plateau difference is large on physiological tuning curves. On the high-frequency side, the wave V tuning curve matches the slope of the psychophysical tuning curve very closely for all subjects. The correspondence between the wave I tuning curve and the psychophysical tuning curve is poorer and highly variable across subjects. Overall, the differences between the wave I tuning curves and psychophysical tuning curves are greater on the high-frequency side than on the low-frequency side. Because the tip regions are not well defined, a quantitative description of sharpness of tuning with a measure such as the Q_{10} is not possible. If a slice is taken at 15 dB above signal level, or 76 dB SPL, and tuning curve bandwidths are measured, the psychophysical tuning curve has the smallest bandwidth, then the wave V curve, and the wave I tuning curve has the largest one. These results are equivocal in that they may indicate little more than energy splatter of the probe, and the fact that off-frequency energy is a critical factor in psychophysical judgments, less so in the generation of wave V, and perhaps not at all for wave I; or they may indicate that sharpening increases at higher levels of the auditory system.

Another factor that should be considered which may affect the relation between wave I and wave V tuning curves is level of the probe signal. Input/output functions (response amplitude versus signal intensity) are different for waves I and V. At low signal levels wave V amplitude is larger than wave I, but at high levels, waves I and V amplitudes are equal. In other words, the growth of wave I amplitude is steeper than wave V. Thus, variation in signal spectra and intensity can have nonlinear effects on the amplitude relations between waves I and V. The signal parameters used in determining the tuning curves thus may dictate many of the differences of similarities of tuning curves of physiological potentials.

Our third purpose was to examine the effects of TTS on psychophysical tuning curves and tuning curves of the auditory nerve and brainstem. The specific details are discussed elsewhere, and are only briefly summarized here (see Klein and Mills, 1981b). The changes observed in the psychophysical tuning curves were qualitatively identical to those shown in Fig. 35 (and Figs. 49 and 50), i.e., the tuning curves were widened by the effects of TTS. While these effects at the level of the auditory brainstem (wave V) were less pronounced than those observed psychophysically, the most prominent feature of the data was the qualitative similarity of the psychophysical results for our four subjects. At the level of the auditory nerve (wave I), however, responses could not even be recorded for two subjects even though wave V was easily recorded. For the others, tuning curves of wave I were significantly wider than the psychophysical or brainstem tuning curves. Thus, wave I is affected much more severely than either of the other measures.

Postexposure amplitude–intensity functions showed that when there were reductions in amplitudes of the evoked responses, the reductions in wave I amplitudes usually exceeded reductions in wave V amplitudes. This finding is similar to observations by Sohmer and Pratt (1975) on the brainstem response recorded from humans after they were exposed to noise. It is also consistent with the findings of Benitez *et al.* (1972) where the wave I from chinchillas exposed to noise was more affected than a scalp-recorded evoked response assumed to arise from the inferior colliculus. Benitez *et al.* suggested that the disruption of wave I was due to a desynchronization of the contributing neural elements by the temporary noise trauma. Little disruption in the brainstem response occurred because less synchrony is required. However, Salvi *et al.* (1979) performed a similar experiment on chinchillas and examined the relationship between behavioral thresholds, wave I thresholds, and features of single-unit responses. Salvi *et al.* found that wave I thresholds to clicks were not only recorded easily but that their thresholds were elevated by an amount equal to the behaviorally measured TTS. The reasons for the contradictory wave I findings in the above studies are unclear. In the present experiments data for two subjects supported the findings of Benitez *et al.* whereas data for two others are consistent with Salvi *et al.* The large range of individual differences encountered makes any one interpretation difficult to support.

The changes seen in psychophysical tuning curves after exposure to noise are in agreement with Feth *et al.* (1979) and with our data on Fig. 35 (also Figs. 49 and 50). These findings are also similar to results from studies of psychophysical tuning curves from humans with permanent hearing impairment of cochlear origin (Wightman *et al.*, 1977; Zwicker and Schorn, 1978; Thornton and Abbas, 1980; Florentine *et al.*, 1980). While we are not aware of other reports describing changes in wave I or wave V tuning curves after exposing humans to noise, Eggermont (1977) reported that wave I tuning curves from humans with Meniere's disease are less sharply tuned to signals in the frequency region of hearing loss than are tuning curves for signals in frequency regions with normal thresholds.

In studies on subjects with permanent hearing impairment the amount of hearing loss is much larger than the amount of TTS observed in our subjects. Regardless, the effects on psychophysical tuning curves and physiological curves seem to be similar. One notable difference in methods between the present study and studies on humans with preexisting hearing impairments is in setting signal level. In the present study, signal SPL was held constant across all conditions and subjects whereas in the other studies signal SPL was adjusted to maintain a constant sensation level (SL) across subjects with different amounts of hearing loss. By keeping SPL constant for pre- and postexposure measurements it is possible that the changes in tuning curves that occurred may in part be due to decreases in signal SL after noise exposure. Change in SL, however, cannot totally account for the changes in psychophysical tuning curves. For example, subjects with virtually identical TTSs had tuning curves that were affected maximally or not at all. To make the story more involved, the amplitudes of wave I and wave V were reduced after the noise exposure in the unmasked condition in some subjects (JW and TS). One can assume that less intense maskers will then be needed to reach criterion threshold (complete elimination of the response) for these subjects. Thus, the "widening" of wave I and wave V tuning curves after noise exposure is confounded by changes in the wave morphology of the physiological potentials.

An examination of the relative changes between psychophysical wave I tuning curves and wave V tuning curves after noise exposure indicates that wave I tuning curves showed larger change from preexposure values than wave V tuning curves or psychophysical curves. Changes in the wave V curves, on the other hand, compared well with changes in the psychophysical tuning curves. The postexposure broader tuning of wave I may be attributed to several factors as mentioned previously, but loss of synchronous firing among primary fibers after exposure to noise is possibly the best bet.

Some insight on additional factors responsible for the widening in the wave I, wave V, and psychophysical tuning curves may be gained by considering single-unit data from animals. In these animal studies, the cochlear lesions produced arc severe and not comparable to temporary cochlear changes in humans briefly exposed to moderate sound levels. Tuning curves of auditory neurons originating from locations in cochleas damaged by intense noise exposure or ototoxins may have several abnormal characteristics such as the disappearance of a sharply tuned tip and the appearance of a hypersensitive tail (Kiang *et al.*, 1976a; Dallos *et al.*, 1977; Liberman and Kiang, 1978; Schmiedt *et al.*, 1980; Cody and Johnstone, 1980). If indeed the wave I tuning curve is a measure which reflects the summated characteristics of the underlying single-unit activity (Dallos and Cheatham, 1976; Harris, 1979; Abbas and Gorga, 1981), then changes seen in wave I tuning curve during TTS may be due to similar changes at the single-unit level. These alterations in tuning at the periphery may be passed on to more central sites. This notion is complicated by the problem of recovery.

Because recovery from TTS begins immediately after the exposure is terminated, the tuning curves were first measured in a state of recovery. Therefore, it is not possible to determine if the larger differences seen for wave I tuning curves compared to wave V and psychophysical tuning curves are the result of a slower rate of recovery for wave I, alterations in synchronized firing among primary fibers (decrement in response amplitude), or real changes in frequency tuning of those fibers. The close correspondence between wave V and psychophysical tuning curves suggests that in addition to wave V providing a good estimate of behavioral threshold, the shifts in psychophysical masking functions (or possibly frequency tuning) induced by TTS are closely followed in magnitude and time by wave V masking functions.

Before offering a summary and some conclusions involving psychophysical

tuning curves under conditions of simultaneous masking, it may be more useful
to examine psychophysical tuning curves under conditions of forward masking,
auditory suppression in forward masking, and the effects of noise on tuning
curves and suppression obtained in forward masking.

V. FREQUENCY SELECTIVITY: TUNING CURVES AND SUPPRESSION IN FORWARD MASKING

A. Introduction

Forward masking has become a very popular phenomenon in the past few
years. This popularity is due to a number of factors including problems inherent
to simultaneous masking such as beats and distortion products, and the inability
to measure suppression effects (Houtgast, 1972). In addition, the analogies of
psychophysically measured tuning curves and suppression to physiologically
measured tuning curves and two-tone rate suppression are just too strong and too
obvious for the psychophysicists to ignore.

A summary of the state of the art of tuning curves and suppression measured in
a forward masking paradigm is a difficult task, perhaps even an impossible task
at this date. There are several sources of difficulty. One, as already discussed, is
individual differences in tuning curves that are apparently unrelated to differences between subjects with respect to auditory sensitivity. A second is related
to ''energy splatter'' of the probe tone. That is, one is necessarily forced to use a
short duration signal, and an arbitrary trade-off must be made between the need
for a spectrally narrow signal and the need to produce a large amount of forward
masking. A third is the need to control the criterion of the subject which forces
the experimenter to use signal-detection paradigms. Signal-detection procedures
are not efficient. Accordingly, the number of subjects in most published papers
rarely exceeds three or four, and oftentimes includes the authors of the paper. It
is noteworthy that the standard error of the mean in some conditions is 10–12 dB
(Jesteadt, 1980), and, accordingly, in many papers data are reported for individuals (for example, see O'Malley and Feth, 1979). It seems that on many
occasions the ability to reach a strong conclusion is not possible or that the
conclusion must be tempered because it is true only for two of three subjects or
two of four subjects.

The experimenter is never really certain of the cues or information used by the
subject to make the judgment (Moore, 1980b; Lufti and Yost, 1980). For example, some subjects may be using a number of cues including pitch, loudness, and
quality. The cues used by a given subject are oftentimes beyond the control of the
experimenter. It is quite likely that the physiological mechanisms underlying
psychophysical tuning curves and suppression measured in a forward masking

paradigm are unusually susceptible to minor pathological changes of the cochlea and auditory nerve, and that measures of auditory sensitivity for pure tones are unaffected by these minor pathological changes (Salvi *et al.*, 1982). In nearly every experiment the only prerequisite for subjects is a "normal" audiogram and the ability to perform the required task reliably. Lastly, the number of papers being published on psychophysical tuning curves is remarkable and quite surprising given the fact that Small's paper appeared in 1959 and not one psychophysical tuning curve paper arrived until the early 1970s. Thus it appears that just as psychophysicists in the 1960s directed their efforts to studies of masking-level differences after Hirsh (1948) and the applications of signal detection theory, psychophysicists in the 1980s will be attacking tuning curves after Small (1959). (If we carry this argument one step further, then someone in 1978 or so must have published a paper which will be discovered in 1992, and the topic will become overwhelmingly popular from about 1995 to 2010. But, we digress.)

Before proceeding to our own experiments we should like to comment on the analogies between psychophysical tuning curves and suppression, and physiological tuning curves and two-tone rate suppression. While we believe that many of the analogies are valid and useful, we believe also that many of the "coincidences" between physiology and psychophysics are overworked. For example, nearly all comparisons are made between psychophysics and physiology at the level of the peripheral auditory system. This is an understandable occurrence but we have always wondered what all those neurons and nuclei of the auditory central nervous system are doing. Similarly, as previously mentioned, it can be shown that gross responses of the auditory nerve (masked action potentials) can be remarkably abnormal, and brainstem responses can be perfectly normal. Apparently, an adequate stimulus for one physiological mechanism can be ineffective for other physiological mechanisms. It follows, therefore, that some physiological data can be "unrelated" to other physiological data and to some psychophysical phenomena. Similarly, some parameters of a signal are critical to certain psychophysical phenomenon and are of no value to certain physiological effects. So called "off-frequency" listening is perhaps the best example. That "off-frequency" information is used by the listener in certain psychophysical tasks is well documented (Leshowitz and Wightman, 1971). Additional documentation comes from human physiological and psychophysical data. For example, Klein (1982b, see Fig. 26, this paper) shows tuning curves of the slow-wave response (SN_{10}) for probe levels covering a range of 50 dB, and that the slow-wave response is frequency specific over this range. For the probe tone used in the SN_{10} study, psychophysical tuning curves (simultaneous masking) could be obtained only for the lowest probe level. At higher probe levels masked thresholds and therefore psychophysical tuning curves could not be obtained. Our interpretation is that the effective portion of the stimulus that produces the slow-wave response is entirely different from the portion of the stimulus used by the observer in the detection task. In different words, the human observer uses both on- and off-frequency information, whereas off-frequency information contributes little to the slow-wave response and to many other physiological responses as well.

B. Experimental Results

In our experiments forward masking was measured by means of the method of adjustment wherein the subject adjusted the frequency of the masker. The level of the masker was fixed for a given judgment. Four to five levels of masker were used to define a tuning curve. Probe level was fixed at 25, 35, 45, or 55 dB SPL. The stimulus paradigm is schematically presented in Fig. 37 and the power spectrum of the probe signal is given in Fig. 1. For a tuning curve at a given probe level, the SPL of the probe was held constant for all observers. In many studies of other investigators the probe is fixed in sesnsation level rather than SPL. The issue of SPL vs SL will be discussed later.

To measure auditory suppression a third signal (the suppressor) was introduced. It was equal in duration to the masker and was gated simultaneously with the masker. At least three suppressor signals differing in frequency were used on

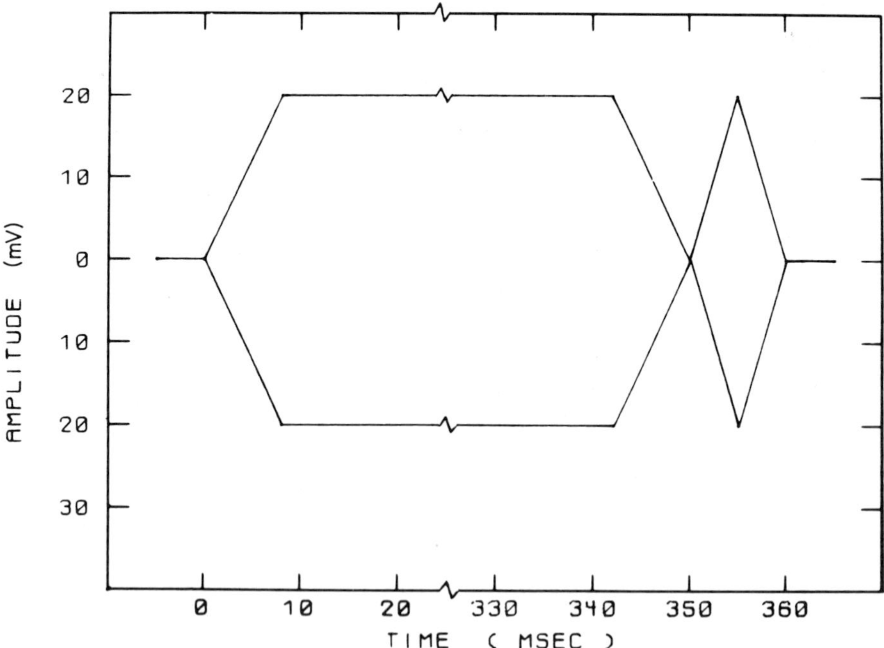

Figure 37 Schematic diagram of the stimulus paradigm used in the forward masking studies. The spectrum of the probe signal is given on Fig. 1.

the high side of a tuning curve and at least four suppressor signals were used on the low side. With the masker about 150 Hz below the frequency of the probe tone and with the masker at a level sufficient to render the probe inaudible (approximately -3 to -5 dB SL), the suppressor was introduced at a sound pressure level of about -10 to $+10$ dB. The subject adjusted the level of the suppressor until the probe signal became audible. This level of suppressor was taken as the lower threshold boundary of suppression. The subject then continued to increase the level of the suppressor until the probe signal was inaudible. This was taken as the upper boundary of suppression. With highly trained subjects, a tuning curve and its associated suppression areas could be measured in 20–25 min with three judgments/condition. Of course, the subjects were kept honest by the insertion of random amounts of attenuation in the suppression task and the use of different starting frequencies in the tuning curve task.

As in the simultaneous masking studies, great care was taken in the selection of subjects. Hearing levels were required to be better than 10 dB HL (re ANSI-53-1969) from 250 to 6.0 kHz. In addition, subjects were required to be able to perform the listening task reliably and efficiently. Over 200 subjects were screened with respect to hearing levels. About 50 survived the screening and received some training in the forward masking task. The 25 best subjects in terms of variance in their judgments and time to obtain a judgment were retained, and used in the forward masking studies. These studies occurred over the period from 1976 to 1981 and are continuing.

Perhaps the most remarkable feature of the tuning curve data is the magnitude of individual differences. Figure 38 shows the median tuning curve and the range of individual differences for probe tones of 0.5, 1.0, 2.0, and 4.0 kHz. It must be noted that the number of subjects per condition varies from 5 at 4.0 kHz, to 16 at 2.0 kHz, to 9 at 1.0 kHz, and to 9 at 500 Hz, and that different groups of subjects were used for each probe frequency. Of course, the ideal design would use the same group of subjects for all conditions; however, the data in Fig. 38 and subsequent figures were collected over a lengthy period and it was not possible to retain subjects. The median tuning curves in Fig. 38 conform in most respects to those reported by others, i.e., steep high-frequency slopes and less steep low-frequency slopes.

Quantitative comparisons to the data of others are difficult because of different experimental conditions, particularly those with respect to the waveform and spectrum of the probe, the interval between the offset of the masker and the offset of the probe, and the large difference in psychophysical methods (method of adjustment whereby the subject adjusts the frequency of the masker versus adaptive forced-choice methods whereby the experimenter varies the level of the masker). Nonetheless, we have tried it anyway. Figure 39 compares averaged data for four subjects reported by Jesteadt (1980) for a 1.0 and a 4.0-kHz probe signal presented at a sensation level of 10 dB, and our median data from Fig. 38.

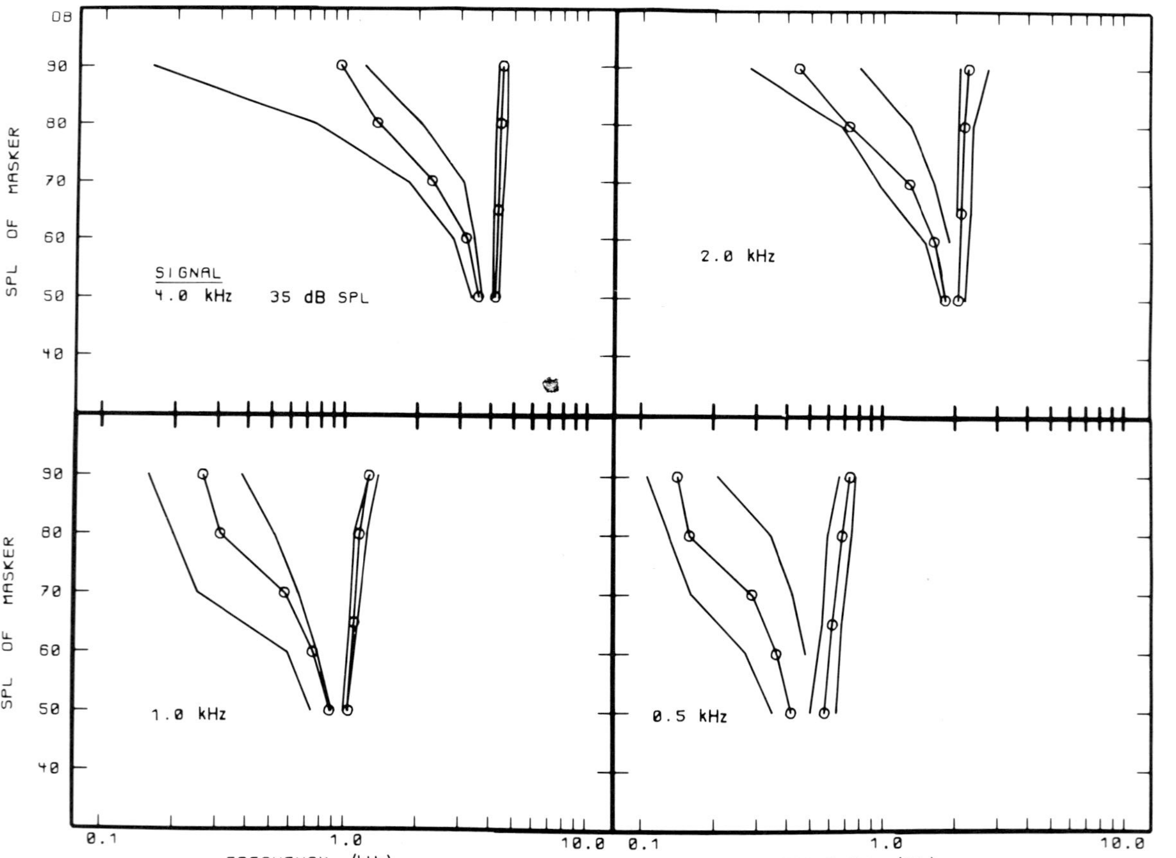

Figure 38 Psychophysical tuning curves obtained by means of forward masking for probe tones of 4, 2, 1, and 0.5 kHz. Probe level is 35 dB SPL. Median data are shown by open circles. The solid lines show the ''narrowest'' tuning curve and the ''widest'' tuning curve exhibited by any subject. $N = 5$ at 4.0 kHz, 16 at 2.0 kHz, 9 at 1.0 kHz, and 9 at 0.5 kHz.

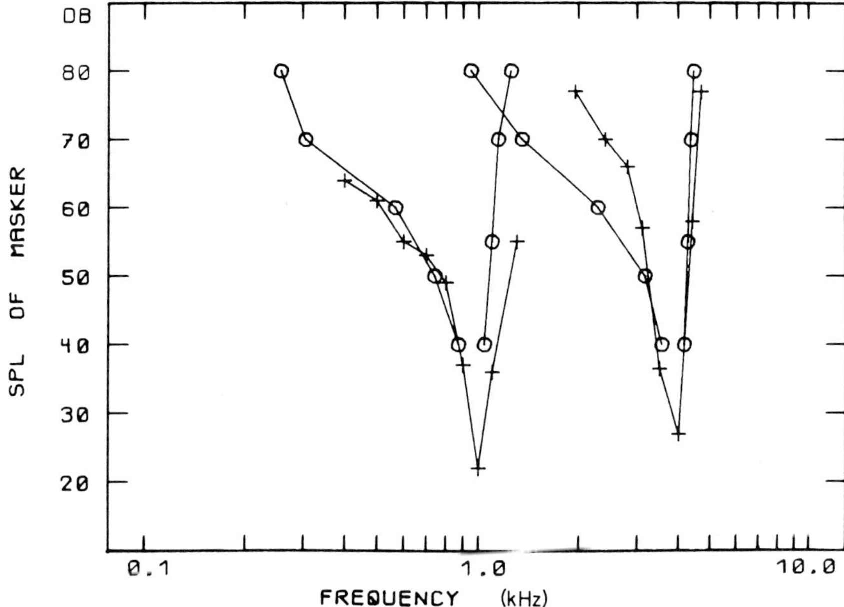

Figure 39   Median data from Fig. 37 (circles) are compared to mean data reported by Jestedt (1980) (crosses) for probe signals of 1.0 and 4.0 kHz. The data from Fig. 37 have been "adjusted" in an effort to equate the level of the probe signals (see text).

Our data were obtained at a sensation level of approximately 18–22 dB. To correct for differences in probe level we have arbitrarily subtracted 10 dB from the masker level. As Fig. 39 indicates, the comparison of our data to Jesteadts is excellent in some instances and there are significant differences in others. The probable reasons for the differences are many and include most of those discussed above. In addition we have found that differences between subjects on the high side of a tuning curve are minimized by adjusting the frequency of the masker (fixed in level) rather than the level of the masker (fixed in frequency). The standard error of our data at 70 dB SPL is 10–30 Hz depending upon probe frequency, whereas Jesteadt (1980) found the standard error of masker levels to be 10–12 dB.

Quantitative descriptions of nearly all psychophysical tuning curves include the high-and low-frequency slopes of the tuning curves, and $Q_{10\ \mathrm{dB}}$. On Fig. 39 the high-frequency slopes of the median tuning curves are only 100–150 dB octave when the slope is calculated over the entire range of the high-frequency side by the equation

$$\text{slope in dB/octave} = \frac{\mathrm{dB}_2 - \mathrm{dB}_1}{3.32 \log_{10} (f_2/f_1)}$$

When a small portion of the tuning curve is selected or when individual subjects are used, then slopes range from less than 80 to as high as 220 dB/octave. In contrast, others report slopes of 402–1325 dB/octave (O'Malley and Feth, 1979) and even 2895 dB/octave (Moore, 1978). It is not clear to us why there should be such large disparities between the high-frequency skirts of the tuning curves of our data and those of others. One possibility is in the method of calculating slope, i.e., over the entire range of the tuning curve versus the steepest portion, over a specified portion, etc. The slope magnitude is extremely sensitive to the range it is measured over because the curve is being differentiated. Thus, any slope measurements *must* be qualified as to the range over which they were obtained. It is nevertheless difficult not to be amazed at the range of the slope of the high-frequency skirts (80–2800 dB/octave). In contrast, in gerbils the high-frequency slopes of peripheral auditory neurons are typically between 300 and 500 dB/octave at 70 dB SPL. At high CFs (above 4.0 kHz) skirts are steeper and may occasionally approach 1000 dB/octave (Schmiedt *et al.*, 1980). Inasmuch as we did not measure the tips of tuning curves, we will not report estimated Q values, tip-to-tail ratios, and bandwidths.

Figure 38 indicates the "widest" and the "narrowest" tuning curves observed for each group, or, in other words, the range of differences between individuals. These differences may be due to a number of factors. We cannot account for all of the factors but we can eliminate some of them. One is auditory sensitivity at the probe frequency. At 4.0 kHz, the difference in auditory sensitivity between the subject with the widest tuning and the subject with the narrowest tuning is less than 3 dB, whereas the differences in tuning on the low side are as large 15–20 dB. Similarly, at probe conditions of 0.5, 1.0, and 2.0 kHz the largest difference in auditory sensitivity between the subjects with the widest and the narrowest tuning curve is 3 dB. Thus, the variability in tuning curves across individual subjects cannot be reduced in a measurable and systematic manner by equating subjects with respect to auditory sensitivity, i.e., the use of sensation level rather than sound pressure level. Repeatability of judgments for a given subject over a period of weeks was excellent regardless of the specific details of their tuning curves.

While large differences between subjects cannot be attributed to the reliability of judgments or to the differences in auditory sensitivity at the probe, it is possible that criterion used by the subjects contributes to the magnitude of the differences. Equally likely is the possibility that the subjects are using different cues such as quality versus pitch or quality versus duration (see Moore, 1980b). Another likely possibility, however, involves the "energy splatter" of the probe signal. Several studies show that tuning curves in forward masking are different when a low-level background noise is presented (O'Malley and Feth, 1979; Nelson and Turner, 1980; Green *et al.*, 1981). This noise presumably affects the side lobes of the spectrum of the probe signal, and, therefore, reduces the effects of ''off-frequency'' listening. Since the amount of information available to the listener is reduced by the low-level background noise, the level of masker used in determining the psychophysical tuning curve is reduced, and the tuning curve becomes wider. The effects of ''off-frequency'' listening become even more apparent for probe levels greater than about 25 dB SL.

Figure 40 shows median tuning curves from Fig. 38 normalized with respect to probe frequency. The lowside of the tuning curve for probes of 0.5, 1, 2, and 4 kHz can be fitted with one line, and the departures of datum points from the fitted line are trivial. On the high-frequency side, the skirt at 4.0 is slightly steeper than at 2.0 kHz and then decreases systematically as probe frequency is decreased to 1.0 and 0.5 kHz. There is a high degree of coincidence between the shapes of the high sides of the normalized tuning curves of Fig. 40 and normalized tuning curves from single auditory neurons (Harris, 1979; Schmiedt *et al.*, 1980) and even tuning curves of the (SN_{10}) slow-wave response recorded from the scalp of human subjects (see Fig. 26).

Figure 41 shows tuning curves at probe frequencies of 4, 2, 1, and 0.5 kHz for probe levels of 35, 45, and 55 dB SPL. Median data are plotted and show that in

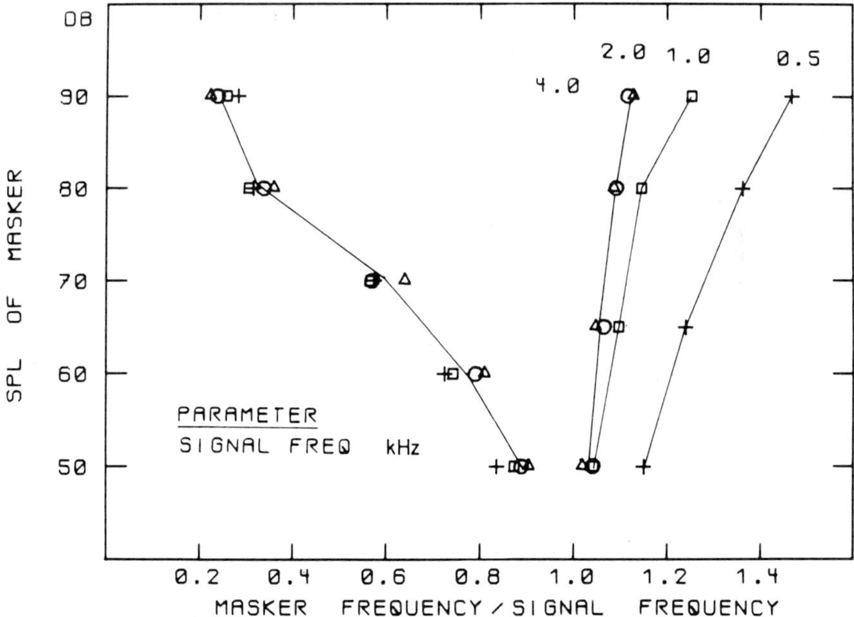

Figure 40 Median psychophysical tuning curves in forward masking from Fig. 38 have been normalized with respect to probe frequency and masker frequency. Note that the low side can be fitted with one line whereas on the high side, the data rank themselves with respect to probe frequency. See Fig. for symbols; circles correspond to the 4.0 kHz data.

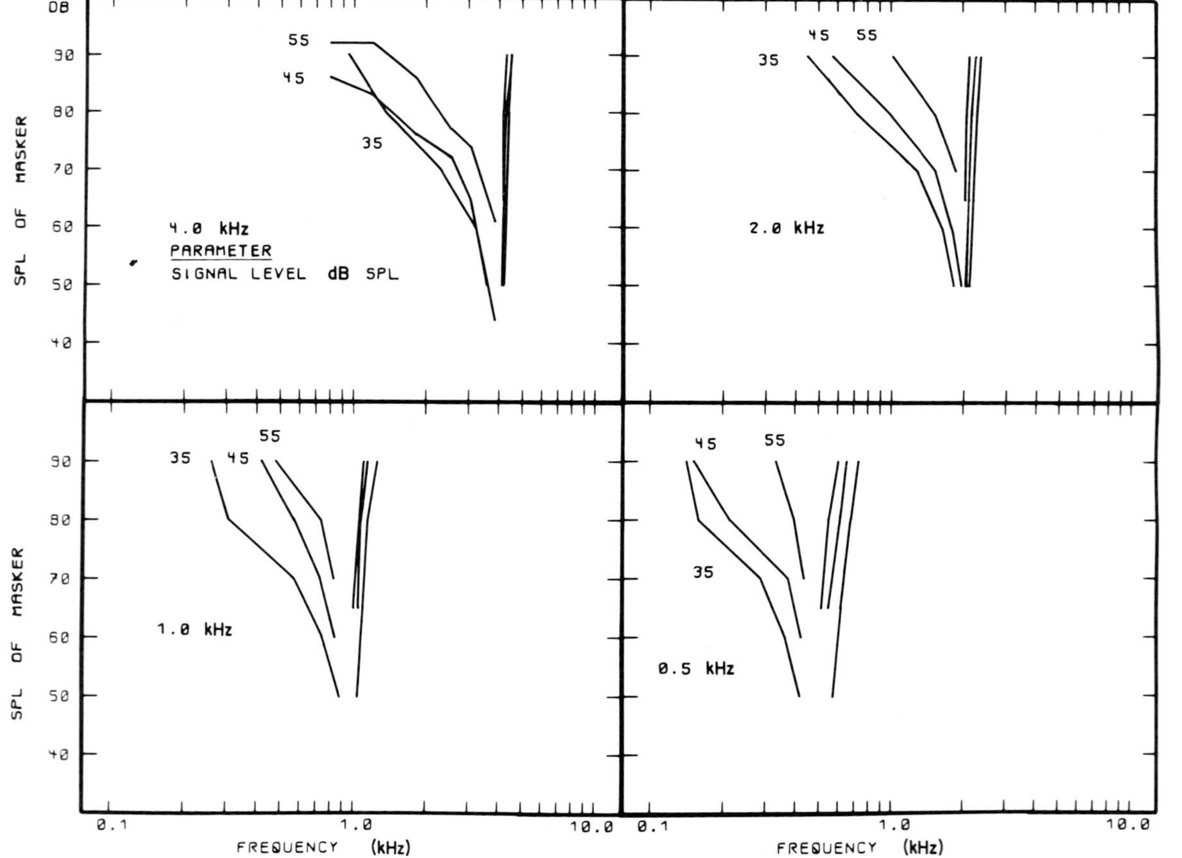

Figure 41   Median psychophysical tuning curves in forward masking at probe frequencies of 4.0, 1.0, 2.0, and 0.5 kHz, and probe levels of 35, 45, and 55 dB SPL. The increased tuning at probe levels of 45 and 55 dB SPL almost surely reflects energy splatter of the probe signal and the fact that side lobes of the spectrum become audible. The result is that masker levels must be increased and the tuning curve therefore appears narrower. Some of the irregularities in the data reflect unequal *N*s and different groups of observers at different conditions. In other words, the interpretation of these data (and that of others) at high probe levels is not a simple task.

most instances as probe level is increased, masker levels must be increased as well. Tuning curves thus become tighter or narrower as probe level is increased. These results particularly at probe levels of 45 and 55 dB SPL are "quasi-artifactual" because of the energy splatter of the probe signal. That is, at probe levels of 25 dB SPL (about 10 dB SL) and 35 dB SPL (about 20 dB SL) the side bands or lobes of the signal are inaudible. Recall from Fig. 1 that the peak of the first lobe of the probe is about −22 dB re the main lobe of the spectrum. At probe levels of 45–55 dB SPL the sidebands would clearly be audible. Accordingly, the subject must raise the level of the masker to mask the spectral peak and sidebands. The result is a narrowing of the tuning curve as is depicted in Fig. 41. As mentioned previously, others have avoided or at least minimized these "off-frequency effects" by presenting a continuous wide-band noise masker at low levels. The effects of this masker are clearly demonstrated—the tuning curves do not become narrower as probe level is increased. Indeed, it appears that the shape of the tuning curve is independent or nearly so of probe level (Green *et al.*, 1981). Why didn't we use a continuous masker? One of our major purposes was to produce temporary threshold shifts at specific frequency locations. We assumed these TTSs could be used to reduce the effects of off-frequency listening

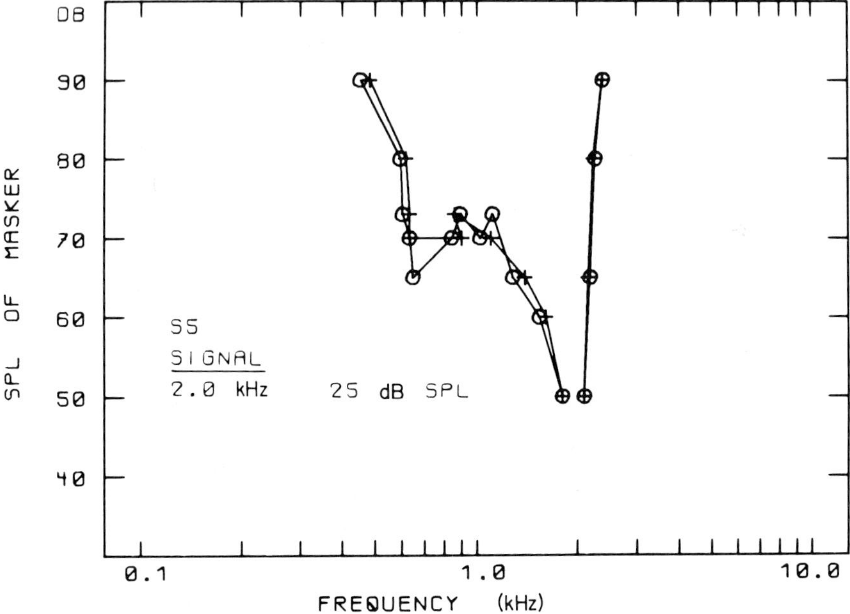

Figure 42 An unusual psychophysical tuning curve in forward masking from one subject. Please note the low side of the tuning curve. Data points are median judgments from several prenoise exposure listening sessions (circles) and 30 days and two noise exposures later (crosses). This subject has suppression on the high side of the tuning curve, but suppression could not be measured on the low side despite repeated efforts.

and thus restrict the effects of energy splatter. TTS results will be discussed later.

Figure 42 shows repeated measurements for one subject at a probe frequency of 2.0 kHz and a probe level of 25 dB SPL. Circles are the medians of five judgments and crosses are the medians of five judgments made 30 days (and two noise exposures) later. This subject has been selected to show an unusually shaped tuning curve on the low-frequency side. Please note the steep slope near a masker frequency of 0.6 kHz and the irregularities in the shape of the tuning curve between masker frequencies of 0.6 and 1.2 kHz. These irregularities were detected when this subject for a 70 dB masker gave judgments that ranged from 600 to 1200 Hz. To obtain the data in Fig. 42 the experimenter set the starting frequency to 300 Hz (± 100 Hz) and the subject "mapped" areas of audibility and inaudibility by changing masker frequency. Then the procedure was repeated at a level of 72 dB SPL. Thus, what appeared to be unreliable judgments were indeed highly reliable but very unusual. The high-frequency side of the tuning curve for this subject is unremarkable. In regard to suppression, this subject had suppression effects on the high-frequency side, but despite our repeated efforts suppression effects could not be shown on the low-frequency side. While we have many other subjects who have shown suppression on the high side but not on the low side, the low side of their tuning curves is unremarkable and unlike the data in Fig. 42. Measurements of suppression are discussed below.

C. Auditory Suppression

Figure 43 shows auditory suppression for probe levels of 35 dB SPL and probe frequencies of 4, 2, 1, and 0.5 kHz. At 4.0 kHz, suppression experiments were completed with only four subjects. All four showed suppression effects on the high side of the tuning curve whereas only two subjects had suppression on the low side. The averaged data for these two individuals are shown in Fig. 43. At 2.0 kHz, median suppression data are shown. The range of suppression is about 35 dB on the high side and 10 dB on the low side. Of 16 subjects 12 had suppression on the high side (range 10–55 dB), whereas only 8 of 16 subjects had suppression on the low side (range 6–15 dB). Peculiar individual differences in suppression have been noted by others (Shannon, 1976; Weber, 1978; O'Malley and Feth, 1979). Suppression data at 1.0 kHz are highly similar to those at

---

Figure 43 Median psychophysical tuning curves in forward masking at 4, 1, 2, and 0.5 kHz (from Fig. 37) and auditory suppression (see text). The ranges of suppression are given by the dotted areas. At 4, 2, and 1 kHz approximately 50% of the subjects showed suppression on both the high and low sides of the tuning curve, about 25% showed suppression on just the high side, and about 25% did not have suppression on either the high side or the low side. Suppression could not be measured at 500 Hz for any subject. Recall that all of these subjects had "normal hearing" according to the most rigorous standards of normal hearing. For an individual, suppression measured on the low side almost guarantees that suppression will be measured on the high side; however, suppression measured on the high side is of little predictive value with respect to the measurement of suppression on the low side.

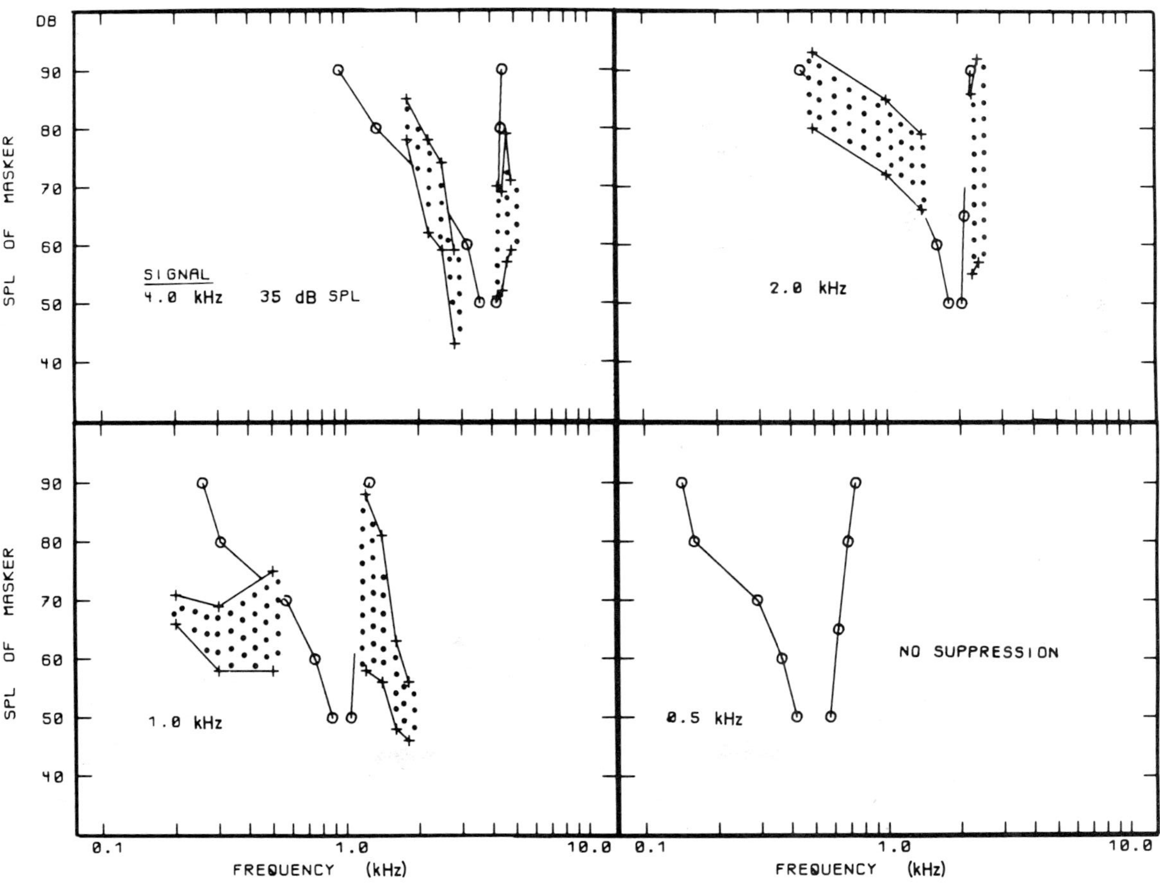

SPL OF MASKER
FREQUENCY (kHz)
SIGNAL
4.0 kHz   35 dB SPL
2.0 kHz
1.0 kHz
0.5 kHz
NO SUPPRESSION

2.0 kHz in terms of magnitude and incidence. The oddly shaped suppression data at 1.0 kHz on the low side reflect the averaging of data across subjects ($N=4$). We were unable to measure suppression at 500 Hz. This was attempted with nine subjects. Each of these nine subjects had shown suppression effects at either 2.0 or 4.0 kHz and on both the high- and low-frequency sides. Additional efforts to show suppression at 500 Hz included increasing the probe to 45 dB SPL and decreasing the probe to 30 dB SPL. To date, not one subject has demonstrated suppression at 500 Hz.

Besides the absence of suppression at 500 Hz, another very striking aspect is individual differences. For reasons unknown to us some subjects do not show suppression effects on either the high or low side of the tuning curve, others show suppression on both the high side and the low side, and others show suppression just on the high side. To date, no subject has shown suppression on the low side but not on the high side. These differences between subjects are clearly not related to measurements of auditory sensitivity for pure tones (the audiogram) nor to differences between subjects with respect to noise-induced TTS. There is also a qualitative correspondence between the data of Fig. 43 and those physiological data in Fig. 24.

D. Effects of Noise on Tuning Curves and Suppression

The effects of exposure to noise on psychophysical tuning curves (forward masking) are complicated for a number of reasons. As we shall see the noise exposure can produce changes in auditory sensitivity at the probe frequency and at adjacent frequencies. Thus, when changes in tuning are observed they can be due to changes in auditory sensitivity (pre- and postexposure probe level is fixed in SPL) at the probe frequency, at the probe and adjacent frequencies, or just at adjacent frequencies. In addition, we have used noise exposures that do not change auditory sensitivity but nevertheless produce minor changes in tuning, and changes in auditory suppression that range from the elimination of suppression to sizable reductions. Thus, when a tuning curve changes shape, is it due to changes in auditory sensitivity or to changes in suppression? Another confounding factor is the spectral characteristics of the probe tone. TTSs at the probe and adjacent frequencies reduce not only auditory sensitivity but some of the problems associated with energy splatter.

Our data on simultaneous masking indicated that a 24-hour exposure to an octave-band noise (CF = 4.0 kHz, skirts of 24 dB/octave) which produced no changes in the audiogram could nevertheless change the shape of the psychophysical tuning curve on the high-frequency side. The low-frequency side and tip region were unaffected, as was a tuning curve in the control ear. We wished to replicate and extend these observations from simultaneous masking to forward masking. At the time (1977) it seemed like a superb idea to use an exposure to a wide-band noise and to monitor tuning curves and suppression at periodic intervals throughout and following the exposure. Accordingly, four subjects were trained and tuning curves and suppression data were obtained for a 4.0 kHz probe at 25 dB SPL. The noise was wide-band with a level of 75 dB(A). Its duration was 48 hours. Tuning curve and suppression data were obtained as planned. Not only were there no measurable TTSs, there were no measurable changes in the tuning curves or in suppression in either the test ear or the control ear. Also, the experimenters were very tired. We then repeated the entire experiment using a 1.0-kHz band of noise with skirts of 24 dB/octave, a duration of 8 hours, and a level of 78 dB SPL. Equivocal changes in tuning and suppression were observed for two of four subjects. We then became aware of an experiment by McFadden and Pasanen (1979) who used a very steep noise as a masker and found effects which occurred over the course of the experiments and which appeared to be persistent. That is, it appeared that the steep skirt of the masking noise may have acutely altered the ear. We decided to use a noise with skirts of 48 dB/octave and repeat some of our earlier experiments that were negative or equivocal in their outcome.

Subjects were two highly trained observers who had been selected for their accuracy and speed in the listening task. They were also homogeneous with respect to auditory sensitivity (±3 dB, 250–4000 Hz) prior to and following exposure to a wide-band noise (TTS ±2 dB). In addition, one of the subjects

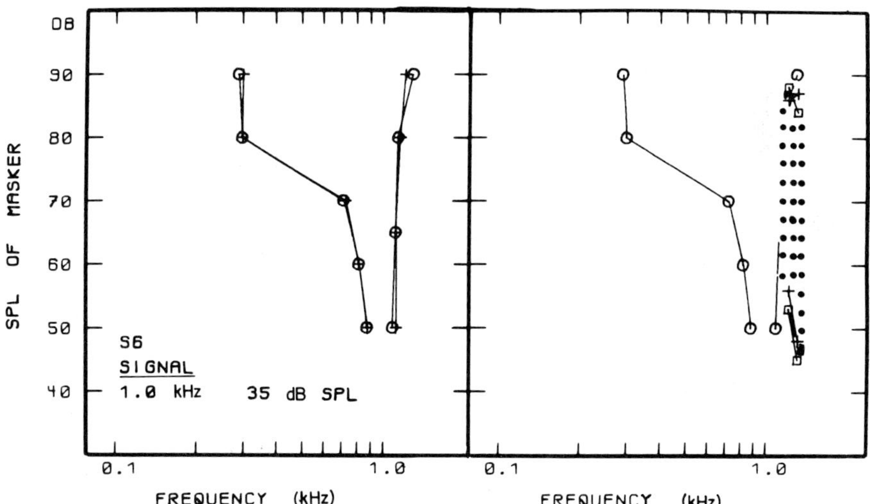

Figure 44 Effects of an 8-hour exposure to noise on psychophysical (forward masking) tuning curves and suppression on one subject who had only high-side suppression. The noise band was 200 Hz wide and centered at 707 Hz with skirts of 48 dB/octave. Pre- (circles) and postexposure (crosses) tuning curves are on the left-hand side of the figure, and pre- (squares) and postexposure suppression data (crosses) are on the right-hand side. For this subject the exposure to noise affected neither the tuning nor the suppression. The dotted area indicates the range of postexposure suppression.

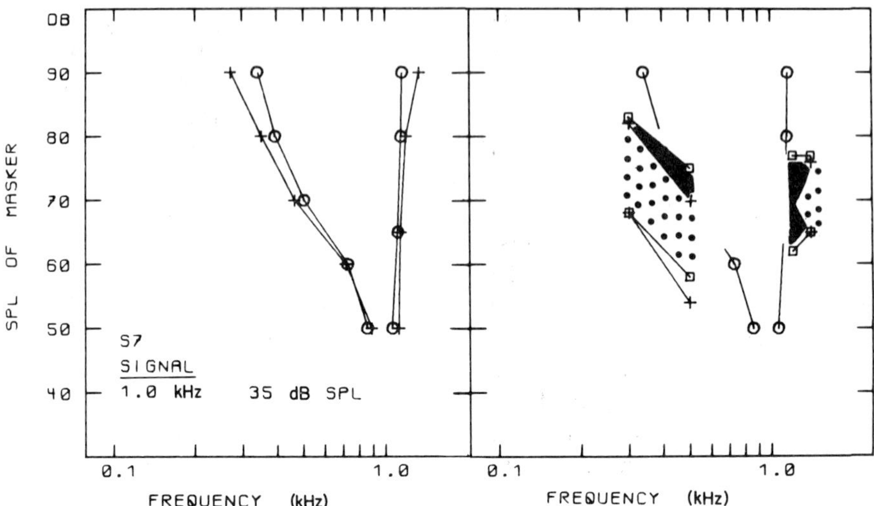

Figure 45   Effects of a 7-hour exposure to noise on psychophysical (forward masking) tuning curves and suppression on one subject who had high- and low-side suppression. Details are as described for Fig. 44. Postexposure data (crosses) at a masker level of 90 dB SPL (left-hand portion of the figure) exceed the range of preexposure judgments. On the right-hand portion of the figure shaded areas indicate losses of suppression. Significant amounts of suppression are still measured as indicated by the dotted areas.

showed suppression on both the high and low sides of the tuning curves, whereas one subject had suppression only on the high side. The latter subject differed from the former with regard to the low side of the tuning curve for a 1.0-kHz probe. As shown in Figs. 44 and 45, both subjects were exposed for 8 hours to a band of noise centered at 707 Hz and with skirts of 48 dB/octave. Auditory thresholds measured about 6 to 12 min after termination of the noise exposure were within ±2 dB of preexposure thresholds over the frequency range from 500 to 2000 Hz.

Figure 44 indicates that the noise exposure had no measurable effects on either the gross or fine shape of the tuning curve or on the suppression areas on the high-frequency side for the latter subject. Note the magnitude of the suppression effects on the high-frequency side. The suppressor signal is effective over a range from 45 to 88 dB SPL. Thus, this subject shows unusual tuning on the low-frequency side, no suppression on the low-frequency side, steep skirts on the high side, and the largest amount of suppression on the high side of all subjects tested. Exposure to noise affected neither the fine structure of the tuning curve nor suppression.

Data for the other subject are plotted in Figs. 45 and 46. Data in Fig. 45 are preexposure data and data collected after 7 hours exposure to the 707-Hz noise. The preexposure tuning curve is unremarkable and suppression is measured on

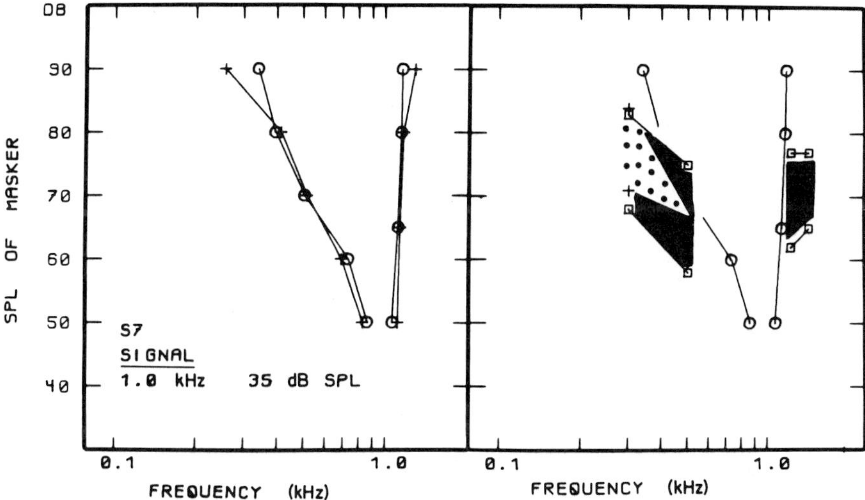

Figure 46 Effects of an 8.5-hour exposure to noise on psychophysical tuning curves and suppression on the subject whose data are described in Fig. 45. The noise exposure and other details are described in Fig. 44. While no TTS was measurable, the tuning curve is shifted measurably on both sides only at masker level of 90 dB SPL. Suppression is eliminated on the high side (shaded area) and reduced on the low side (see text).

both the high and low sides of the tuning curve. After 7 hours of noise exposure TTS was ±2 dB from 500 to 2000 Hz; however, tuning curves are widened only for masker levels of 90 dB SPL, and suppression is reduced (shaded areas) on both sides of the tuning curve. Some suppression remains (dotted areas).

Figure 46 shows the data for the same subject after 8.5 hours of exposure. There are only small changes on both the high and low sides of the tuning curve occurring at the highest level of masker used. On the one hand, these changes in tuning barely exceed measurement error and thus one is inclined toward deemphasizing them. On the other hand, the change is over 100 dB/octave in high-frequency slope, again pointing out the sensitivity of slope measures to small changes in the tuning curve slope. Are we thus dealing with trivia or with a 100 dB effect? In regard to suppression, note its elimination on the high side and a small residual (dotted area) on the low side. The low-side suppression was measured 20–25 min after the tuning curve and 10–15 min after the high-side suppression. As we shall show later, recovery of suppression can be extremely rapid. Thus, we believe that during the measurement of the tuning curve, suppression was eliminated on both the low and high sides of the tuning curve. If this is not the case, then this would be the first time we have observed suppression on the low side of a tuning curve with no suppression measured on the high side. The points we should like to make from Figs. 45 and 46 are that the gross shape of the tuning curve is essentially unaffected by the noise exposure, the fine

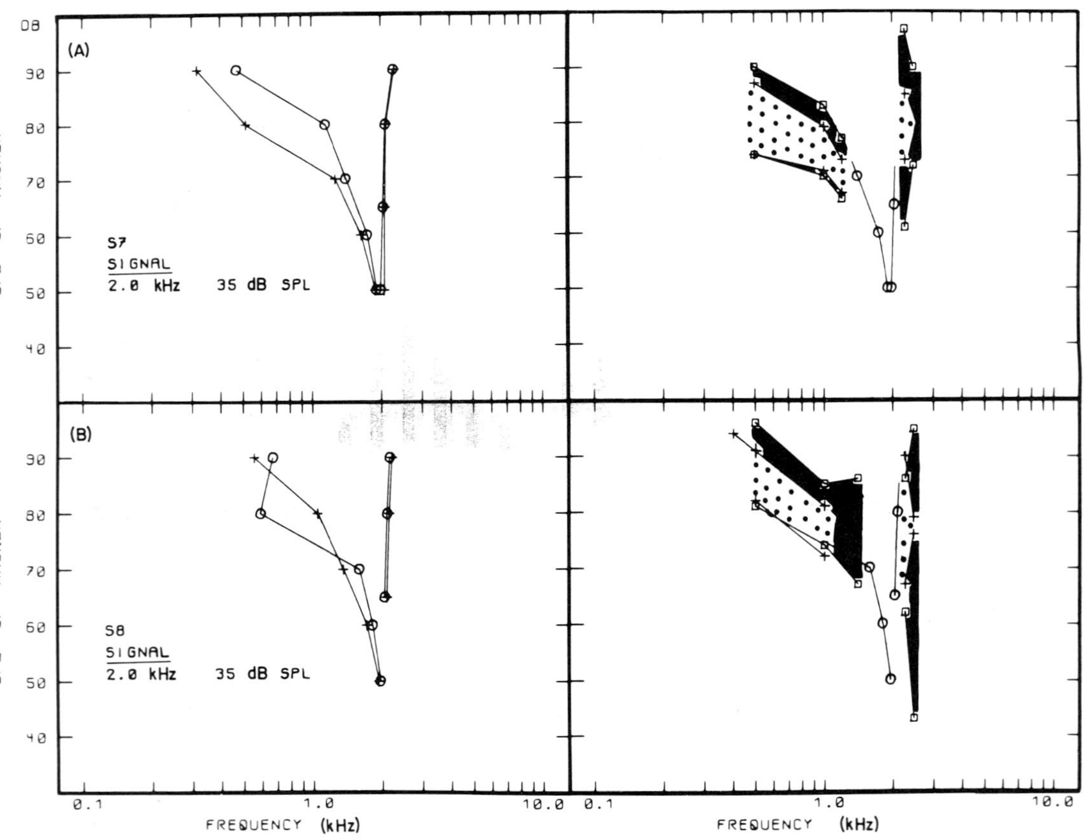
(A)
SPL OF MASKER
S7
SIGNAL
2.0 kHz   35 dB SPL
(B)
S8
SIGNAL
2.0 kHz   35 dB SPL
FREQUENCY (kHz)
FREQUENCY (kHz)

structure is altered by a barely measurable amount, but suppression is reduced and even eliminated on the high side. All of these changes occurred in the absence of measurable changes in auditory sensitivity.

Whereas the data in Figs. 45 and 46 show results on tuning and suppression in the absence of a measurable TTS, Figs. 47 to 50 show effects on tuning and suppression that were measured during time when TTS ranged from 5 to 20 dB. The major result of these latter data is that in the presence of TTS at the probe frequency, the low side of the tuning curve is shifted downward (lower level maskers are needed) and the high side is unaffected, unless auditory suppression on the high side is eliminated completely. Even when small amounts of suppression are measurable on the high side there is little or no change in the high side of the tuning curve. When there was no measurable TTS at the probe frequency but 10–15 dB TTS at adjacent frequencies, there were no measurable effects on tuning or on suppression.

In Fig. 47, tuning curves are affected (TTSs of 8–12 dB from 1.5 to 2.5 kHz) only on the low side, and differently for each observer. The high-side tuning is unaffected. Suppression is reduced (shaded areas) on both sides but significant amounts of suppression are still measured (dotted areas). We do not know why these two subjects differ on the low side with respect to the effects on tuning. Apparently, the reason is unrelated to suppression as the suppression data for these two subjects are qualitatively and quantitatively similar. On the high side, we should like to stress the fact that while tuning was unaffected and suppression effects were reduced, there were *still* measurable regions of suppression.

Figure 48 shows data for four subjects exposed to two separate bands of noise. The strategy was to produce 0 TTS at the probe frequency and 5–15 dB TTS at adjacent frequencies. For two subjects, shown in Fig. 48A and B, our strategy was unsuccessful in that TTS was 5–8 dB at the probe frequency and 10–15 dB at 1.5 and 2.5 kHz. For both of these subjects, the effects of TTS at the probe and adjacent frequencies are to produce small but measurable changes on the low side of the tuning curve, to have no effects on the high side of the tuning curve, and to have reduced suppression on both sides (S6) or just the high side (S9, suppression was not measurable on the low side either pre- or postexposure). For the other two subjects, our strategy was successful (S8, S5, Fig. 48C and D). TTS was ±2 dB at the probe frequency and decreased to 10–12 dB at 1.5 and 2.5 kHz. Tuning curves were not changed. Suppression areas increased on the high

---

Figure 47 Effects of noise on psychophysical tuning curves (forward masking) and suppression. Symbols are described in Figs. 44 and 45. The noise was a narrow band (400 Hz) centered at 1.4 kHz. It was presented at 90 dB SPL for 8 hours. TTSs measured 3–8 min after termination of the exposure were 8 dB at 1.5 kHz, 12 dB at 2.0 kHz, and 10 dB at 2.5 kHz for subject S7(A), and 8 dB at 1.5 kHz, 8 dB at 2.0 kHz, and 8 dB at 2.5 kHz for subject S8 (B). Although auditory sensitivity for the probe signal is reduced by 10–15 dB, only the low side of the tuning curve is affected. The high side is unaltered. Suppression on the high side is reduced but still measurable. On the low side suppression is reduced for both subjects; however, the tuning curve narrows for one subject (S8) and increases for the other (S7).

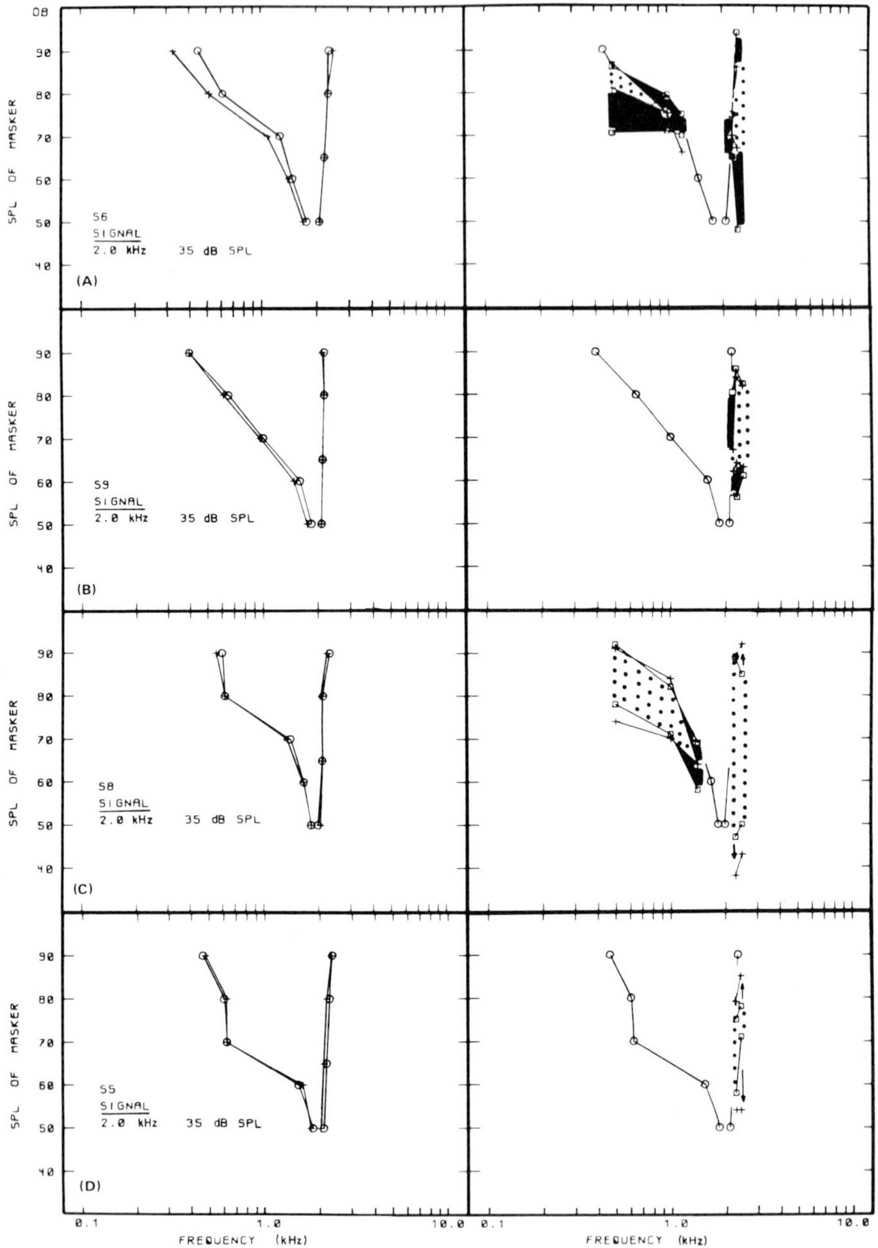

Figure 48 Effects of a 16-hour noise on psychophysical tuning curves (forward masking) and suppression for four subjects (A–D). The noise was an octave band centered at 500 Hz (89 dB SPL) and an octave band centered at 2.0 kHz (83 dB SPL). Skirts were 24 dB/octave and the octave-band levels of each noise were set to produce TTSs from 500 to 1800 Hz and 2400 to 4.0 kHz. Previous TTS data suggested that we could expose subjects to this two-band noise and produce 0 TTS at the probe frequency and 5–15 dB TTS in adjacent frequency regions. For some subjects this procedure was successful. Symbols are as described for Figs. 44 and 45. Arrows in (C) and (D), right-hand side, indicate postexposure increases in the range of suppression.

side for both subjects. For subject S8 low-side suppression was affected minimally if at all. The increase in suppression areas is difficult to explain. On the one hand it may reflect a narrowing of the spectrum of the probe because of TTS at frequency regions adjacent to the spectral peak. When a background noise is used to mask energy splatter of the probe, suppression effects increase; however, the tuning curve also changes shape (O'Malley and Feth, 1979). Thus, observed increases in suppression unaccompanied by changes in tuning curve shape may be unrelated to the energy splatter problem. Again, we should like to emphasize that for all the subjects in Fig. 48, the high side of the tuning curve is unaffected by TTS and that, while suppression areas may have increased or decreased, it was still measurable.

Figure 49 contains both forward and simultaneous masking data for the same subject using identical signals. First, we will discuss the forward masking data. TTS was 16 to 25 dB when the data in Fig. 49A were obtained. The low-frequency side of the tuning curve was lowered, the high side was not changed significantly (i.e., postexposure data were within the range of preexposure data), and suppression (Fig. 49A, right) was reduced but measurable. Measurements in Fig. 49B were made when TTS was 7–13 dB with a 25 dB SPL probe. Note that the forward masking tuning curve is altered on both the low side and the high side. On the high side measurable changes in tuning occur for a masker level of 80 dB SPL. At a masker level of 65 dB, postexposure tuning is equal to preexposure tuning. Note as well that suppression (Fig. 49B, right) is not measurable.

Data in Fig. 50 are like those in Fig. 49 with a notable exception: the high side of the tuning curve is unaffected and suppression is measurable. The forward-masking data in Figs. 49 and 50 thus support the contention that the high side of the tuning curve is unaffected by TTS *unless* the suppression mechanism is *completely* inoperative. When suppression is not measurable, the tuning curve on the high side is then broadened. Tuning on the low side appears to decrease when TTS is present and this decrease in tuning occurs independently of changes in the high side of the tuning curve or in suppression measured on either the high side or low side.

Data from Figs. 49 and 50 have been replotted on Fig. 51 to emphasize a point. Note that whereas the SPL of the probe signal is 25 or 35 dB SPL, the sensation level of the probe varies from 5 to 22 dB. Over this range of sensation levels the low sides of the curves are clearly different, but perfectly rank-ordered with respect to sensation level. That is, as sensation level is increased from 5 to 22 dB SL the tuning curve becomes narrower. On the high side the striking feature is the similarity of the data regardless of the shape of the low side of the tuning curve and the SL of the probe signal. There is one aberrant data point ($\triangle$, Fig. 51A). However, this is the example from Fig. 48 where high-side suppression was eliminated. It would thus appear that for probe tones covering a range of at least 22 dB or so (probably greater) the high-side slope is invariant, providing the mechanism responsible for suppression has not been rendered totally inoperative. The shape of the low side of the tuning curve is determined by the (effec-

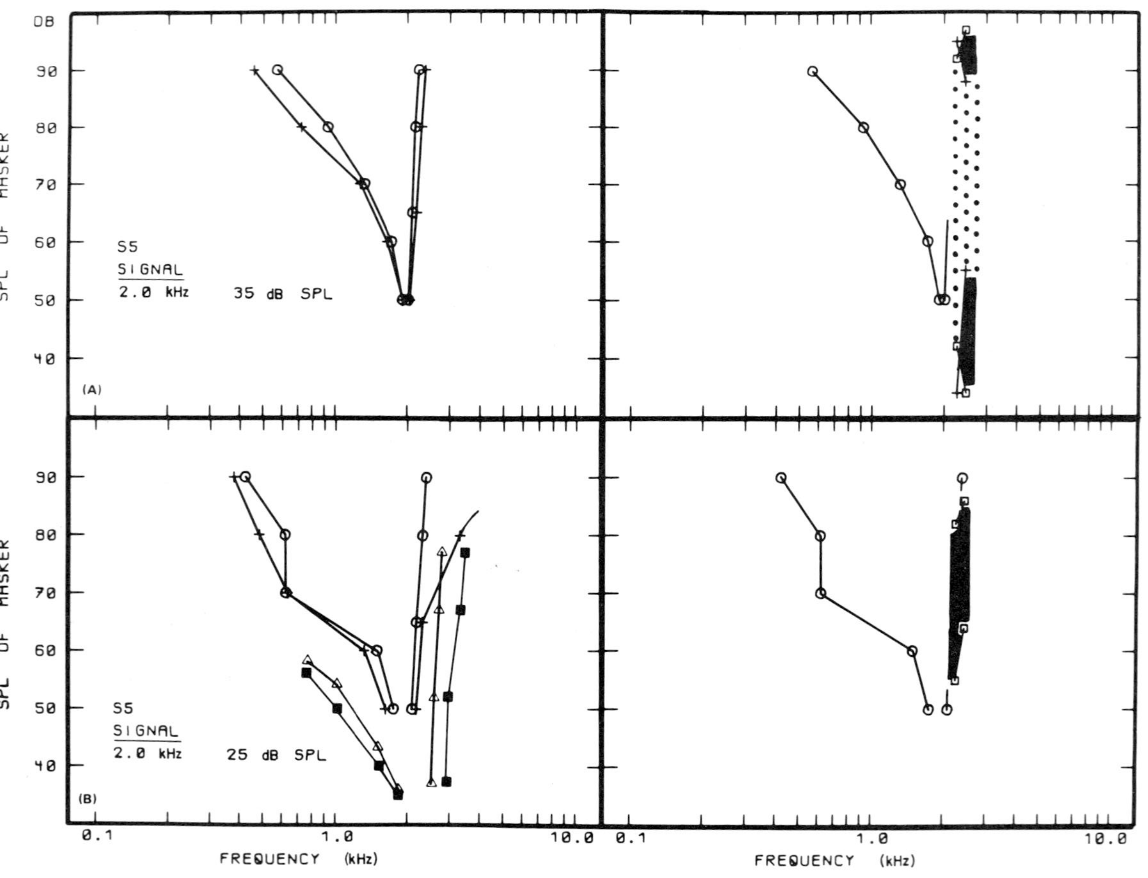

DB
90
80
70
60
50
40
SPL OF MASKER
S5
SIGNAL
2.0 kHz
35 dB SPL
(A)
90
80
70
60
50
40
SPL OF MASKER
S5
SIGNAL
2.0 kHz
25 dB SPL
(B)
0.1
1.0
10.0
FREQUENCY (kHz)
0.1
1.0
10.0
FREQUENCY (kHz)

tive) level of the probe signal. Data from Figs. 49 through 51 support this conclusion as do most of the data from Figs. 47 and 48. In addition, we believe physiological data reported by Bauer (1978) provide excellent qualitative agreement (see Fig. 23). In Fig. 23, note the invariance of the high side of the tuning curve for probes over a 20–dB range, and that the low side is determined by the level of the probe. In other psychophysical experiments, however, data suggest that when the effects of energy splatter are controlled by presenting a wide-band masker the shape of the tuning curve is independent of probe level on both the high and low side (Nelson and Turner, 1980; Green *et al.*, 1981). We cannot resolve these differences between our psychophysical data and data of others.

When temporary changes are produced in tuning or in suppression, the validity of these changes can be judged by following the time course of the recovery of the change. Figure 52 shows the recovery of the high side of the psychophysical tuning curve to preexposure values. Note that recovery can be complete in 2 hours (or less), or it may require less than 16 hours. For S6 (crosses) we show in Fig. 53 that recovery of suppression at 2.4 kHz is rapid and nearly returns to preexposure values in 2 hours. If our explanation of high-side tuning is correct, i.e., tuning on the high side is invariant providing the mechanism for suppression is in any way operative, then the tuning curve on the high side should return to its preexposure state prior to the return of suppression to its preexposure state. The data in Figs. 51 and 52 (S6) provide only equivocal support for this notion.

With many subjects, an attempt was made to assess the changes in tuning and in suppression as a function of the duration of the exposure or the time after the exposure. This proved to be a difficult task. For some subjects when changes in tuning or suppression occurred we had selected the inappropriate suppressor frequency or masker level. In others, we monitored the low side, and all changes occurred on the high side. In many subjects, we monitored the high side, and no changes in tuning were measured. Lastly, in some subjects we produced TTSs at the probe frequency that were too large (25–35 dB), and the subjects could not detect the 25 or 35 dB SPL probe. Thus, the few data obtained are in Figs. 52 and 53.

Figure 49 Effects of exposure to noise on psychophysical tuning curves and suppression of one subject. Forward masking with a probe level of 35 dB SPL is shown in A (left), and suppression is shown in A (right). B (left) shows both simultaneous and forward masking for a 25 dB SPL probe. Suppression in forward masking for a 25-dB probe is shown in B (right). Simultaneous masking is shown by a filled square (postexposure) or unfilled triangle (preexposure). Other symbols are as described for Figs. 44 and 45. The noise exposure was a narrow-band noise centered at 1.4 kHz, and was presented at 90 dB SPL for 24 hours. Data in (A) were obtained 8–25 min after a 20-hour exposure (TTS = 16 to 25 dB from 1500 Hz to 3.0 kHz). Data in (B) were obtained 1.5 hours after 24-hour exposure (TTS = 7 to 13 dB from 1500 Hz to 3000 kHz). Note in B (right) that suppression is eliminated and the high side of the tuning curve in forward masking (B, left) is changed.

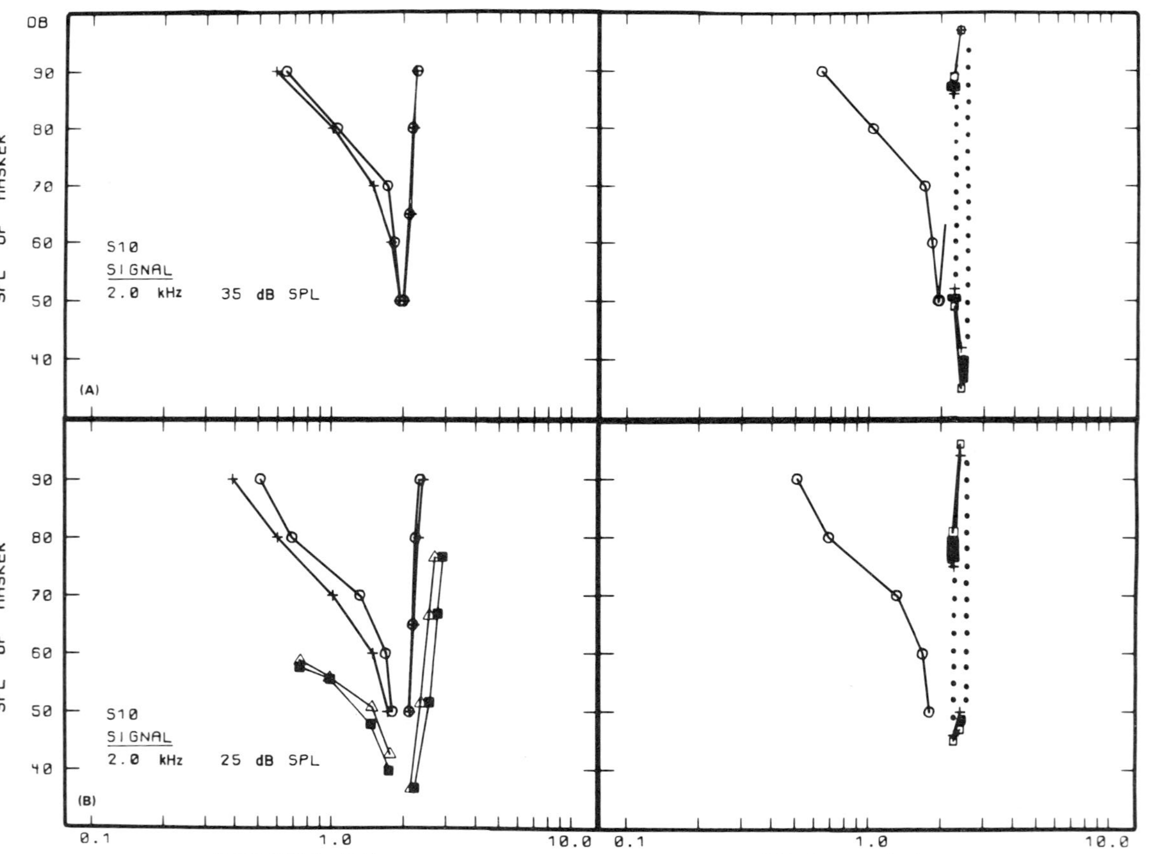

Figure 50   As for Fig. 48 except the data were obtained from another subject. (A) Tuning curves and suppression measured at postexposure times of 8–25 min after a 20-hour exposure. TTSs were 12–26 dB from 1.5–3.0 kHz. (B) Same, but after a 24-hour exposure and at recovery times of 1–1.5 hours. TTSs were 6–12 dB from 1.5 to 3.0 kHz.

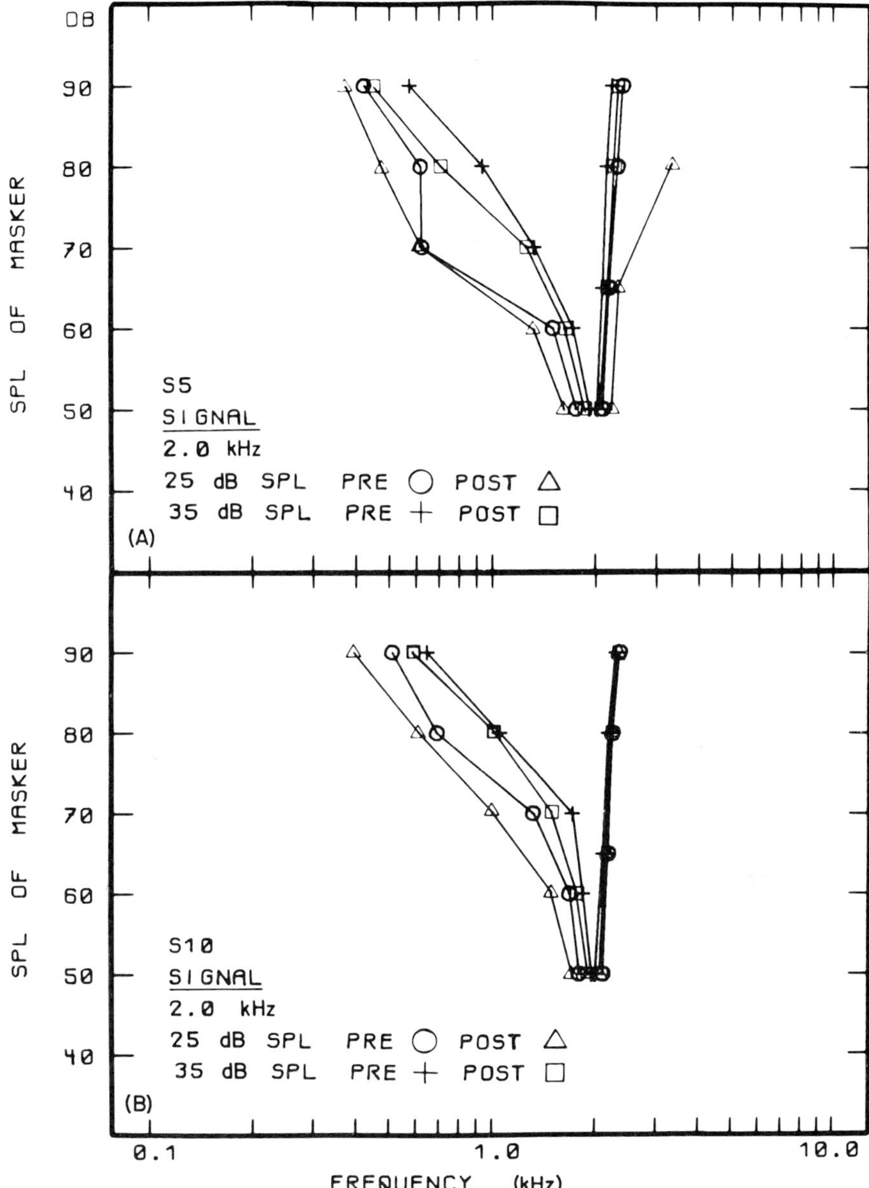

Figure 51 Pre- and postexposure forward masking data for 25 and 35 dB SPL probe signals from Fig. 49 are replotted in A and the data from Fig. 50 are replotted in B. For both subjects the low sides of the tuning curves show considerable variation. This variation is correlated perfectly with the estimated sensation level of the probe signals, i.e., as the estimated sensation level increases, higher masker levels are required, thereby narrowing the tuning curve. On the high side essentially one line fits all the data with one exception, S5, 25 dB SPL postexposure. Recall from Fig. 49 that for this condition and subject, suppression on the high side was totally eliminated by the noise exposure.

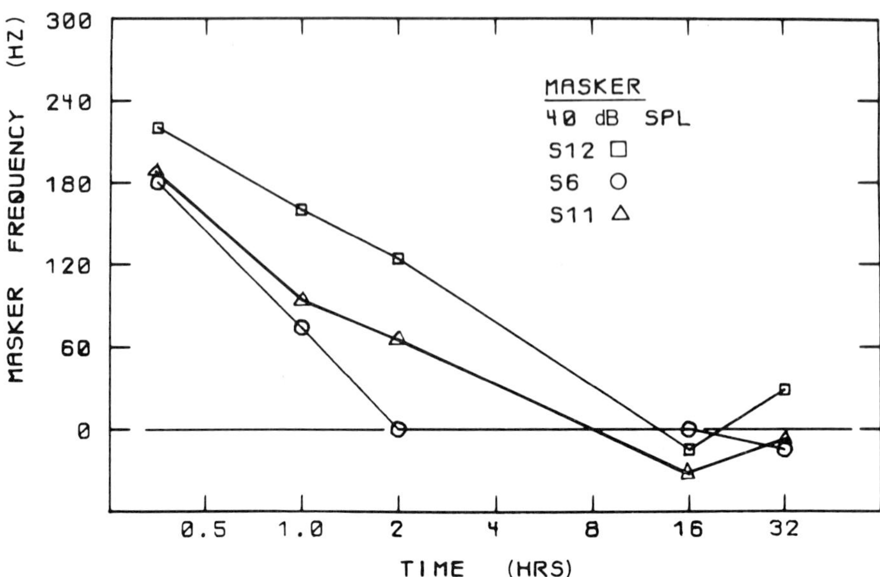

Figure 52 Recovery of the high side of the psychophysical tuning curve (forward masking) to preexposure values for three subjects. Ordinate is the shift in the masker frequency from its preexposure value.

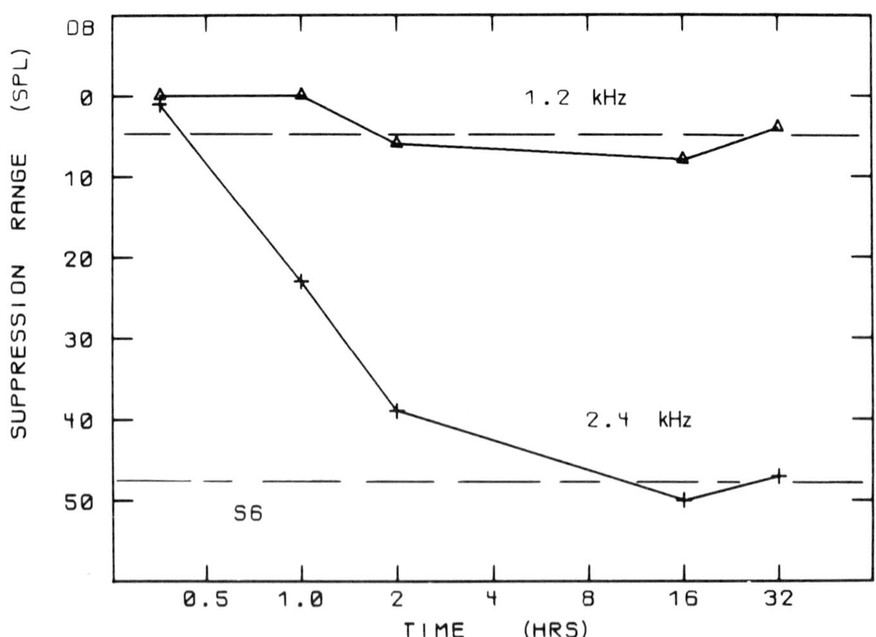

Figure 53 Recovery of suppression on the low side (1.2 kHz) and high side (2.4 kHz) of the psychophysical tuning curves (forward masking, 2-kHz probe). Ordinate is the range of suppression at either 1.2 or 2.4 kHz. Dashed lines indicate preexposure values.

VI. DISCUSSION

One of the reasons behind our psychophysical and physiological studies with humans was to find indices of auditory function that were more sensitive to injury of the ear than the pure tone audiogram and other traditional clinical measurements of hearing. From the data discussed, there appear to be several measurements which are more sensitive than the audiogram. These are (1) low side and high side of the tuning curve in simultaneous masking; (2) confounding of the tuning curve in simultaneous masking by the effects of the combination tone $(2f_1 - f_2)$; (3) evoked responses (ear canal recordings), especially the whole-nerve action potential of the auditory nerve; (4) the high side of the tuning curve in forward masking; and (5) auditory suppression in forward masking. In some instances we believe the information to be gained is of questionable merit and is difficult to interpret. For example, poor recordings of the whole-nerve action potential can be attributed to poor recording conditions or to a decrease in synchronous neural firing. Also, less than 200 missing outer hair cells in the base of the cochlea apparently can have disastrous effects on synchronous neural activity (Eldredge *et al.*, 1973). As evoked responses arising from the auditory nerve are difficult to obtain and to interpret, so too is the measurement of tuning curves and suppression in forward masking. With young, alert, normal hearing subjects, it is a difficult task. With patients it is probably too difficult a listening task and there is probably too little time available for training. This leaves us with simultaneous masking. We suggest that the major clinical dividend from tuning-curve studies will be in the application of the simultaneous masking paradigm for tuning curves. Moreover, we suggest that the high side be assessed by adjusting the frequency of a masker which is fixed in level, and that the low side be assessed by adjusting the intensity of a masker which is fixed in frequency. Beats can be avoided by maintaining an appropriate frequency separation between the masker and signal. Moreover, the confounding effects of combination tones or the absence of such effects can be assessed as well. Lastly, the entire procedure can be automated including the use of a forced-choice, adaptive psychophysical method. We would predict significant correlations between tuning curve data as described and other measures of auditory function. That the measurement of simultaneous masking with patients can yield dividends has been shown previously (see Martin and Picket, 1970; Thornton and Abbas, 1980). Such data in combination with "ear canal" measurements of acoustic distortion products, particularly of the cubic tone, may prove to be clinically useful.

Another measure of auditory function that has remained mysterious is frequency discrimination. For example, in persons with sensorineural hearing loss frequency discrimination is highly variable. It ranges from normal to clearly abnormal. Indeed, we have been puzzled by the many sets of data. Brandt (1967), for example, shows that after exposure to noise, frequency discrimination was unaffected in frequency regions of TTS, but was abnormal at lower frequency regions where TTS was negligible. Similarly, Weir *et al.* (1977) in an extensive study of frequency discrimination in normal-hearing subjects show that the frequency difference limen is dependent on both signal intensity and signal frequency. In addition, at frequencies of 200 and 800 Hz, the function relating the frequency difference limen to the frequency of the signal was nonmonotonic. That is at sensation levels ranging from 5 to 20 dB, the difference limen was larger at 800 Hz than at 1.0 or 600 Hz. Weir *et al.* state "available models . . . based on current knowledge of the peripheral auditory system appear to have difficulty accounting for the interactions found between the frequency difference limen, sensation level, and signal frequency."

We may have gained some insight into the mechanism of frequency discrimination. Originally in our measurement of a psychophysical tuning curve the *level* of the masker was adjusted on both the high and low sides. This proved to be a difficult task on the high side and a quite simple one on the low side. We then continued this procedure on the low side but adjusted frequency of the masker on the high side (masker fixed in level). This proved to be a simple task for most (but not all subjects) in simultaneous masking. In forward masking, frequency is adjusted on both sides. Casual, almost incidental observations of pilot data indicated that variance changed dramatically when one compared low-level maskers to high-level maskers. In addition, one of us (JHM) had little difficulty at 1.0 kHz, but considerable difficulty at 4.0 kHz, with low-level maskers. This subject has normal frequency discrimination at 1.0 kHz but well below average frequency skills at 4.0 kHz for low-level signals. Our laboratory-verbal explanation was that "some listeners have steep skirts and use them very well. Others have poor skirts and have little to use." It also raised the issue of the high-frequency slope of a physiological tuning curve and the question of a dependence on signal level and characteristic frequency. Was it possible that the frequency difference limen with its dependence on frequency and sensation level could be explained by the high-frequency slopes of tuning curves with their dependence on CF and level?

Figure 54 shows the high-frequency slope of a tuning curve (dB/octave) as a function of the sound pressure level (dB) of the signal (*not* the sensation level). These data are from Fig. 5. There are some irregularities in the figure which are due to the stochastic process of obtaining automated tuning curves. Also, a measurement error of a "few" Hertz can change the calculated slope from 1000 to 500 dB/octave. Here, we wish to emphasize two points. One is that the slope changes dramatically as the signal level is increased by 10 dB from the threshold of the unit. The other is that, in gerbils, fibers with CFs of 6.4 and 13 kHz achieve nearly all of the change in slope over about a 10-dB range in signal,

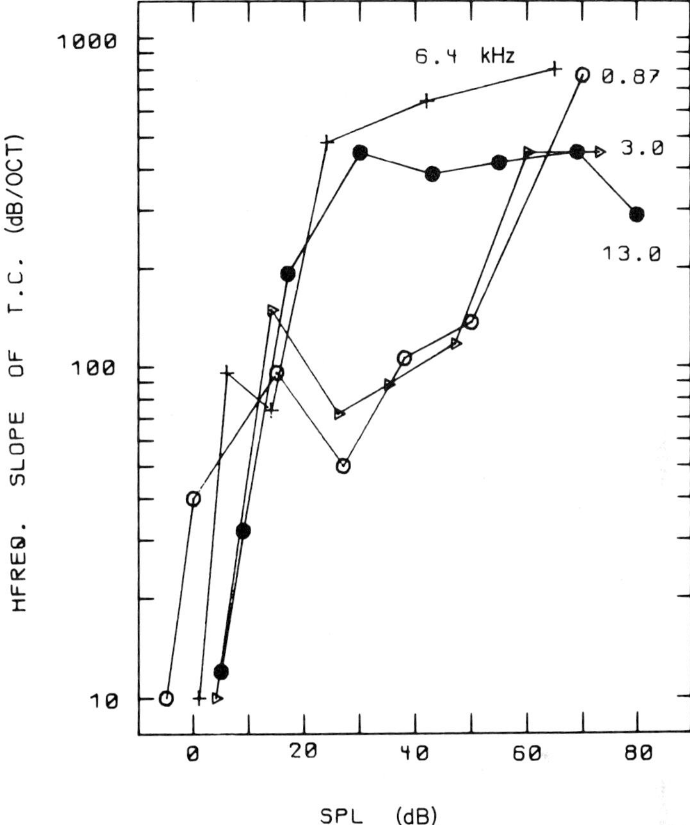

Figure 54 Slopes of the high-frequency side of physiological tuning curves obtained from single-unit recordings of primary auditory neurons of gerbil. Raw data are shown in Fig. 5. Slopes were calculated over level intervals of 10 dB, and the resulting slopes are plotted at the levels corresponding to the midpoints of the respective intervals. The slope at CF (0 dB) was taken to be zero. Please note that for units with CFs of 870 Hz to 3.0 kHz the slope of the high side of the tuning curve increases from 10 dB/octave at low sound pressure levels to about 150 dB/octave from 15 to 50 dB SPL, and then increases to 600–800 dB/octave at levels above about 65 dB SPL. Please note as well that the slopes for units with CFs of 6 and 13 kHz differ significantly from units with CFs of 0.87 and 3.0 kHz, especially over the range from 20 to 60 dB SPL.

whereas the change in lower frequency fibers occurs over a wider range of levels. Thus, the high-frequency skirt is dependent upon level and CF. Currently, we are examining single-unit data from cats, gerbils, and chinchillas. The strategy is to find for each species a number of fibers with CFs covering the low-, mid-, and high-frequency regions. When their respective thresholds at CF are normalized, our prediction is that averaged single-unit data will provide a data-bound explanation of frequency discrimination in psychophysics. In other words, we believe the dependence of frequency discrimination on signal frequency and sensation level will be explained on the basis of peripheral auditory physiology, particularly the high-frequency slope of a tuning curve. Even the nonmonotonic behavior observed by Weir *et al.* (1977) may be explained. For example, at frequencies below 1.0 kHz, high-frequency slopes of tuning curves often display irregularities particularly at signal levels of 5–20 dB SL. An alternative explanation might involve an interaction between a temporal mechanism with peak efficiency near 600 Hz and a spectral mechanism with its effectiveness decreasing below 1.0 kHz. This argument attributes frequency discrimination below 500 Hz to temporal information. Additional comments await our reanalysis of our own data and the data of other investigators.

Given the hypothesis on frequency discrimination and both the psychophysical and physiological data which show that the high-frequency slope is altered only when high-side suppression is eliminated, it follows that auditory suppression is a significant factor in frequency discrimination. Is it possible that the unusual high-frequency skirts shown in Fig. 30 (1.0 kHz, simultaneous masking) and Fig. 33 (4.0 kHz, simultaneous masking, postexposure) reflect the elimination of the suppression mechanism? We are reluctant to speculate on this point inasmuch as suppression effects are supposed to be minimal in simultaneous masking.

At this point we are somewhat puzzled about what to do with the low side of a tuning curve and the small amounts of suppression that one can measure psychophysically. If one adopts our hypothesis about the functional significance of high-side tuning and suppression, then the low-side tuning and suppression are unnecessary for frequency selectivity. What do they do? Our current speculation is that the low side of the tuning curve with its shallow slopes and low-side suppression plays more of a role in intensity discrimination and in temporal processing (including phase-locking) than in frequency selectivity. Conversely, the high-frequency side of tuning and suppression contribute little to intensity and temporal processing but, as stated earlier, are probably responsible in large part for frequency selectivity. The coupling of low-side tuning and high-side tuning is very loose, barely existent, and so is the coupling of low-side tuning to low-side suppression. Similarly, the coupling of high-side suppression to low-side suppression is loose as well. In other words, the ear has the best of two worlds—the world of sharp frequency selectivity and the world of excellent intensity discrimination (which is essentially independent of frequency) and temporal resolving power. As stated in Section I, in the physical world excellent temporal resolving power is usually achieved at the expense of spectral information, and keen frequency resolving power is usually achieved at the expense of temporal information. In the ear, however, we can use one filter for spectral information, and we can use another, nearly independent one for temporal and intensity information. The tip of the tuning curve provides excellent auditory sensitivity by exploiting both filters. These speculations are probably too simplistic to be correct. On the other hand, when explanations are very complicated, they are often incorrect.

Acknowledgments

Original psychophysical and human physiological data reported here were obtained with grant support from the National Institute of Environmental Health Sciences (NIEHS, ES-01301). Larry Kulish was heavily involved in the psychophysical studies. Original physiological data from animals were obtained with a South Carolina Biomedical Research Grant. Preparation of the manuscript was supported in part by the NIEHS grant, in part, by a contract from National Institutes of Neurological and Communicative Disorders and Stroke (N01-NS-1-2381), and in part by a grant from NSF. Nancy Topham, Janet Simmons, and Donna Ostrander spent many hours on the preparation of the manuscript. Their assistance is appreciated and gratefully acknowledged.

References

Abbas, P. J., and Gorga, M. P. (1981). AP responses in forward-masking paradigms and their relationship to responses of auditory-nerve fibers. *J. Acoust. Soc. Am.* **69**, 492–499.

Allen, J. B. (1977). Cochlear micromechanics—a mechanism for transforming mechanical to neural tuning within the cochlea. *J. Acoust. Soc. Am.* **62**, 930–939.

Allen, J. B. (1980). Cochlear micromechanics—A physical model of transduction. *J. Acoust. Soc. Am.* **68**, 1660–1670.

Anderson, D. J., Rose, J. E., Hind, J. E., and Brugge, J. F. (1971). Temporal position of discharges in single auditory nerve fibers within the cycle of a sinewave stimulus: frequency and intensity effects. *J. Acoust. Soc. Am.* **49**, 1131–1139.

Anderson, S. D., and Kemp, D. T. (1979). The evoked cochlear mechanical response in laboratory primates. *Arch. Otorhinolaryngol.* **224**, 47–54.

ANSI (1969). "Specifications for Audiometers." S3, 6-1969 Am. Natl. Stan. Inst., New York.

Bauer, J. W. (1978). Tuning curves and masking functions of auditory-nerve fibers in cat. *Sensory Processes* **2**, 156–172.

Békésy, G. v. (1928). Zur Theorie des Hörens; die Schwingungsform des Basilarmembrans. *Physiol. Z.* **29**, 793–810.

Békésy, G., v. (1947). The variation of phase along the basilar membrane with sinusoidal vibrations. *J. Acoust. Soc. Am.* **19**, 452–460.

Békésy, G., v. (1958). Funneling in the nervous system and its role in loudness and sensation intensity on the skin. *J. Acoust. Soc. Am.* **30**, 399–412.

Békésy, G., v. (1959). Similarities between hearing and skin sensation. *Psychol. Rev.* **66**, 1–22.

Békésy, G., v. (1960). "Experiments in Hearing." McGraw-Hill, New York.

Benitez, L. D., Eldredge, D. H., and Templer, J. W. (1972). Temporary threshold shifts in chinchilla: electrophysiological correlates. *J. Acoust. Soc. Am.* **52**, 1115–1123.

Bode, H. W. (1945). "Network Analysis and Feedback Amplifier Design." Van Nostrand Reinhold, Princeton, New Jersey.

Boer, E., de, and Bouwmeester, J. (1974). Critical bands and sensorineural hearing loss. *Audiology* **13**, 263–259.

Brandt, J. F. (1967). Frequency discrimination following exposure to noise. *J. Acoust. Soc. Am.* **41**, 448–457.

Brugge, J. F., Anderson, D. J., Hind, J. E., and Rose, J. E. (1969). Time strcture of discharges in single auditory nerve fibers of the squirrel monkey in response to complex periodic sounds. *J. Neurophysiol.* **32,** 386–401.

Butterworth, S. (1930). On the theory of filter amplifiers. *Exp. Wireless* **7,** 536–541.

Carlson, A. B. (1968). "Communication Systems: An Introduction to Signals and Noise in Electrical Communication." McGraw-Hill, New York.

Carterette, F. C., Friedman, M. P., and Lovell, J. D. (1969). Mach bands in hearing. *J. Acoust. Soc. Am.* **45,** 986–998.

Chistovich, L. A. (1957). Frequency characteristics of masking effect. *Biofizika* **2,** 743–755.

Cody, A. R., and Johnstone, B. M. (1980). Single auditory neuron response during acute acoustic trauma. *Hear. Res.* **3,** 3–16.

Cohen, M. F. (1982). Detection threshold microstructure and its effect on temporal integration data. *J. Acoust. Soc. Am.* **71,** 405–409.

Dallos, P., and Cheatham, M. A. (1976). Compound action potential (AP) tuning curves. *J. Acoust. Soc. Am.* **59,** 591–597.

Dallos, P., and Cheatham, M. A. (1977). Analog of two-tone suppression in whole nerve response. *J. Acoust. Soc. Am.* **62,** 1048–1052.

Dallos, P., and Harris, D. (1978). Properties of auditory nerve responses in absence of outer hair cells. *J. Neurophysiol.* **41,** 365–383.

Dallos, P., Ryan, A., Harris, D., McGee, T., and Ozdamar, O. (1977). Cochlear frequency sensitivity in the presence of hair cell damage. *In* "Psychophysics and Physiology of Hearing" (E. F. Evans and J. P. Wilson, eds.), pp. 249–258. Academic Press, New York.

Dallos, P., Harris, D. M., Ozdamar, O., and Ryan, A. (1978). Behavioral, compound action potential and single unit thresholds: relationship in normal and abnormal ears. *J. Acoust. Soc. Am.* **64,** 151–157.

Dallos, P., Harris, D. M., Relkin, E., and Cheatham, M. A. (1980). Two-tone suppression and intermodulation distortion in the cochlea: Effect of outer hair cell lesions. *In* "Psychophysical, Physiological, and Behavioral Studies in Hearing" (G. van den Brink and F. A. Bilsen, eds.), pp. 242–249. Delft Univ. Press, Delft, The Netherlands.

Davis, H. (1976). Electric response audiometry. *Ann. Otol. Rhinol. Laryngol. Suppl. 28,* pp. 5–96.

Davis, H., and Hirsh, S. K. (1979). A slow brain stem response for low-frequency audiometry. *Audiology* **18,** 445–461.

Davis, H., Derbyshire, A. J., Kemp, E. H., Lurie, M. H., and Upton, M. (1935). Functional and histological changes in the cochlea of the guinea pig resulting from prolonged stimulation. *J. Gen. Psychol.* **12,** 251–278.

Duifhuis, H., and Van deVorst, J. J. W. (1980). Mechanics and nonlinearity of hair cell stimulation. *Hear. Res.* **2,** 493–504.

Eggermont, J. J. (1977). Compound action potential tuning curves in normal and pathological human ears. *J. Acoust. Soc. Am.* **62,** 1247–1251.

Ehmer, R. H. (1959). Masking patterns of tones. *J. Acoust. Soc. Am.* **31,** 1115–1120.

Eldredge, D. H., Mills, J. H., and Bohne, B. A. (1973). Anatomical, behavioral, and electrophysiological observations on chinchillas after long exposures to noise. *Adv. Oto-Rhino-Laryngol.* **20,** 64–81.

Evans, E. F. (1975a). The sharpening of cochlear frequency selectivity in the normal and abnormal cochlea. *Audiology* **14,** 419–442.

Evans, E. F. (1975b). Cochlear nerve and cochlear nucleus. *In* "Physiology" (W. D. Keidel and W. D. Neff, eds.), Vol. 5, Part II, Ch. 1, Springer-Verlag, Berlin and New York.

Evans, E. F., and Wilson, J. P. (1973). The frequency selectivity of the cochlea. *In* "Basic Mechanisms In Hearing" (A. Moller, ed.), pp. 519–551. Academic Press, New York.

Evans, E. F., and Wilson, J. P. (1975). Cochlear tuning properties: Concurrent basilar membrane and single nerve fiber measurements. *Science,* **190,** 1281–1221.

Festen, J. M., and Plomp, R. (1981). Relations between auditory functions in normal hearing. *J. Acoust. Soc. Am.* **70**, 356–369.

Feth, L. E., Oesterie, E. C., and Kidd, G. (1979). Frequency selectivity after noise exposure. *J. Acoust. Soc. Am. Suppl. 1,* **65**, S118.

Fletcher, H. (1940). Auditory patterns. *Rev. Mod. Phys.* **12**, 47–65.

Florentine, M., Buss, S., Scharf, B., and Zwicker, E. (1980). Frequency selectivity in normally-hearing and hearing impaired observers. *J. Speech Hear. Res.* **23**, 646–669.

Fourier, J. B. J. (1829). La theorie analytique de la chaleur. *Acad. Sci. Paris Mem. Acad. R. Sci.* **8**, 581–622.

Galambos, R., and Davis, H. (1943). The response of single auditory-nerve fibers to acoustic stimulation. *J. Neurophysiol.* **6**, 39–57.

Galambos, R., and Davis, H. (1944). Inhibition of activity in single auditory nerve fibers by acoustic stimulation. *J. Neurophysiol.* **7**, 287–304.

Galambos, R., and Davis, H. (1948). Action potentials from single auditory-nerve fibers? *Science* **108**, 513.

Gardner, M. B. (1947). Short duration auditory fatigue as a method of classifying hearing impairment. *J. Acoust. Soc. Am.* **19**, 178–190.

Geisler, C. D., Rhode, W. S., and Kennedy, D. T. (1974). Responses to tonal stimuli of single auditory nerve fibers and their relationships to basilar membrane motion in the squirrel monkey. *J. Neurophys.* **37**, 1156–1172.

Green, D. M. (1976). "An Introduction to Hearing." Erlbaum, Hillsdale, New Jersey.

Green, D. M., Shelton, B. R., Picardi, M. C., and Hafter, E. R. (1981). Psychophysical tuning curves independent of signal level. *J. Acoust. Soc. Am.* **69**, 1758–1762.

Greenwood, D. D. (1971). Aural combination tones and auditory masking. *J. Acoust. Soc. Am.* **50**, 502–543.

Hall, J. L. (1977a). Spatial differentiation as auditory "second filter": assessment in a non-linear model of the basilar membrane. *J. Acoust. Soc. Am.* **61**, 520–524.

Hall, J. L. (1977b). Two-tone suppression in a nonlinear model of the basilar membrane. *J. Acoust. Soc. Am.* **61**, 802–810.

Hall, J. L. (1980). Cochlear models: Two-tone suppression and the second filter. *J. Acoust. Soc. Am.* **67**, 1722–1728.

Harris, D. M. (1979). Action potential suppression, tuning curves and thresholds: Comparison with single fiber data. *Hear. Res.* **1**, 133–154.

Harris, D. M., and DAllos, P. (1979). Forward masking of auditory nerve fiber responses. *J. Neurophysiol.* **42**, 1083–1107.

Harris, J. D., and Rawnsley, A. I. (1953). Patterns of cochlear adaption in three frequency regions. *J. Acoust. Soc. Am.* **25**, 760–764.

Harris, J. D., Rawnsley, A. I., and Kelsey, P. (1951). Studies in short-duration auditory fatigue: I. Frequency differences as a function of intensity. *J. Exp. Psychol.* **42**, 430–436.

Harrison, R. V. (1981). Rate-versus-intensity functions and related AP responses in normal and pathological guinea pig and human cochleas. *J. Acoust. Soc. Am.* **70**, 1036–1044.

Helmholtz, H. L. F. (1863). Die Lehre von den Tonempfindungen als physiologische Grundlage fur die Theorie der Musik. *In* "On the Sensations of Tone" (A. J. Ellis, trans. 1885). Reprinted by Dover, New York, 1954.

Henderson, D., Onishi, S., Eldredge, D. H., and Davis, H. (1969). A comparison of chinchilla auditory evoked response and behavioral response thresholds. *Percept. Psychophys.* **5**, 41–45.

Hensen, V. (1863). Morphologic der Schnecke des Menschen und der Saugethiere. *Z. Wiss. Zool.* **13**, 481–512.

Hind, J. E., Anderson, D. J., Brugge, J. F., and Rose, J. E. (1967). Coding of information pertaining to paired low-frequency tones in single auditory nerve fibers of the squirrel monkey. *J. Neurophysiol.* **30**, 794–816.

Hirsh, I. J. (1948). The influence of interaural phase on interaural summation and inhibition. *J. Acoust. Soc. Am.* **20**, 536–544.

Hirsh, I. J., and Bilger, R. C. (1955). Auditory threshold recovery after exposures to pure tones. *J. Acoust. Soc. Am.* **27**, 1186–1194.

Holton, T. (1980). Relations between frequency selectivity and two-tone rate suppression in lizard cochlear-nerve fibers. *Hear. Res.* **2**, 21–38.

Houtgast, T. (1972). Psychophysical evidence for lateral inhibition in hearing. *J. Acoust. Soc. Am.* **51**, 1885–1894.

Houtgast, T. (1973). Psychophysical experiments on 'tuning curves' and 'two-tone inhibition'. *Acoustica* **29**, 168–179.

Houtgast, T. (1974). Masking patterns and lateral inhibition. *In* "Facts and Models in Hearing" (E. Zwicker and E. Terhardt, eds.), pp. 258–265. Springer-Verlag, Berlin and New York.

Javel, E. (1981). Suppression of auditory nerve responses. I: Temporal analysis, intensity effects and suppression contours. *J. Acoust. Soc. Am.* **69**, 1735–1745.

Jerger, J. (1955). Influences of stimulus duration on the pure tone threshold during recovery from auditory fatigue. *J. Acoust. Soc. Am.* **27**, 121–125.

Jerger, J. F., Tillman, T. W., and Peterson, J. L. (1960). Masking by octave bands of noise in normal and impaired ears. *J. Acoust. Soc. Am.* **32**, 385–390.

Jesteadt, W. (1980). Frequency analysis in normal and hearing impaired listeners. *Ann. Otol., Rhinol., Laryngol.* **89** Suppl. 74, 88–95.

Jesteadt, W., Bacon, S. P., and Lehman, J. R. (1982). Forward masking as a function of frequency, masker level, and signal delay. *J. Acoust. Soc. Am.* **71**, 950–962.

Jewitt, D., and Williston, J. (1971). Auditory-evoked for fields averaged from the scalp of humans." *Brain* **94**, 681–696.

Johnson, D. H. (1980). The relationship between spike rate and synchrony in responses of auditory-nerve fibers to single tones. *J. Acoust. Soc. Am.* **68**, 1115–1122.

Johnson-Davies, D., and Patterson, R. (1979). Psychophysical tuning curves: Restricting the listening band to the signal region. *J. Acoust. Soc. Am.* **65**, 765–770.

Johnstone, B. M., and Boyle, A. J. F. (1967). Basilar membrane vibration examined with the Mossbauer technique. *Science* **158**, 389–390.

Kemp, D. T. (1978). Stimulated acoustic emissions from within the human auditory system. *J. Acoust. Soc. Am.* **64**, 1386–1391.

Kemp, D. T. (1979). Evidence of mechanical nonlinearity and frequency selective wave amplification in the cochlea. *Arch. Otorhinolaryngol.* **224**, 37–45.

Kemp, D. T. (1982). Cochlear echoes: Implications for noise-induced hearing loss. *In* "New Perspectives on Noise-Induced Hearing Loss" (R. Hamernik, D. Henderson, and R. Salvi, eds.), pp. 189–208. Raven, New York.

Khanna, S. M., and Leonard, D. G. B. (1982). Basilar membrane tuning in the cat cochlea. *Science* **215**, 305–306.

Kiang, N. Y. S., and Moxon, E. C. (1974). Tails of tuning curves of auditory-nerve fibers. *J. Acoust. Soc. Am.* **55**, 620–630.

Kiang, N. Y. S., Watanabe, T., Thomas, E. C., and Clark, L. F. (1965). "Discharge Patterns of Single Fibers in the Cat's Auditory Nerve." MIT Press, Cambridge, Massachusetts.

Kiang, N. Y. S., Moxon, E. C., and Levine, R. A. (1970). Auditory-nerve activity in cats with normal and abnormal cochleas. *In* "Sensorineural Hearing Loss" (G. Wolstenholme and J. Knight, eds.), pp. 241–268. Churchill, London.

Kiang, N. Y. S., Liberman, M. C., and Levine, R. A. (1976a). Auditory-nerve activity in cats exposed to ototoxic drugs and high-intensity sounds. *Ann. Otol. Rhinol. Laryngol.* **85,** 752–768.

Kiang, N. Y. S., Moxon, E. C., and Kahn, A. R. (1976b). The relationship of gross potentials recorded from the cochlea to single unit activity in the auditory nerve. *In* "Electrocochleography" (J. Ruben, C. Elberling, and G. Salomon, eds.), pp. 95–116. Univ. Park Press, Baltimore, Maryland.

Kim, D. O., and Molnar, C. E. (1975). Cochlear mechanics: Measurements and modesl. *In* "The Nervous System, Vol. 3, Human Communication and its Disorders" (D. Tower, ed.). Raven, New York.

Kim, D. O., and Molnar, C. E. (1979). A population study of cochlear nerve fibers: comparison of the spatial distributions of average data and phase locking measures of responses to single tones. *J. Neurophysiol.* **42,** 16–30.

Kim, D. O., Molnar, C. E., and Pfeiffer, R. R. (1973). A system of nonlinear differential equations modeling basilar-membrane motion. *J. Acoust. Soc. Am.* **54,** 1517–1529.

Kim, D. O., Molnar, C. E., Matthews, J. W., and Neely, S. T. (1980). Cochlear mechanics: nonlinear behavior in two-tone responses as reflected in cochlear-nerve-fiber responses and in ear-canal sound pressure. *J. Acoust. Soc. Am.* **67,** 1704–1721.

Klein, A. J. (1983a). Properties of the brain-stem response slow-wave component. I. Latency, amplitude and threshold sensitivity. *Arch. Otolaryngol.,* **109,** 6–12.

Klein, A. J. (1983b). Properties of the brain-stem response slow-wave component. II. Frequency specificity. *Arch. Otolaryngol.,* **109,** 74–78.

Klein, A. J., and Mills, J. H. (1981a). Physiological (waves I and V) and psychophysical tuning curves in human subjects. *J. Acoust. Soc. Am.* **69,** 760–768.

Klein, A. J., and Mills, J. H. (1981b). Physiological and psychophysical measures from humans with temporary threshold shift. *J. Acoust. Soc. Am.* **70,** 1045–1053.

Kreyszig, E. (1962). "Advanced Engineering Mathematics." Wiley, New York.

Lathi, B. P. (1965). "Signals, Systems and Communication." Wiley, New York.

Lathi, B. P. (1968). "Communication Systems." John Wiley and Sons, New York.

LePage, E. L., and Johnstone, B. M. (1980). Nonlinear mechanical behaviour of the basilar membrane in the basal turn of the guinea pig cochlea. *Hear. Res. 2,* 183–189.

Leshowitz, B. (1978). Measurements of the auditory stimulus. *In* "Handbook of Perception" (E. Carterette and M. Friedman, eds.), pp. 84–123. Academic Press, New York.

Leshowitz, B., and Lindstrom, R. (1977). Measurement of nonlinearities in listeners with sensorineural hearing loss. *In* "Psychophysics and Physiology of Hearing" (E. F. Evans and J. P. Wilson, eds.), pp. 27–30. Academic Press, New York.

Leshowitz, B., and Wightman, F. L. (1971). On-frequency masking with continuous sinusoids. *J. Acoustic Soc. Am.* **49,** 1180–1190.

Liberman, M. C. (1978). Auditory-nerve response from cats raised in a low-noise chamber. *J. Acoust. Soc. Am.* **63,** 442–455.

Liberman, M. C. (1980). Morphological differences among radial afferent fibers in the cat cochlea: An electron-microscopic study of serial sections. *Hear. Res. 3,* 45–63.

Liberman, M. C. (1982). The cochlear frequency map for the cat: Labeling auditory-nerve fibers of known characteristic frequency. *J. Acoust. Soc. Am.* **72,** 1441–1449.

Liberman, M. C., and Kiang, N. Y. S. (1978). Acoustic trauma in cats. *Acta Otolaryngol. Suppl.* **358.**

Liberman, M. C., and Mulroy, M. J. (1982). Acute and chronic effects of acoustic trauma: Cochlear pathology and auditory nerve physiology. *In* "New Perspectives on Noise-Induced Hearing Loss" (R. Hamernik, D. Henderson, and R. Salvi, eds.), pp. 105–136. Raven, New York.

Lufti, R. A., and Yost, W. A. (1980). Two-tone unmasking in the forward-masking procedure: suppression or perceptual cueing? *J. Acoust. Soc. Am.* **68,** 700–702.

Luscher, E., and Zwislicki, J. (1947). The decay of sensation and the remainder of adaptation after short pure-tone impulses on the ear. *Acta Oto-Laryngol.* **35**, 428–445.

Luscher, E., and Zwislocki, J. (1949). Adaptation of the ear to sound stimuli. *J. Acoust. Soc. Am.* **21**, 135–139.

McFadden, D., and Pasanen, E. G. (1979). Permanent changes in psychophysical tuning curves following exposure to weak steep-sided noise. *J. Acoust. Soc. Am.* **65**, (Suppl. 1), S118.

McGee, T., Ryan, A., and Dallos, P. (1976). Psychophysical tuning curves of chinchillas. *J. Acoust. Soc. Am.* **60**, 1146–1150.

Manley, G. A. (1978). Cochlear frequency sharpening—A new synthesis. *Acta Oto-Laryngol.* **85**, 167–176.

Margolis, R. M., and Goldberg, S. M. (1980). Auditory frequency selectivity in normal and presbycusic subjects. *J. Speech Hear. Res.* **23**, 603–613.

Martin, E. S., and Pickett, J. M. (1970). Sensorineural hearing loss and upward spread of masking. *J. Speech Hear. Res.* **13**, 426–437.

Mills, J. H., and Schmiedt, R. A. (1982). A possible physiological correlate of frequency discrimination. *J. Acoust. Soc. Amer.* **72**, S90.

Mills, J. H., Gengel, R. W., Watson, C. S., and Miller, J. D. (1970). Temporary changes of the auditory system due to exposure to noise for one or two days. *J. Acoust. Soc. Am.* **48**, 524–530.

Mills, J. H., Gilbert, R. M., and Adkins, W. Y. (1979). Temporary threshold shifts in humans exposed to octave bands of noise for 16–24 hours. *J. Acoust. Soc. Am.* **65**, 1238–1248.

Mills, J. H., Adkins, W. Y., and Gilbert, R. M. (1981). Temporary thresholds shifts produced by wideband noise. *J. Acoust. Soc. Am.* **70**, 390–396.

Moore, B. C. J. (1978). Psychophysical tuning curves measured in simultaneous and forward masking. *J. Acoust. Soc. Am.* **63**, 524–532.

Moore, B. C. J. (1980a). Mechanism and frequency distribution of two-tone suppression in forward masking. *J. Acoust. Soc. Am.* **68**, 814–824.

Moore, B. C. J. (1980b). Relation between pitch shifts and MMF shifts in forward masking. *J. Acoust. Soc. Am.* **69**, 594–597.

Munson, W. A., and Gardner, M. B. (1950). Loudness patterns—A new approach. *J. Acoust. Soc. Am.* **22**, 177–190.

Nelson, D. A., and Turner, C. W. (1980). Decay of masking and frequency resolution in sensorineural hearing-impaired listeners. *In* "Psychophysical, Physiological, and Behavioral Studies in Hearing" (G. van den Brink and F. A. Bilsen, eds.), pp. 175–182. Delft Univ. Press, Delft, The Netherlands.

Nomoto, M., Suga, N., and Katsuki, Y. (1964). Discharge pattern and inhibition or primary auditory nerve fibers in the monkey. *J. Neurophysiol.* **27**, 768–787.

Ohm, G. S. (1843). Ueber die Definition des Tones, nebst, daran geknüpfter Theorie der Sirene und ahnlicher Tonbildener Vorrichtungen. *Ann. Physiol.* **59**, 497–565.

O'Malley, H., and Feth, L. L. (1979). Relationship between psychophysical tuning curves and 'suppression.' *J. Acoust. Soc. Am.* **66**, 1075–1087.

Papoulis, A. (1962). "The Fourier Integral and its Application." McGraw-Hill, New York.

Peake, W. T., and Ling, A., Jr. (1980). Basilar-membrane motion in the alligator lizard: Its relation to tonotopic organization and frequency selectivity. *J. Acoust. Soc. Am.* **67**, 1736–1745.

Pfeiffer, R. R., and Kim, D. O. (1973). Considerations of nonlinear response properties of single cochlear nerve fibers. *In* "Basic Mechanisms in Hearing" (A. Moller, ed.), pp. 555–591. Academic Press, New York.

Pfeiffer, R. R., and Kim, D. O. (1975). Cochlear nerve fibers responses: Distribution along the cochlear partition. *J. Acoust. Soc. Am.* **58**, 867–890.

Pick, G. F., Evans, E. F., and Wilson, J. P. (1977). Frequency resolution in patients with hearing loss of cochlear origin. *In* "Psychophysics and Physiology of Hearing" (E. F. Evans and J. P. Wilson, eds.). Academic Press, New York.

Rabinowitz, W., Bilger, R. C., Trahiotis, C., and Nuetzel, J. (1980). Two-tone masking in normal hearing listeners. *J. Acoust. Soc. Am.* **68**, 1096–1106.

Ratliff, F. (1965). "Mach Bands. Quantitative Studies on Neural Networks in the Retina." Holden-Day, San Francisco, California.

Rhode, W. S. (1971). Observations of the vibrations of the basilar membrane in squirrel monkeys. *J. Acoust. Soc. Am.* **49**, 1218–1231.

Rhode, W. S. (1973). An investigation of post-mortem cochlear mechanics using the Mossbauer effect. *In* "Basic Mechanisms in Hearing" (A. Moller, ed.), pp. 49–68. Academic Press, New York.

Rhode, W. S. (1978). Some observations on cochlear mechanics. *J. Acoust. Soc. Am.* **64**, 158–176.

Rhode, W. S. (1980). Cochlear partition vibration—Recent views. *J. Acoust. Soc. Am.* **67**, 1696–1702.

Robertson, D., and Johnstone, B. M. (1979). Aberrant tonotopic organization in the inner ear damaged by kanamycin. *J. Acoust. Soc. Am.* **66**, 466–469.

Robertson, D., and Johnstone, B. M. (1981). Primary auditory neurons: Nonlinear responses altered without changes in sharp tuning. *J. Acoust. Soc. Am.* **69**, 1096–1098.

Robertson, D., Johnstone, B. M., and McGill, T. J. (1980). Effects of loud tones on the inner ear: A combined electrophysiological and ultrastructural study. *Hear. Res.* **2**, 39–53.

Rose, J. E., Brugge, J. F., Anderson, D. J., and Hind, J. E. (1967). Phase locked response to low-frequency tones in single auditory nerve fibers of the squirrel monkey. *J. Neurophysiol.* **30**, 769–793.

Russell, I. J., and Sellick, P. M. (1977). Tuning properties of cochlear hair cells. *Nature (London)* **267**, 858–860.

Russell, I. J., and Sellick, P. M. (1978). Intracellular studies of hair cells in the guinea pig cochlea. *J. Physiol.* **284**, 261–290.

Sachs, M. B. (1969). Stimulus-response relation for auditory-nerve fibers: Two-tone stimuli. *J. Acoust. Soc. Am.* **45**, 1026–1036.

Sachs, M. B. and Kiang, N. Y. S. (1968). Two-tone inhibition in auditory-nerve fibers. *J. Acoust. Soc. Am.* **43**, 1120–1128.

Salvi, R. J., Henderson, D., and Hamernik, R. P. (1979). Single auditory nerve fiber and action potential latencies in normal and noise-treated chinchillas. *Hear. Res.* **1**, 237–251.

Salvi, R., Perry, J., Hamernik, R., and Henderson, D. (1982). Relationships between cochlear pathologies and auditory nerve and behavioral responses following acoustic trauma. *In* "New Perspectives on Noise-Induced Hearing Loss" (R. Hamernik, D. Henderson, and R. Salvi, eds.). Raven, New York.

Scharf, B. (1970). "Foundations of Modern Auditory Theory" (J. V. Tobias, ed.), Vol. 1, pp. 157–202. Academic Press, New York.

Schmiedt, R. A. (1982a). Characteristics of auditory-nerve activity in gerbil: Similarities to cat data. Abstracts of the midwinter research meeting of the Association for Research in *Otolaryngology* **5**, 12–13.

Schmiedt, R. A. (1982b). Boundaries of two-tone rate suppression of cochlear-nerve activity. *Hear. Res.* **7**, 335–351.

Schmiedt, R. A. (1982c). Differential effects of kanamycin and impulse-noise exposure on responses of auditory-nerve fibers. *In* "New Perspectives on Noise-Induced Hearing Loss" (R. Hamernik, D. Henderson, and R. Salvi, eds.), pp. 153–163. Raven, New York.

Schmiedt, R. A., and Adams, J. C. (1981). Stimulated acoustic emissions in the ear canal of the gerbil. *Hear. Res.* **5**, 295–305.

Schmiedt, R. A., and Zwislocki, J. J. (1980). Effect of hair-cell lesions on responses of cochlear nerve fibers. II. Single- and two-tone intensity functions in relation to tuning curves. *J. Neurophysiol.* **43,** 1390–1405.

Schmiedt, R. A., Zwislocki, J. J., and Hamernik, R. P. (1980). Effects of hair cell lesions on responses of cochlear nerve fibers. I. Lesions, tuning curves, two-tone inhibition and responses to trapezoidal-wave patterns. *J. Neurophysiol.* **43,** 1367–1389.

Schubert, E. D. (1978). History of research on hearing. *In* "Handbook of Perception" (E. Carterette and M. Friedman, eds.), pp. 41–75. Academic Press, New York.

Schuknecht, H. F., and Woellner, R. C. (1955). An experimental and clinical study of deafness from lesions of the cochlear nerve. *J. Laryngol.* **69,** 75–97.

Sellick, P. M., and Russell, I. J. (1979). Two-tone suppression in cochlear hair cells. *Hear. Res.* **1,** 227–236.

Shannon, R. V. (1976). Two-tone unmasking and suppression in a forward masking situation. *J. Acoust. Soc. Am.* **59,** 1460–1470.

Siebert, W. M. (1970). Frequency discrimination in the auditory system: place or periodicity mechanism. *Proc. IEEE* **58,** 723–730.

Small, A. M. (1959). Pure-tone masking. *J. Acoust. Soc. Am.* **31,** 1619–1625.

Smith, R. J. (1966). "Circuits, Devices, and Systems." Wiley, New York.

Smith, R. L. (1977). Short-term adaptation in single auditory nerve fibers: Some post stimulatory effects. *J. Neurophysiol.* **40,** 1098–1112.

Smith, R. L. (1979). Adaptation, saturation, and physiological masking in single auditory nerve fibers. *J. Acoust. Soc. Am.* **65,** 166–178.

Smoorenburg, G. F. (1980). Effects of temporary threshold shift on combination-tone generation and on two-tone suppression. *Hear. Res.* **2,** 347–355.

Smoorenburg, G. F., and van Heusden, E. (1979). Effects of acute noise traumata on whole-nerve and single unit activity. *Arch. Otorhinolaryngol.* **224,** 117–124.

Sohmer, H., and Pratt, H. (1975). Electrocochleography during noise-induced temporary threshold shifts. *Audiology* **14,** 130–134.

Stevens, S. S. (1951). "Handbook of Experimental Psychology." Wiley, New York.

Stevens, S. S., and Davis, H. (1938). "Hearing: Its Psychology and Physiology." Wiley, New York.

Strelioff, D., Sitko, S. T., and Honrubia, V. (1976). Role of inner and outer hair cells in neural excitation. *Trans. Am. Acad. Ophthalmol. Otolaryngol.* **82,** 322–327.

Tasaki, I. (1954). Nerve impulses in individual auditory nerve fibers of guinea pig. *J. Neurophysiol.* **17,** 97–122.

Tasaki, I., Davis, H., and Legouix, J. P. (1952). The space-time pattern of the cochlear microphonics (guinea pig) as recorded by differentiate electrodes. *J. Acoust. Soc. Am.* **24,** 502–519.

Thornton, A. R., and Abbas, P. J. (1980). Low-frequency hearing loss: perception of filtered speech, psychophysical tuning curves and masking. *J. Acoust. Soc. Am.* **67,** 638–643.

Vogten, L. L. M. (1974). Pure-tone masking: A new result from a new method. *In* "Facts and Models in Hearing" (E. Zwicker and E. Terhardt, eds.), pp. 142–155. Springer-Verlag, Berlin and New York.

Volkmann, A. W. (1844). Neurophysiology. *In* "Handwörterbuch der Physiologie, II" (R. Wagner, ed.), pp. 521–526.

Weber, D. L. (1978). Suppression and critical bands in band-limiting experiments. *J. Acoust. Soc. Am.* **64,** 141–150.

Weber, D. L., and Green, D. M. (1978). Temporal factors and suppression effects in backward and forward masking. *J. Acoust. Soc. Am.* **64,** 1392–1399.

Weber, D. L., and Green, D. M. (1979). Suppression effects in backward and forward masking. *J. Acoust. Soc. Am.* **65,** 1258–1267.

Weber, D. L., and Moore, B. C. J. (1981). Forward masking by sinusiodal and noise maskers. *J. Acoust. Soc. Am.* **69**, 1402–1409.

Wegel, R. L., and Lane, C. E. (1924). The auditory masking of one pure-tone by another and its probable relation to the dynamics of the inner ear. *Physiol. Rev.* **23**, 266–285.

Weir, C. C., Jesteadt, W., and Green, D. M. (1977). Frequency discrimination as a function of frequency and sensation level. *J. Acoust. Soc. Am.* **61**, 178–184.

Weiss, T. F., Peake, W. T., Ling, A., Jr., and Holton, T. (1978). Which structures determine frequency selectivity and tonotopic organization of vertebrate nerve fibers? Evidence from the alligator lizard. *In* "Evoked Electrical Activity in the Auditory Nervous System" (R. Naunton and C. Fernandez, eds.). Academic Press, New York.

Weissing, H. (1968). Relation of threshold shift to noise in the human ear. *J. Acoust. Soc. Am.* **44**, 610–615.

Wever, E. G. (1949). "Theory of Hearing." Wiley, New York (republished by Dover, New York, 1970).

Wiederhold, M. L. (1970). Variations in the effects of electrical stimulation of the crossed olivocochlear bundle on cat single auditory-nerve-fiber responses to tone bursts. *J. Acoust. Soc. Am.* **48**, 966–977.

Wightman, F. L. (1982). Psychoacoustic correlates of hearing loss. *In* "New Perspectives on Noise-Induced Hearing Loss" (R. P. Hamernik, D. Henderson, and R. Salvi, eds.). Raven, New York.

Wightman, F. L., McGee, T., and Kramer, M. (1977). Factors influencing frequency selectivity in normal and hearing impaired listeners. *In* "Psychophysics and Physiology of Hearing" (E. F. Evans and J. P. Wilson, eds.). Academic Press, New York.

Wilson, J. P., and Johnstone, J. R. (1975). Basilar membrane and middle-ear vibration in guinea pig measured by capacitive probe. *J. Acoust. Soc. Am.* **57**, 705–723.

Yamamoto, T., Koichi, T., Shoji, H., and Yoneda, H. (1970). Critical band with respect to temporary threshold shift. *J. Acoust. Soc. Am.* **48**, 978–987.

Zurek, P. M. (1981). Spontaneous narrowband acoustic signals emitted by human ears, *J. Acoust. Soc. Am.* **69**, 514–523.

Zwicker, E. (1974). On a psychoacoustical equivalent of tuning curves. *In* "Facts and Models in Hearing" (E. Zwicker and E. Terhardt, eds.). Springer-Verlag, Berlin and New York.

Zwicker, E., and Manley, G. (1981). Acoustical responses and suppression-period patterns in guinea pigs. *Hear. Res.* **4**, 43–52.

Zwicker, E., and Schorn, K. (1978). Psychoacoustical tuning curves in audiology. *Audiology* **17**, 120–140.

Zwislocki, J. J. (1946). Über die mechanische Klangandyse des Ohres. *Experientia* **2**, 415–417.

Zwislocki, J. J. (1948). Theorie der Schneckenmechanik: Qualitative and quantitative Analyse. *Acta Oto-Laryngol Suppl* **72**.

Zwislocki, J. J. (1950). Theory of the acoustical action of the cochlea. *J. Acoust. Soc. Am.* **22**, 778–784.

Zwislocki, J. J. (1953). Review of recent mathematical theories of cochlear dynamics. *J. Acoust. Soc. Am.* **25**, 743–751.

Zwislocki, J. J. (1960). Theory of temporal auditory summation. *J. Acoust. Soc. Am.* **32**, 1046–1060.

Zwislocki, J. J. (1965). Analysis of some auditory characteristics. *In* "Handbook of Mathematical Psychology" (R. Luce, R. Bush, and E. Galanter, eds.), Vol. II, pp. 1–98. Wiley, New York.

Zwislocki, J. J. (1978). Masking: Experimental and theoretical aspects of simultaneous, forward, backward and central masking. *In* "Handbook of Perception Vol. IV. Hearing" (E. C. Carterrette and M. O. Friedman, eds.). Academic Press, New York.

Zwislocki, J. J. (1981). Sound analysis in the ear: A history of discoveries. *Am. Sci.* **69,** 184–192.

Zwislocki, J. J., and Kletsky, E. J. (1979). Tectorial membrane: A possible effect on the frequency analysis in the cochlea. *Science* **204,** 639–641.

Zwislocki, J. J., and Pirodda, E. (1952). On the adaptation, fatigue and acoustic trauma of the ear. *Experientia* **8,** 279–284.

Index